APPLIED SPORTS
MEDICINE FOR
COACHES

JAMES H. JOHNSON, PhD
Department of Exercise and Sport Studies
Smith College
Northampton, Massachusetts

ESTHER M. HASKVITZ, PhD, PT, ATC
Department of Physical Therapy
The Sage Colleges
Troy, New York

BARBARA A. BREHM, EdD
Department of Exercise and Sport Studies
Smith College
Northampton, Massachusetts

 Wolters Kluwer | Lippincott Williams & Wilkins
Health
Philadelphia • Baltimore • New York • London
Buenos Aires • Hong Kong • Sydney • Tokyo

Acquisitions Editor: Emily Lupash
Developmental Editor: Jennifer P. Ajello
Marketing Manager: Christen Murphy
Production Editor: Beth Martz
Design Coordinator: Terry Mallon
Compositor: Maryland Composition

Library of Congress Cataloging-in-Publication Data

Johnson, James H. (James Harmon), 1942-
  Applied sports medicine for coaches / James H. Johnson, Esther M. Haskvitz, Barbara Brehm-Curtis.
    p. ; cm. ; cm.
  Includes bibliographical references.
  ISBN 978-0-7817-6549-7
  1. Sports medicine. 2. Coaches (Athletics) I. Haskvitz, Esther M. II. Brehm-Curtis, Barbara. III. Title.
  [DNLM: 1. Athletic Injuries—prevention & control. 2. Athletic Performance—physiology. 3. Athletic Performance—psychology. 4. Sports Medicine—methods. QT 261 J67a 2009]
  RC1210.J58 2009
  617.1'027--dc22

                                                             2008011143

DISCLAIMER

Care has been taken to confirm the accuracy of the information present and to describe generally accepted practices. However, the authors, editors, and publisher are not responsible for errors or omissions or for any consequences from application of the information in this book and make no warranty, expressed or implied, with respect to the currency, completeness, or accuracy of the contents of the publication. Application of this information in a particular situation remains the professional responsibility of the practitioner; the clinical treatments described and recommended may not be considered absolute and universal recommendations.

The authors, editors, and publisher have exerted every effort to ensure that drug selection and dosage set forth in this text are in accordance with the current recommendations and practice at the time of publication. However, in view of ongoing research, changes in government regulations, and the constant flow of information relating to drug therapy and drug reactions, the reader is urged to check the package insert for each drug for any change in indications and dosage and for added warnings and precautions. This is particularly important when the recommended agent is a new or infrequently employed drug.

Some drugs and medical devices presented in this publication have Food and Drug Administration (FDA) clearance for limited use in restricted research settings. It is the responsibility of the health care provider to ascertain the FDA status of each drug or device planned for use in their clinical practice.

To purchase additional copies of this book, call our customer service department at **(800) 638-3030** or fax orders to **(301) 223-2320**. International customers should call **(301) 223-2300**.

Visit Lippincott Williams & Wilkins on the Internet: http://www.lww.com. Lippincott Williams & Wilkins customer service representatives are available from 8:30 am to 6:00 pm, EST.

Dedication

For my favorite team: Carolyn, Cheryl, Scott, and Luke.
—J.J.

For my family and friends who have helped me go the distance.
—E.H

For my favorite athletes, Ian and Adam Curtis, who have taught me about the power of sport.
—B.B.

Reviewers

Randall Deere, DA
Assistant Dean
WKU College of Health and Human Services
Bowling Green, Kentucky

M.L. DeFuria, PhD
Adjunct Instructor
Department of Exercise Science
Syracuse University
Syracuse, New York

Phillip L. Henson, PhD
Coordinator of Coaching Education
Indiana University at Bloomington
Bloomington, Indiana

Sally Paulson, PhD
Assistant Professor
Department of Exercise Science
Shippensburg University
Shippensburg, Pennsylvania

Brian Phillips, MA, CSCS
Instructor
Department of Physical Education, Health and Sport Studies
Oxford, Ohio

Jeff Seegmiller, PhD
Assistant Professor
School of Recreation and Sport Sciences
Ohio University
Athens, Ohio

Enza Steele, BS, MS
Associate Professor
Lynchburg College
Lynchburg, Virginia

Linn Stranak, PhD
Department Chair
Department of Physical Education, Wellness, and Sport
Union University
Jackson, Tennessee

Preface

At Smith College we have specialized in the education of coaches for more than 20 years. Our program is recognized nationally for its excellence, and is the only institution to have received Level IV accreditation from the National Association for Sport and Physical Education. One of our goals is to translate theory into practice. What do coaches need to know to successfully prepare athletes for competition, prevent injury, and keep their athletes healthy? Programs in coaching education are often varied, but with a few exceptions they require their students to take a course in athletic injuries. Such sports medicine courses are usually oriented to the care and prevention of athletic injuries, and coaching education students are mixed in with students intending to be athletic trainers. But students in coaching education programs are preparing for a career in coaching, not athletic training.

Sports medicine for coaches is far more than the care and prevention of injuries. Coaches structure the training of athletes and prepare their teams for athletic contests. Coaches must do all they can to structure training cycles and daily practices in ways that both prevent injury *and* help their athletes achieve peak performance. By understanding the common causes of sports injuries, coaches can design effective practices that reduce injury risk. By improving motor skills, muscle balance, and physical fitness, coaches can help athletes prevent noncontact anterior cruciate ligament (ACL) injuries. Understanding the physiology of recovery processes, coaches can help their athletes walk the fine line between training and overtraining, and prevent overuse injuries while at the same time building physical fitness. While coaches must respond appropriately to emergency situations, they do not diagnose injury or prescribe treatment. However, they do welcome recovering athletes back to play and work with health care professionals to understand returning athletes' limits and training needs. Coaches should understand common athletic injuries in order to communicate effectively with their athletic trainers and help athletes return safely to play.

For some time we have been aware that a textbook that specifically addresses what a coach needs to know about sports medicine does not exist in this country. There are a number of excellent athletic injury books, but they are written for the licensed health care professionals who diagnose and care for athletes who have been injured. We believe it is time for a text that specifically addresses what coaches need to know about sports medicine and that is why we wrote this book.

Who Should Read this Book?

Any student entering the field of coaching will find this book interesting and relevant. In addition, current coaches may find this book a welcome addition to traditional athletic injury texts. Coaches will no longer have to weed through unnecessary information to find out what they need to know about training athletes appropriately for peak performance and injury prevention. Indeed, we believe that anyone interested in coaching may benefit from this text.

Highlighted Topics

Written for the Coach. One of the main highlights of this text is that it is specifically written for coaches. We have pared down sports medicine knowledge to what coaches need to know. Each chapter has specific recommendations for the coach's role. We are well aware of the time constraints placed upon coaches. Therefore, one of our goals is the integration of optimal performance training with injury prevention. The properly trained athlete is the best defense against injury.

Overtraining. Sport in the United States is more competitive than ever. As a consequence, athletes often train year round for competition in one sport. Young athletes often specialize early in their careers, training to compete in only one sport. As a result, overtraining injuries have become more common. This book includes a chapter on overtraining, examining various causes and symptoms of overtraining, and spells out what the coach can do to prevent overtraining.

ACL Injury Prevention. The anterior cruciate ligament is frequently injured in a number of sports. This is particularly true for female athletes. Interestingly, most ACL injuries do not happen during contact but when an athlete stops, turns, or lands. Recent work at several institutions has shown promising results for the reduction of such injuries. We have instituted such a program at Smith College with great success. The program simultaneously develops power, balance, and agility; qualities necessary for many sports. We have included a chapter on how to institute an ACL injury prevention program.

Psychology of Injury. As sport psychology has become a significant part of sport, so has the psychology of injury. When athletes are injured, the psychological symptoms are often as important as the physical ones. Fear, depression, and anxiety are commonly associated with athletic injury and affect an athlete's quality of life, rate of recovery, and return to competition. What do you do with the athlete who receives a serious injury in the beginning of the season? Are some athletes more prone to injury? Our chapter on psychology and injury will help answer such questions.

Pedagogical Features

Chapter Objectives. Each chapter begins with a list of objectives. We hope the information provided in the chapter will help readers achieve each of the listed objectives.

Case Studies. Each chapter opens with a case study designed to illustrate a standard problem related to the material in the chapter. These interesting and compelling cases demonstrate the importance of information in the chapter.

Focal Point. These chapter boxes provide additional anecdotes, brief cases, hot topics, and current debates that support text material.

From the Athletic Training Room. These boxes present interesting medical information on various sports medicine topics. Information in these boxes gives the reader more scientific background in relevant areas and enhances the coach's understanding of important material.

Additional Resources

Applied Sports Medicine for Coaches includes additional resources for both instructors and students that are available on the book's companion website at http://thePoint.lww.com/Johnson.

Instructors. Approved adopting instructors will be given access to the following additional resources:

- PowerPoint presentations
- Image bank
- WebCT and Blackboard Ready Cartridge

The PowerPoint presentations were created by Randy Deere of Western Kentucky University.

Students. Purchasers of the text can access the searchable Full Text On-line by going to the *Applied Sports Medicine for Coaches* website at http://thePoint.lww.com. See the inside front cover of this text for more details, including the passcode you will need to gain access to the website.

When people are asked to give examples of peak experiences from their lives, they often mention their involvement in sport. Sport provides people with opportunities to develop self-discipline, physical fitness, the ability to work with others, and to have fun. Good coaches help to set the scene for great sport experiences. Coaches who are well-educated and knowledgeable about proper training and injury prevention help to promote a positive regard for sport in our society and peak experiences for their athletes. We hope that this book helps to increase your confidence in addressing sports medicine issues in your work, and the satisfaction you find in your coaching career.

James H. Johnson
Esther M. Haskvitz
Barbara A. Brehm

Acknowledgments

During the past 25 years numerous students have completed our coaching education program. These students now range far and wide, coaching all manner of sports. Our students have challenged us to do our best to make information clear and applicable to sport. This challenge has continually pushed us to reconsider our course content and teaching methods in order to more fully engage our coaching education students, and we wish to thank our students for their diligence. Likewise, we have worked with many excellent coaches who expect us to understand coaching, to appreciate the responsibilities of the coach, and to understand the power of sport. Coaches have kept our feet on the ground and we appreciate their candor.

Specifically, we wish to thank the following coaches and athletic trainers for spending the time to participate in numerous interviews and question sessions: Dave Allen, Tim Bacon, Karen Balter, Kim Bierwert, Deb Coutu, Chris Davis, Liz Feely, Karen Klinger, Kris Martini, Bonnie May, E. J. Mill, Lynn Oberbillig, Phil Nielsen, Kelli Steele, and Andy Whitcomb.

At Lippincott Williams & Wilkins, we wish to think our developmental editors, Jennifer Ajello and Karen Ruppert; art director, Jennifer Clements; and our acquisitions editor, Emily Lupash, for her belief in this project.

Contents

PART III: SPORTS INJURIES

INJURY PREVENTION

Coaches' Role in Sports Medicine

Upon reading this chapter, the coach should be able to:

1. Understand the different roles coaches play in the area of sports medicine.
2. Understand how they can facilitate the athlete during rehabilitation.
3. Develop a method of open communication with training room personnel.
4. Identify methods of achieving trust between the coach and the athletic trainer.
5. Understand that the role of the coach goes beyond the playing field and that coaches serve as important resources for athletes, faculty, and staff.

Jake was on the football squad at a small New England college. He had always had some shoulder problems, but it wasn't until his senior year that the athletic trainers told him his career was over. He was devastated. Jake was a good student and very motivated to succeed in school, but football had been a huge part of his identity for the better part of 10 years and he didn't want to give it up. Jake's coach knew he loved the game and didn't want him to lose his spirit. He asked Jake to help direct some of the drills and to work with some of the lesser skilled players on technique. Jake was back to being part of the team and ended the season with enthusiasm. Jake started thinking he might like to coach.

Bonnie was in a similar situation at her Division II school. She was looking forward to her best year yet when she entered her senior year. A soccer goalie, she had played organized soccer for 17 years. It was the third game of the year when she was knocked unconscious while diving for a ball. This was her third concussion and the symptoms lasted for more than a week. After consulting with the athletic trainer, her parents, and the team doctor, she was advised to discontinue playing. Her coach told her she was sorry to lose her but accidents happen. Bonnie walked home thinking about all the speeches the coach had made about teamwork. "Where was the teamwork now?" Bonnie felt like she had been betrayed.

Coaches quickly learn that their responsibilities go far beyond offense and defense. With regard to sports medicine, coaches are the first line of defense against injury. They become responsible for the physical as well as mental health of their players. Coaches (Fig. 1.1) are often the first adult an athlete will approach with a problem. Coaches are often emulated and their behaviors frequently copied. Indeed, coaches have profound effects on the development of young people. Fortunately, these effects are largely positive, leaving athletes with fond memories and positive behaviors as the result of their athletic activities. However, there are occasions (as with the case of Bonnie's coach) when an athlete becomes embittered because of their athletic experience.

We believe strongly in the student-athlete model encouraged in our schools. But we also believe that athletics are an extracurricular experience; an experience designed to enhance the development of young people. Student-athletes should leave the scholastic athletic experience with a healthy sports experience.

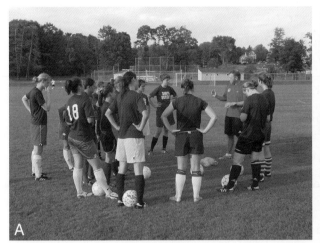
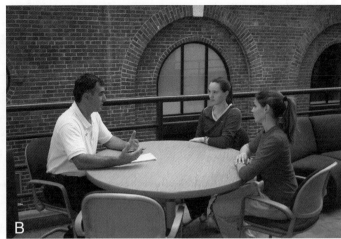

■ **FIGURE 1.1 A.** Coaches teach technique, tactics, and strategy. **B.** Coaches often counsel athletes on a wide variety of subjects.

The coach's role in sports medicine is a unique one, and the knowledge and attitude of the coach is one key to achieving this goal. We also believe that coaches should have a firm philosophical foundation regarding the place of athletics in the development of the individual. Coaches need knowledge in exercise physiology, biomechanics, sport psychology, and motor learning. Coaches should have a firm pedagogical base and awareness of the sociocultural basis of sport. Coaches should never stop learning.

In preparation for this text, and specifically for this chapter, we set out to learn some of the "Best Practices" presented by a wide variety of successful and respected coaches. We selected new as well as seasoned coaches from a variety of sports and institutions. We conducted personal interviews with each coach regarding their role in sports medicine, problem solving, and establishing a working relationship with the athletic trainer. We learned that coaches are resource persons for students and faculty. In addition, we also interviewed athletic trainers to get their side of the picture. We wanted to know the best way for athletic trainers and coaches to work together to do what's best for the athlete. The following is a summary of the questions and answers we gathered.

FOCAL POINT

Excerpts from an Interview with E. J. Mills, Amherst College Football Coach

Q: With regard to sports medicine, how do you see your role?

A: Ultimately, we have a great medical staff. I trust them and in almost all cases I defer to the medical staff. I never, ever question their judgment when they tell me an athlete cannot play. As the head coach I have to create an environment where athletes feel comfortable going to the athletic trainer. We do a pretty good job with this. My golden rule is that I try to coach the team as if I was coaching my own children. How would I want them to be treated? I put a lot of faith and trust in the medical staff. We have a great situation with two full-time athletic trainers, a general practitioner who is here almost daily, and an orthopedic surgeon who is routinely in attendance. I believe the athletic trainers act in the best interest of the athletes. We have a united front.

Q: What is the best way to establish communication with the training room staff?

A: We're fortunate with one athletic trainer assigned exclusively to us. We play on Saturday afternoons and have a clinic starting at noon on Sunday with all medical staff. Sometimes athletes feel fine after the game and then something may swell during the night. I meet with the doctors and athletic trainer on Sunday afternoon to review each athlete. I meet every day with the athletic trainer at 11:30 and go over what each athlete can do. There's a lot of communication. You can almost set your watch by our meetings.

(continues)

Excerpts from an Interview with E. J. Mills, Amherst College Football Coach (continued)

Q: Is there ever conflict between you and the athletic trainer?

A: To me it's pretty clear. If an athlete is hurt they should go to the training room. If they're not hurt they shouldn't be in there. I don't want the athlete to hide in the training room and I'll talk to the athletic trainer if that happens. But if an athlete says they are hurt, who am I to tell them they're not.

Q: What happens when an athlete receives a serious injury during the season? Do you have a plan to maintain contact with the athlete?

A: If an athlete has to go to the hospital, I'm right there with them as soon as practice is over. I do whatever it takes at that point. Athletes normally use practice time to get treatment and rehab since school pressures here are quite tough. But I try to boost them up and encourage them to keep working. I do try to get the athletes to maintain contact and encouragement. I know it's devastating for many athletes and I think they often get very down when they go back to their room. But let's face it; I still have about 60 other athletes to deal with. This is a very tough situation for coaches and athletes.

THE COACH'S ROLE IN SPORTS MEDICINE

The common theme identified by our coaches was injury prevention. "My most important role in sports medicine is to prevent the injury from happening. Let's face it; the best way to treat an injury is to prevent it from happening in the first place." The last thing coaches want to do is hurt their athletes. "Do no harm" was a commonly mentioned position. Many factors are involved in injury prevention (see Chapter 2). Injuries can be caused by such factors as poor technique, poor training, bad equipment, or unsafe practices. For example, one of our swimming coaches indicated that, "One of my main responsibilities is to determine if the athlete is doing anything that will predispose them to injury. When an athlete first comes to our program I find out what injuries they have had, what kind of treatment they received, and what did they do about it?"

Teaching technique and training athletes are two of the main jobs of the coach, as well as two of the most effective measures of defense against injury. "I try to make sure that everyone is properly trained and not overtrained. I try to keep everyone healthy." As one of the soccer coaches said, "I'm responsible in our practice program for knowing what the most common injuries are and how to prevent them. I'm very careful with those athletes who start the season unprepared. This is especially true for new athletes. They just don't know what's in store for them and how to prepare. This is one reason why I do fitness testing at the beginning of the year. I know that I have to ease some athletes in if their fitness is low and they are more susceptible to injury. I spend considerable time and attention teaching athletes the system before they leave school. It's the new athletes who seem to be the most vulnerable."

The coach is often immediately involved when an athlete is injured. In many of the smaller colleges and high schools an athletic trainer is not present during practice. In such cases we recommend that schools adopt a procedure for prompt communication between coach and athletic trainer. If an athlete gets hurt on the field, do you wait to send them to the training room or send them immediately? If an athlete sprains an ankle during practice they may frequently continue to play on it. The prior exercise has an analgesic effect and the athlete doesn't feel too bad. However, continued exercise with an injured ankle simply facilitates blood flow (and swelling) to the area. That extra 30 minutes of practice may not be worth it in the long run. What do you do when athletes hit heads and one loses consciousness? All coaches should be First Aid and CPR certified but we believe these certifications are minimal at best. Coaches need more.

②The second most common role mentioned is to facilitate the rehabilitation process. When athletes get injured they are normally assigned to treatment and rehabilitation. The athletic trainer's goal is to put a healthy athlete back onto the field as quickly as possible. But the athletic trainer may be dealing with athletes from as many as 5 teams, as well as some out of season athletes. As one of the volleyball coaches said, "The trainers have to contend with 300 athletes; I only have 15. My job is to follow up with the trainer's advice. Is the athlete doing what she's supposed to do to get back on the court? I don't direct the rehab work but I do make sure they're doing it." The coach is the ultimate person the athlete reports to. Normally, athletic trainers have little control over the athletes and coaches have to be involved. The athlete should also know that the coach continues to be interested in them and that they are important to the team.

Coaches are occasionally involved with some specifics of the rehabilitation process. If the athletic trainer understands the functional requirements of the sport, they can rehabilitate the athlete to satisfy those requirements. Some athletic trainers may not be fully aware of a sport. Many times coaches are not allowed to work with students out of season because of national and/or conference regulations. One of the best practices we learned involved an athletic trainer and an out of season athlete. "We were rehabilitating an athlete to return to basketball but she was really nervous about performing some of the drills. We asked the coach to demonstrate the various drills the athlete would need to perform. He provided us with a drill packet and demonstrated the various drills involved. We then worked with the athlete until she was confident that she could perform those same drills."

WORKING WITH THE ATHLETIC TRAINER

Every coach we interviewed indicated that communication is the key to a good working relationship with the athletic trainer. Face-to-face is the most desirable form of communication. Questions can be asked and answered and misunderstandings are reduced. Our coaches routinely informed us that they do not want to receive injury information from the athlete; athletic trainer to coach is the appropriate line of communication. Our coaches and athletic trainers agreed that the responsibility for communication is equal between coach and athletic trainer. Occasionally, part of the problem is that athletic trainers tend to be less mobile than coaches. Since most of their work is limited to the training room, we learned that it is usually best for the coach to visit the athletic trainer. Coaches should adopt a policy of routinely visiting the athletic trainer at a time when the athletic trainer is not so busy. An athlete may have been injured and not notified the coach. The athletic trainers must adopt some system to notify a coach that they have seen an injured athlete. In all cases, communication between coach and athletic trainer should be private. When athletes are seriously injured, our coaches suggested that the coach, athletic trainer, and athlete should all meet together to discuss treatment and rehabilitation. The athlete should be a part of the process.

The attitude of the coach toward the athletic trainers is an important one for athletes. Athletic trainers want athletes to play; sending an athlete to the training room is the best way to care for and prevent further injury. As our athletic trainers suggested, "Coaches need to present a mindset at the beginning of the season that it is acceptable to seek treatment; that it is often better to seek treatment for a minor injury rather than wait until it is more serious, resulting in extensive time lost to practice and competition. Athletes should not need permission to seek treatment."

When an Athlete is Injured

When an athlete has been injured the coach needs to know the specifics. What can the athlete do? What are the limits? Are they out for the day, the week? Whether the athlete can practice or not is an important question. This is where communication is vitally important. Coach and athlete have to agree on what the athlete can do. One good suggestion that we repeatedly heard was that coaches should discuss their practice plans with the athletic trainer. In this way the athletic trainer can help the coach decide which drills or activities are appropriate. Since maintaining contact with the team is an important part of rehabilitation, encourage the athlete and athletic trainer not to use the entire practice time to conduct rehabilitation.

Coaches who have an understanding of tissue injury and recovery have a better idea of what athletes can and cannot do. Certain injuries routinely take a certain amount of time to recover and attempts to hurry that process often result in additional lost time. It is well known that athletes who have been injured are more susceptible to that same injury (1–3). This is especially true if the athlete has not recovered and continues to play or practice. Let's look at an obvious example of an acute injury that the coach wants to rush. An athlete has been injured and takes 3 days off for treatment and rehab. The athletic trainer wants the athlete to rest for one more day but the coach insists that the athlete start practicing on the fourth day. If the athlete gets hurt again, the injury will probably be more serious and the initial 3 days have been wasted. One extra day off may make a huge difference.

Athletes who have been injured during competition (Fig. 1.2) are immediately seen by the athletic trainer. In some sports a physician is also on duty on the sidelines.

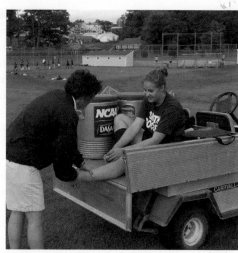

■ **FIGURE 1.2** An NATA certified athletic trainer evaluates an injured athlete on the field.

The athletic trainer has the final decision whether the athlete can continue to play. Occasionally, the athlete can be brought into these conversations. For example, our coaches and athletic trainers were willing to be a bit less conservative with older, more experienced athletes. Experienced athletes know their bodies and know their limits, and this knowledge should be considered. The basic question is whether the athlete will be placed at risk. If additional risk is involved, the athlete should not play.

Establishing Trust

The best practice is for the athletic trainer and coach to have mutual trust. Once again, communication is one key to this trust and should start prior to the season. The athletic trainer needs to trust the coach to do the right thing and the coach needs to believe that the athletic trainer wants the athletes to play. Coaches need to take time to talk to the athletic trainer other than about specific athletes and injuries. When coaches ignore the advice of the athletic trainer trust is reduced. One of our athletic trainers presented the following example: "The coach stopped by and we agreed on the practice schedule for one of the injured athletes. Apparently the coach got angry that day and decided to really hammer this athlete, pushing him far beyond what we agreed. I decided at that point that I would be extra conservative the next time the coach asked. I didn't trust him to do the right thing."

Coaches must respect the athletic trainer and believe they are working in the best interest of the athlete. Coaches should include the athletic trainer in their plans and seek their advice. Athletic trainers spend considerable time observing sport and are very good at it. They will often spot unsafe practices before the coach does. Coaches often feel more comfortable if the athletic trainer understands their sport and athletic trainers need to work to acquire a basic understanding of each sport. Although the responsibilities of the coach and athletic trainer are fairly distinct, there is considerable overlap in knowledge and responsibility. A good mutual relationship is therefore critical.

Knowledge is one way to improve trust. Coaches should stay abreast of the latest information on their sport; discussing this information with the athletic trainer keeps open the line of communication. Coaches should know what injuries are most frequent and the best way to prevent those injuries. Pushing athletes until they drag into the training room on a daily basis is not a good example. Punishing athletes by administering excessive exercise is another poor example. Professional meetings often include sports medicine information in addition to sport technique, strategy, etc. Coaches need to be well-read across the spectrum. Ignorance does not enhance trust.

The New Coach and the Athletic Trainer

Establishing trust is particularly important for the new coach. Even though the coach may have considerable experience, they are still unknown to the athletic trainer. As one coach said, "Don't make the assump-

From the Athletic Training Room: Certified Athletic Trainers

The National Athletic Trainers' Association (NATA) was founded in 1950 in Kansas City. About 200 athletic trainers attended this first meeting. The NATA now has a membership of approximately 30,000 with a rigorous and well structured certification process. To become a certified athletic trainer a degree from an accredited athletic training curriculum is required. Athletic trainers typically earn a bachelor's degree and many have advanced degrees. Athletic trainers must pass a myriad of courses including such topics as injury and illness prevention, acute care of injury and illness, clinical examination, rehabilitation, therapeutic modalities, nutrition, pharmacology, and psychosocial intervention and referral. Classroom learning is enhanced through extensive clinical experience under the supervision of a certified athletic trainer. Certification is only acquired after completing all academic and clinical requirements in addition to a comprehensive certification examination. Once athletic trainers are certified they use the designation "ATC" or "CAT." Athletic trainers must participate in continuing education throughout their careers. Since that first meeting in 1950, the NATA has come a long way to establish a group of well educated and qualified athletic trainers for our athletes.

tion that things will work the same way as your last school. Take some time and adapt to the system and then suggest for change to happen if you feel it necessary." New coaches should start communication with the athletic trainers before the season begins; get to know the staff early. Remember that the athletic trainers probably know the athletes better than you do. New coaches should go through the roster with the athletic trainers to find out what problems athletes have had.

MONITORING STRESS

Training and competing in sport presents significant stress to the athlete. When athletes cannot adapt to stress they tend to underperform and start a downward spiral that is difficult to stop (see Chapter 6). Student athletes are particularly vulnerable as they must deal with the stress of academics and athletics. In addition, family and social life may present problems that have negative impact on athletes. Coaches are normally aware of the stress of training and competition, but the stress on an athlete is the accumulation of training and nontraining stressors. Coaches see athletes for 2 to 3 hours a day but many things can happen to an athlete during the remaining parts of the day that have significant effect. We asked our coaches if they have a way of monitoring their athletes on and off the field.

Many of our coaches relied on training room staff to assist with such problems. "We're the bartenders of the gym," one of our athletic trainers said. Athletes often come to us with problems, but we also overhear students talking. "I believe athletes think we cannot hear," one of our athletic trainers said. "Many of the complaints are the familiar ones. 'I'm sore. I don't feel like practicing.' But occasionally I hear something that needs to be addressed and bring the coach into my confidence." Another good source of information is the senior athlete. "I rely heavily on my captains for information. They know what's going on in school and they frequently see the other players around campus. They usually know more than I do. However, if I ask an athlete to stop by my office I never suggest that I heard something from someone. I want them to think it's my idea."

Over the years we have found that coaches are great observers. They often know when an athlete seems overly fatigued or is underperforming. Coaches then need to follow up to determine what seems to be the problem. "This is difficult to do but we always have a 'sum up' for the team at the end of practice. I look for outward signs of excess fatigue, depression, hanging heads. When I see this I make a note to watch that player a little more carefully the next day. I might find a time to ask him or her how they are doing. This may be all that's needed to determine what's wrong. I ask them if they've been sleeping well. Did they miss a meal that day? I never ask athletes about their weight. Practice plans are flexible. If I notice an athlete lagging a bit, I try to adjust his workout."

End of year meetings also help plan for the future. One basketball coach suggested that the end of year meeting was one key to a good season. "We had a fairly small squad that year and our kids had to play a lot. We were rebuilding and I knew we would have a small squad again next year. I realized after meeting with each athlete after the season that they were simply tired. I knew that I had to change my schedule and decided to give them one day off a week. I may have sacrificed some technique but we were more energetic at game time and I think we played better. I don't think I would have known this without those meetings."

THE COACH AS A RESOURCE

Every coach we interviewed indicated their role as a resource person for athletes, faculty, staff, and parents. For this reason we greatly encourage coaches to be knowledgeable about more than just their sport. In our opinion the coach who only knows their individual sport misses out on some wonderful opportunities to assist with the development of young people. Interestingly, we found that those coaches who have the least education are also utilized the least as resources. Athletes quickly learn who is a good resource and who isn't. "Go ask the athletic trainers," is not always a satisfactory answer.

Many high school athletes go through some difficult developmental years. They undergo rapid physical, emotional, and social changes. They are wondering what life has in store for them. They occasionally have difficulty talking to their parents. Frequently, they only have one parent. Coaches are one resource. College coaches often face similar challenges. As one field hockey coach said, "I feel a tremendous responsibility to my players. Parents drop off a 17- or 18-year-old player that I've recruited. I want to see her succeed. I'm here to help to her."

"There seems to be no limit on what an athlete will ask me. Every once in a while I think I've heard it all, but I continue to be surprised," said one coach with 25 years of experience. We found that the range of questions is very broad. Nutrition and weight loss (Chapters 9 and 10) are two of the most common questions asked of coaches. Coaches need to develop competency in these subjects. Since coaches are often role models for their athletes, we strongly encourage appropriate fitness and nutrition behaviors by coaches. Leading by example is important. Most athletes are also interested in year-round fitness. "I try to get them to do new things, cross-train a little, learn a new sport. Normally, I cannot work with them out of season but I can give them good advice."

Student athletes often have time juggling the responsibilities of school and sport. Many athletes also work part-time. One of the most frequent questions is related to time management. Coaches can be of great help here since good time management is something all coaches need. But coaches also need to know their boundaries, to know what is beyond their expertise. Coaches need to be knowledgeable about resources available to the athlete. Most colleges and high schools have a counseling service and coaches should encourage the use of these personnel. Don't be afraid to say that something is beyond your knowledge.

Coaches are also important resources of information for faculty, staff, and parents. "Weight training and weight loss," are the two most common questions. "If I'm working out somewhere I often get asked about the best exercise for this or that." Aches and pains are also frequent questions asked of coaches. Normally, recreational athletes do not have access to the athletic trainer and often figure that coaches know a lot about injury.

Developing your Resource Ability

Certainly, education is one of the main ways to improve your ability to provide good information. As a result of our interviews we have learned that coaches are wonderful resources. We also learned the breadth of information and experiences of each coach. Sharing such information is a great way to learn and we strongly encourage coaches to get together. Coaching meetings should not be just about the routine duties of the athletic staff.

We strongly encourage coaches in schools to go beyond the gymnasium and athletic fields. Get involved in what is going on at the school. Several of the coaches we interviewed participate in programs for faculty and staff. This is a great way to promote your sport. We also found some coaches who participate in retirement programs offered at their schools. The wide variety of experiences and knowledge that coaches have should be shared with others.

SUMMARY

- Coaches need to present a mindset at the beginning of the season that injuries need to be cared for in the training room.
- Coaches should encourage their athletes to go to the training room when necessary.
- The prevention of athletic injuries is primarily the responsibility of the coach.
- The treatment of athletic injuries is primarily the responsibility of the athletic trainer.
- Coaches need to help motivate athletes during their rehabilitation process.
- Communication between coach and athletic trainer is one key to providing the best care for athletes.
- Face to face, private communication is best. Coaches should not receive injury information from the athlete but from the athletic trainer.
- Coaches and athletic trainers must trust each other to work in the best interest of the athlete. Coaches should not overstep their roles.
- Trust is gained by education and by working together.
- New coaches must learn to adapt to the sports medicine procedures of the new school. New coaches should establish lines of communication early in their appointment.
- Coaches are important resources for athletes, faculty, and staff and should develop their ability to give good advice.
- Coaches must continue to stay abreast of current trends in training and sports medicine.

Suggested Readings

Anderson MK, Hall SJ. *Foundations of Athletic Training*, 3rd ed. Philadelphia: Lippincott Williams & Wilkins, 2004.

Arnheim DD, Prentice WE. *Principles of Athletic Training*, 10th ed. Boston: McGraw-Hill, 2000.

Baechle TR, Earle RW. *Essentials of Strength Training and Conditioning*, 2nd ed. Champaign: Human Kinetics, 2000.

Flegel MJ. *Sport First Aid*, 3rd ed. Champaign: Human Kinetics, 2004.

Kraemer WJ, Hakkinen K. *Strength Training for Sport*. Oxford: Blackwell Science, 2002.

Hillman SK. *Introduction to Athletic Training*. Champaign: Human Kinetics, 2000.

Starkey C, Johnson G. *Athletic Training and Sports Medicine*, 4th Ed. Sudbury: Jones and Bartlett Publishers, 2006.

References

1. Arnason A, Sigurdsson S, Gudmundsson A, et al. Risk factors for injuries in football. *Am J Sports Med* 2004;32(1):S5–16.
2. McKay GD, Goldie PA, Payne WR, et al. Ankle injuries in basketball: injury rate and risk factors. *Br J Sports Med* 2001;35:103–108.
3. Beynnon BD, Murphy DF, Alosa DM. Predictive factors for lateral ankle sprains: a literature review. *J Athl Train* 2002;37(4):376–380.

The Prevention of Athletic Injuries

Upon reading this chapter, the coach should be able to:

1. Describe how preparing an athlete for competition is not dissimilar from preparing for injury prevention.

2. Summarize the factors that can be controlled by the coach to prevent injury.

3. Explain the relationship between strong muscles and strong joints.

4. Know the proper way to warm up an athlete for competition and practice.

5. Be able to develop an eccentric strength training program to prevent hamstring injuries.

6. Know the difference between flexibility and flexibility training.

7. Discuss the controversy of pre-event stretching and injury prevention.

8. Be able to design a balance program to prevent ankle injuries.

9. Know the basic factors involved in overuse injuries.

10. Describe how motor skills can be best taught in a distributed fashion with periods of planned rest.

11. List the criteria for a safe playing environment.

Melissa is a 28-year-old teacher and soccer coach in Florida. An excellent and avid athlete who enjoys the thrill of competition, her ability to participate in most sports is over. Arthritis and chronic knee pain are her constant companions. Her soccer career started at 5 but she also played Little League baseball, basketball, volleyball, and ran track. Other than a broken leg at 14 she completed high school in good health; good enough to receive an athletic scholarship, she headed to the east coast to play soccer. Under the direction of the school's strength and conditioning coach she became a fitness fanatic, training beyond what was necessary. An irregular menstrual cycle and stress fractures in her tibia were the result. "I thought I was OK but everyone kept telling me to slow down," she said.

She transferred to a college in Michigan during her sophomore year. That summer, while playing semipro soccer in Chicago, she suffered her first major knee injury—ACL, MCL, and meniscus tears (a.k.a, the "Unhappy Triad") to her left leg. Determined, she worked 3 hours a day to rehabilitate her leg. That winter she tore her right PCL (posterior cruciate ligament) playing indoor soccer, with no surgery but another rehab. Senior year started and she was voted captain of her team. She felt great during the preseason and started the season strongly, but chronic pain interfered with her play. By the end of the season she struggled with the pain. It was endless.

Graduate school and an assistant soccer coaching job followed. During warm-up for a semipro game she suffered the Unhappy Triad to her right leg—another surgery, another rehab. Following graduation she moved to Florida to teach and coach. While playing around in her front yard she slightly twisted her knee and felt a little twinge. "It wasn't much," she said, but the next day her right knee was quite swollen. She had lost stability in her right leg. After making the rounds to multiple orthopedic surgeons, she decided to take their advice and undergo a third major knee surgery, another ACL replacement, and extensive cleanup work. Following 3 months of bracing, intense pain, and rehabilitation, the doctors told her the surgery was a failure.

"My knees feel like they are full of razor blades and I can never straighten out my right leg because it tends to hyperextend," she said. When asked if it was worth it, she laughed a little and said, "Yes."

IS IT POSSIBLE TO PREVENT ATHLETIC INJURIES?

Melissa's situation is not unique, but a great testament to why injury prevention should be a part of all athletic programs. Consider that millions of high school and college athletes play sports almost daily. Additional millions play recreationally in parks, clubs, and backyards all over the country. Although we generally consider participation in sport to be beneficial, the expense and discomfort resulting from sports injuries is staggering. In high school football alone, Powell (1) reported approximately six million high school football injuries a year, accounting for around 500,000 doctor visits and 30,000 hospitalizations. Additionally, games are won or lost because of sport injuries. Many sport injuries can be devastating to young athletes causing considerable physical and emotional distress. Athletic careers end and some athletic injuries cause a lifetime of discomfort resulting in a decreased life quality (2).

Fortunately, many of these injuries are preventable. *Moreover, the strategies and practices adopted to prevent injury are not dissimilar from the preparation of athletes for performance.* Athletes who are well trained, rested, motivated, skilled, healthy, and properly protected are less susceptible to injury. Injury prevention is not a waste of time but a plan to elicit the best possible performance. The techniques we recommend for injury prevention also enhance performance. Properly trained athletes play better and are at less risk.

Unfortunately, there is an absence of high quality research on injury prevention in athletics. For example, Parkkari et al reported on the lack of randomized controlled trials conducted on injury prevention (3). Prevention research is difficult to control and conduct. Researchers face the ethical dilemma of utilizing a prevention technique for one group while withholding it for another. Historical precedent also interferes with such studies. If athletes believe that a particular technique helps reduce injury, they resist eliminating that strategy. For example, many athletes believe that stretching prior to participation helps prevent injury. Athletes (and their coaches) are then reluctant to participate in a study in which they are asked not to stretch. Animal models help researchers answer basic questions, but eventually studies must be conducted with athletes. As a result of these problems, coaches must often rely on anecdotal information

FOCAL POINT

Knee Osteoarthritis and Knee Injury

Swedish researchers studied female soccer players 12 years after they had received an injury to the anterior cruciate ligament (ACL). The subjects underwent knee radiography to determine radiographic symptoms of osteoarthritis and about half of the athletes had radiographic symptoms. More importantly, 75% reported having symptoms that affected their quality of life. The researchers suggested that the very high prevalence of osteoarthritis in these young women, as well as the functional limitations observed, suggest a strong rationale to focus on injury prevention.

Lohmander LS, Ostenberg A, Englund M, et al. High prevalence of knee osteoarthritis, pain, and functional limitations in female soccer players 12 years after anterior cruciate ligament injury. *Arthritis Rheum* 2004;50(10):3146–3152.

and prior practice. Fortunately, there appears to be increased interest in prevention research, allowing coaches to establish prevention methods based on research and not historical precedent.

Many Athletic Injuries are Preventable

Athletes occasionally suffer single catastrophic events that cannot be prevented. As one of our coaches said, "When a 220 pound athlete runs full speed into a knee that is fixed to the ground, the knee loses." Regardless of conditioning, equipment, and skill level, athletic injuries occur. But many athletic injuries result from several variables, many of which can be manipulated to reduce risk (3). Sports medicine literature often presents extrinsic (outside the individual) and intrinsic (within the individual) variables related to injury. For example, an intrinsic cause might be an athlete's gender, age, or anatomical alignment. Although some of these factors may affect the athlete's risk, the coach has little control over these variables. Typical extrinsic variables are training volume, equipment, and technique. For the purposes of this text, we prefer to present injury prevention as those variables (Table 2.1) the coach can modify. Some variables are more adjustable than others. Coaches have reasonable control over conditioning, fatigue, and equipment, but less control over technique, body weight, and nutrition. Coaches cannot control the weather but they can reduce heat illness by manipulating training in the heat. The key to injury prevention is for the coach to recognize and implement strategies to protect the athlete.

Table 2.2 indicates five different types of athletic injuries along with prevention strategies. From Table 2.2 we can see that three common strategies for injury prevention are strength training, warm-up, and flexibility training. These three treatments vary in their effectiveness.

STRENGTH TRAINING AND ATHLETIC INJURIES: HOW DOES MUSCLE STRENGTH PROTECT JOINTS?

Exercise science texts routinely point out that athletes need to be strong. Injury prevention is universally mentioned as a primary benefit of strength training. In fact, both ligaments and muscles work to stabilize joints. Ligaments attach one bone to another across a joint. Ligaments guide joint movements and also stabilize joints by limiting their range of motion. Ligaments can get stronger with exercise but, unlike muscles, they do not have contractile properties. Muscles also cross joints but have contractile properties, allowing them to shorten. When muscles contract to cause movement, part of the force of contraction also works to stabilize the joint. Figure 2.1 illustrates how the force caused by the quadriceps muscles (through

TABLE 2.1   Modifiable Variables in Injury Prevention
Insufficient Warm-Up
Protective Equipment
Conditioning
Technique
Overuse
Fatigue
Excess pressure to win
Muscle Strength Imbalance
Playing Surface
Flexibility
Playing Opponent
Illegal Play

TABLE 2.2	Athletic Injuries and Preventive Techniques	
Type of Injury	**Tissue Damage**	**Methods of Prevention**
Sprain	Sprains are a stretching or tearing injury of a ligament and depending on the severity can cause disruption of a joint. The injury can affect other soft tissue around the joint including the joint capsule and muscle tendons. Severity ranges from mild to very severe.	Strength Training Bracing (e.g., ankle wraps) Proprioceptive Training (practice landing, jumping, hopping, etc.) Warm up Stretching*
Strains	Strains occur to the muscle, tendon, or to the muscle-tendon junction. As with sprains they range in severity.	Warm up Eccentric training Strength Training Symmetrical training of opposing muscles (e.g., quadriceps and hamstrings) Stretching*
Overuse	Overuse injuries include tendinopathy (tendon conditions arising from overuse) and more serious damage to the bone-tendon junction. Stress fractures are also included in this category.	Sufficient rest between practices. Reduce mass training (e.g., high repetitions of the same activity) Periodized training Improve technique (form) allowing individual joint stress to be reduced. Proper footwear. Female athletes need to maintain a regular menstrual cycle.
Contact	Contact injuries are the result of collisions between players as well as with objects. Contact injuries include lacerations, bruises, fractures, and joint damage. They also include concussions and damage to teeth and eyes. Contact injuries can also cause joint sprains.	Protective equipment that fits. Proper playing surface. Limit excessive contact during practice. Schedule opponents of equal skill and size. Proper technique (example: proper blocking and tackling technique in football) Legal play.
Heat Injuries	Heat exhaustion is the most common of these injuries usually resulting in excessive fatigue and weakness. Heat stroke is a serious heat illness and can result in death.	Acclimatization Appropriate fluid replacement Proper clothing Careful monitoring of the environment. Schedule practice according to environmental conditions.

*Stretching remains a controversial technique in injury prevention.

the patella tendon) actually tends to rotate plus stabilize the joint. Since the force acting on the tendon is not perpendicular to the actual movement, one component of the force acts to *rotate* the tibia while a second, *stabilizing component*, acts to pull the tibia toward the femur. In this manner, contraction of the quadriceps muscles actually stabilizes the knee joint as it rotates the knee. This configuration of muscle to joint is evident throughout the body. *Muscle contraction stabilizes joints.* Naturally, stronger muscles contract with more force, providing a greater stabilizing component. This is why strong muscles result in strong joints.

Increasing the strength of the quadriceps muscle group does not necessarily result in better knee stability. The muscle group on the opposite, contralateral, side of the knee must also work to stabilize the knee. Therefore, if an athlete only strengthens the quadriceps, without simultaneous strengthening of the hamstrings, the knee may actually be less stable. As will be pointed out in Chapter 3, excessive quadriceps strength (without associated hamstring strength) is a risk factor for knee injury.

Equal strength development does not mean equal strength. Many muscle groups, because of their large cross-section and mechanical advantage, will always be stronger than the antagonistic group. Equal strength development means that resistance exercises are applied equally around the joint. Athletes must train for extension as well as flexion, abduction as well as adduction, and inward as well as outward rotation. Do not simply assign exercises that imitate the anticipated movements for a particular sport or activity. Rowers need strong lower backs but they also need good abdominal muscles to help stabilize the spine. Chapter 8 presents strength training methods including the need for symmetrical development.

Strength alone is not sufficient to stabilize joints. Athletes must use their strength in a coordinated manner. Sport movements normally occur at high speed, in fact much faster than resistance exercises performed in the weight room. Athletes must be able to stop quickly, to turn in a coordinated manner, and to land smoothly and softly from a jump. Such coordinated movements can only be learned on the field of play by participating in these activities at speeds replicated in competition. Therefore, resistance exercises must be accompanied by whole body exercises such as plyometrics, agility drills, jumping drills, balance drills, sprinting, medicine ball throws, and hill running. Chapter 3 presents a series of drills designed to improve muscle coordination and proprioception.

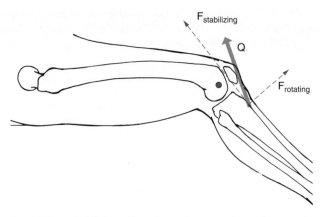

■ **FIGURE 2.1** Stabilizing effect of muscle contraction. When muscles contract part of the force stabilizes the joint. (Modified from Oatis CA. *Kinesiology—The Mechanics and Pathomechanics of Human Movement.* Baltimore: Lippincott Williams & Wilkins, 2004.)

Eccentric Training Helps Prevent Muscle Strains

Muscle strains are one of the most frustrating injuries to athletes and coaches. The hamstring (there are 3 hamstring muscles all performing action at the hip and knee joint) strain is particularly challenging since healing can be very slow and persistent. The reinjury rate for hamstring injuries is fairly high; in fact, the biggest predictor of incurring a hamstring injury is a prior hamstring injury (4,5). Once you tear a hamstring muscle or tendon there is a good chance you will do it again. Preventing these injuries should be a priority for athletes involved in sports involving running and sprinting. Football, soccer, and track athletes are particularly susceptible.

FOCAL POINT

Quadriceps Versus Hamstrings

Go into any weight room and observe how many people exercise their knee extensors versus their knee flexors and you'll find that people tend to train their quadriceps more than their hamstrings. Why? Maybe it's because it's easy to see your quadriceps. It is a little awkward to get into position to strengthen your hamstrings. Athletic trainers tell athletes to strengthen both muscle groups but the quads always seem to win out. The quadriceps muscle group is naturally stronger than the hamstring. There are four (quad) quadriceps while there are only three hamstrings. Plus, the hamstrings are all bi-articular (cross two joints) while only one of the quadriceps (rectus femoris) is bi-articular. All athletes need good hamstring strength. Hamstrings protect the knee during deceleration activities such as landing from a jump. Hamstrings are particularly important for athletes who must move backward quickly such as defensive players, racket sports athletes, and fencers. Prietto and Caiozzo found that the average hamstring to quadricep ratio for typical males was 36.8%. Lieshout tested a group of top level badminton players and found that the male players had a hamstring to quadricep ratio of 60.1% while females had a ratio of 57.5%.

Prietto C, Caiozzo V. The in vivo force-velocity relationship of the knee flexors and extensors. *Am J Sports Med* 1989;17:607–611.
Lieshout K. *Physiological profile of elite junior badminton players in South Africa* [MPhil]. Johannesburg, South Africa: Sport and Movement Studies, Rank Afrikaans University; 2002.

One key to preventing muscle strains is to understand the typical mechanism. The hamstring is vulnerable because of its complicated actions at the knee and hip. During running, the hamstring contracts eccentrically to decelerate the lower leg as it swings forward. During this phase the three hamstring muscles are all getting longer but with enough tension to decelerate the extending leg. Immediately after knee extension is completed the hamstring then contracts rapidly in a concentric fashion to extend the hip (6). These contractions are fairly strong and happen in a very rapid fashion, especially when the athlete is running at high speed. Excellent coordination is essential. Studies suggest that hamstring strains occur during this eccentric phase of muscle contraction (7). One suggestion is that eccentric training of the hamstring may help reduce the frequency of hamstring strain (7).

Swedish researchers conducted a very interesting study in which they specifically trained soccer players eccentrically prior to the soccer season (7). Extra training was performed 1 to 2 times a week during the preseason using a device designed to place an eccentric overload on the hamstrings. The results showed that the incidence of hamstring injury was significantly reduced in those players (3 injuries out of 15 players) than in the group that performed the normal preseason protocol (10 injuries out of 15). In addition, the eccentrically trained group also increased speed and hamstring strength. Although this study was conducted on only 30 players, the use of eccentric training to reduce muscle strains shows potential. From a functional point of view, it would appear that improving musculature, by utilizing the identical form of contraction that causes the injury, makes good sense.

Eccentric training of the hamstrings is easy to implement, fast, and can be conducted without expensive equipment. Figure 2.2 demonstrates a procedure that can be easily used on the field or gym. Athletes work in pairs with one athlete kneeling on the ground or gym mat while a partner anchors them at the ankle. The kneeling athlete then extends at the knee, keeping the entire body in a straight line, and moves toward the ground until just before the resistance becomes too great. Then they return to the original position and repeat 8 to 10 times.

The gastrocnemius (calf) is another muscle commonly strained. Similar to the hamstring group, the gastrocnemius works at the knee as well as the ankle. The contraction and relaxation of this powerful muscle must occur quickly and fluidly during high speed running. Figure 2.3 demonstrates an easy eccentric calf exercise.

WARM-UP

Warming up prior to athletic competition or practice is probably the most common injury prevention technique utilized in sport. Concurrently, the benefit of warming up as an ergogenic (work) aid is widely believed. In fact, studies on the benefit of warm-up have been conducted for over 50 years. For example, in 1945 Swedish researchers found that when muscle temperature is raised, individuals can perform short-term high power activities much faster (8). Bishop reviewed 66 research studies on warm-up and concluded that while there is a scarcity of well-controlled studies on warm-up, active warm-up tends to improve performance (9).

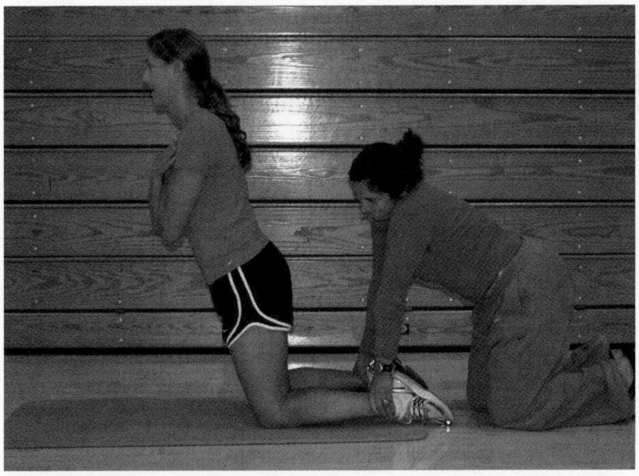

■ **FIGURE 2.2** An eccentric exercise for the hamstrings. From a kneeling position, slowly extend at the knee. Stop prior to failure.

With regard to the relationship between warm-up and injury prevention, the classic study by Safran et al in 1988 using laboratory animals is often utilized as one basis for the role of warm-up in muscular injury (10). They tested muscle tears in muscles that were either prestimulated (warmed-up) or not. They found that those muscles that were warmed by prestimulation were more resistant to muscle tears than muscles that had not been previously stimulated. Warming muscles by repeated contractions helped prevent muscle tears.

Increasing the temperature of muscles has the physiological effect of improving the speed of muscle contraction and relaxation (Table 2.3) plus beneficial effects on metabolism.

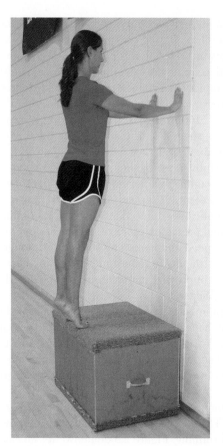 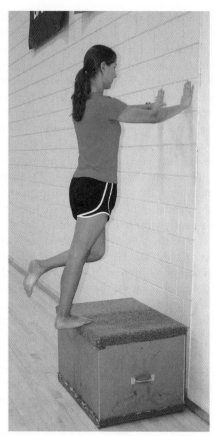

■ **FIGURE 2.3** An eccentric exercise for posterior lower leg muscles. Stand on the corner of a bench and plantar flex both feet followed by controlled lowering on one leg.

Preliminary exercise dilates capillary beds and increases cardiac output (9–11). Warm-up techniques are typically classified as passive or active. Passive warm-up involves such procedures as whirlpool baths, hot packs, and diathermy. Active warm-up is far more popular and can be related or unrelated. General warm-up includes such activities as calisthenics and jogging while related warm-up involves participating in the exact activities one intends to perform while playing. Related warm-up often follows general warm-up. Related warm-up is typically preferred over general warm-up because the exact muscles utilized in performance are heated. Warm-up also has a strong psychological effect. Athletes become familiar with the competitive environment and have time to practice and to fine-tune themselves for the activity at hand. They become motivated for competition.

TABLE 2.3   Benefits of Warm-Up
Muscles contract faster.
Muscles relax faster.
Decrease muscle stiffness.
Economy of movement is improved.
Metabolism is enhanced because of the increased temperature of muscle tissue.
Muscle blood flow is increased.
Provides a last minute practice session
Athletes prepared psychologically for performance.

Related warm-up is particularly important for high velocity, ballistic activities. Javelin throwers must throw the javelin a few times and jumpers must perform a few jumps of increasing intensity. Athletes need to warm up the exact muscle fibers they intend to utilize in performance. Not only does this increase muscle temperature but the athlete can practice the upcoming activity.

The duration and intensity of warm-up is important. Further, the recovery period (time between warm-up and performance) is very important. Warm-up must be of sufficient duration to increase muscle temperature but not so strenuous that the athlete fatigues. Warm-up must also be individualized to the fitness level of the participant. Muscle temperature rises quickly during the first 3 to 5 minutes of warm-up and plateaus around 10 to 20 minutes (9). Start the warm-up slowly and increase the intensity as game time approaches. End the warm-up several minutes before competition to allow for a slight recovery period. Make sure the athletes are warm but recovered prior to the start of a game. Warm-up lasts for a while and an athlete who is well-clothed can remain warm for about 30 minutes. Bishop makes the following points in his review (9).

- Warm-up should last from 5 to 20 minutes. Longer warm-ups are unnecessary and may fatigue the athletes.
- Warm-ups should be moderately vigorous at about 40% to 60% of maximal capacity (heart rate of around 120 to 140).
- Calisthenics alone do not provide sufficient warm-up.
- Highly fit athletes take a little longer to warm up.
- Athletes performing high speed activities need to practice the exact activities with increasing intensity.
- The recovery period following a warm-up should be at least 5 minutes.

SUBSTITUTIONS AND HALF-TIME

Occasionally you will see athletes running back on the field or court because their coach has talked during the entire half-time break. These athletes are more at risk. Athletes need a brief warm-up prior to the second half. Muscle stiffness is common following activity and a brief rewarming reduces stiffness. Research has shown that early second half injuries are reduced when athletes are required to warm up as little as 3 minutes following the halftime break (12). Schedule time for your athletes to warm up prior to the second half and make sure they do.

Imagine sitting on a hard bench for an hour when the coach tells you, "Mike, go in for Frank." You're stiff from sitting more than half the game. You warmed up earlier but the effects are long gone. You're not ready for full-speed play. On the other hand, if your coach says, "Mike, start getting ready. You're going in for Frank," you have some time to prepare yourself for play. While substitutions to replace an injured player are unexpected, the typical substitution is not for emergencies. If you intend to substitute a player, give the athlete ample notice to get ready to play. Although they will probably not be able to perform a related warm-up, they can usually jog, run in place, or ride a stationary cycle to get ready. Extended periods of inactivity occasionally happen during practice when some players are scrimmaging and others are watching. Whether it's a game or a practice, give athletes time to get ready for movement. This additional time will make for better performance and help reduce injury.

FLEXIBILITY TRAINING AND INJURY PREVENTION: A CONTROVERSIAL SUBJECT

About 30 years ago there were reports of football programs hiring coaches whose main job was to design and implement stretching programs. Athletes would spend 20 to 30 minutes performing extensive static stretching exercises prior to games and practice. Newspaper articles expounded the benefits of stretching and athletes wouldn't even think of performing without first stretching. The belief was that flexibility of a muscle-tendon unit improved performance and reduced injury. The premise was that increased flexibility would decrease muscle-tendon stiffness and make the unit more compliant to stretching, reducing the injury potential for muscle strains. A thorough review of the literature in 1999 conducted by Shrier has challenged this claim (13). In fact, there is little evidence that flexibility training (primarily static stretching procedures) prior to exercise reduces the frequency of athletic injury (14). Moreover, the effect of pre-event stretching on performance has been recently questioned. Flexibility training is now a subject of confusion and controversy.

One confusing aspect relates to flexibility training as opposed to flexibility. A review of terms may clarify this discussion:

- *Pre-event stretching* is normally composed of static stretching activities performed some time during warm-up and prior to performance. Occasionally you will see athletes performing more dynamic types of stretching such as high kicks, skipping, and vigorous arm swings. These are often a favorite of track and field athletes.
- *Flexibility* is often considered the simple range of motion (ROM) through which an athlete can move a limb. Flexibility may or may not be related to training since some athletes are naturally flexible without performing any flexibility exercises.
- *Flexibility training* is the deliberate attempt to increase the ROM of various movements. Flexibility training generally occurs during practice and is particularly evident during preseason. Flexibility training usually involves some form of static stretching. Many athletes now accompany static stretching with some form of dynamic stretches as described below.

FOCAL POINT

Does Static Stretching Reduce Injury

There is no clear evidence that performing a static stretch reduces the incidence of injury. However, there is increasing evidence that pre-event stretches similar to Figure A below, performed for extended periods, may reduce power and strength. Static stretching may be better placed at the end of practice. Dynamic stretching (Fig. B) may be a better alternative prior to performance.

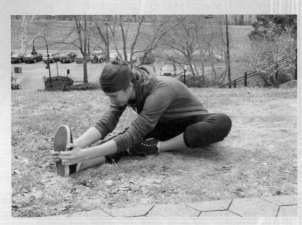

Figure A

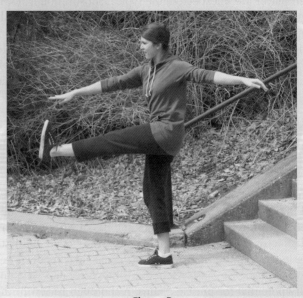

Figure B

Pre-event Stretching: Should Athletes Stretch Before Performing?

The evidence for the use of pre-event stretching to reduce injury is inconclusive. For example, in a recent review of research on this subject the authors concluded that there is insufficient evidence to endorse or discourage routine stretching prior to performance (15). Research on this subject has been difficult to conduct as subjects are frequently noncompliant. Athletes often believe that stretching is beneficial and they are going to do it whether planned or not. We believe the emphasis of pre-event activities should be on warming up the athlete and specifically preparing them for performance. Extensive time spent stretching may also compromise the warm-up. Stretching exercises should never take the place of warm-up, and a few toe touches and hamstring stretches does not prepare an athlete for performance.

Although there is no good evidence that pre-event stretching reduces the risk of injury, there is recent evidence that pre-event stretching may compromise performance. In fact, pre-event stretching has been shown to reduce strength, power, and strength endurance (muscular endurance) activities (16–19). Extensive static stretching prior to performance reduces power and strength. Since many sports require strength and power, static stretching may inhibit performance. Although the evidence is still somewhat unclear, pre-event stretching only seems to affect those activities that require speed, strength, and power. These activities are often typical of the stretch-shortening cycle required in high speed activities like jumping, throwing, and sprinting. One suggestion is that acute stretching reduces stiffness and may reduce the ability of the muscle to transmit force to the skeleton (19,20). Researchers have also determined that pre-event stretching causes a decrease in muscle activation (possibly from fatigue), therefore reducing the ability of the muscle to perform (18,21,22).

We recommend that athletes in high power sports should limit (if not eliminate) pre-event stretching (specifically static stretching) and focus more on entering performance in a rested state following a warm-up highly related to the upcoming activities. Athletes who participate in sports that involve lower power (such as distance running) and are more repetitive may perform pre-event stretching if they wish. However, each athlete is different and their state of mind is highly important for performance. If an athlete feels they will perform better after a few stretching exercises, they probably will.

Does Increased Flexibility Prevent Injury?

Research on flexibility training and injury prevention is most frequently related to the effect of pre-event stretching and performance. Although we know this to be a topic of contention, does routine stretching reduce the incidence of injury? Unfortunately, there are very few good studies in this area. The study most quoted was conducted with military trainees undergoing basic training (23). The researchers incorporated a hamstring flexibility training routine for one group while a second group did not perform the specific exercises. The hamstring trained group had fewer lower extremity injuries than the control group. One study on 306 football players found that hamstring flexibility was not related to hamstring injury but groin strains were related to less flexible hip adductor muscles (24). A third study on professional soccer players in England found that those players who performed a regular hamstring stretching program had reduced hamstring strains (25).

Considering the many years that coaches and athletic trainers have advocated the use of flexibility training to reduce injury, the evidence is rather limited. As Shrier indicated, one of the problems with flexibility research is that some people are naturally flexible and never stretch while others remain inflexible regardless of training. To complicate matters further, the effect of stretching is also specific to the individual. Shrier also presents one common argument for why stretching exercises may be unrelated to injury prevention. Typically, muscle strains do not occur during extreme ranges of motion (26). Extreme range of movement by most athletes appears unnecessary.

The amount of flexibility training needed should be specific to the sport and to the individual. The appropriate ROM required for sport is specific to the activities required by that sport. Gymnasts, divers, hurdlers, and swimmers are just a few examples of athletes who need very good ROM and need to spend more time developing flexibility. In fact, without very good ROM these athletes will not perform well. But only moderate ROM is needed for sports such as basketball, football, field hockey, and soccer. Some sports, such as distance running and rowing, may tend to make athletes less flexible. The highly repetitive nature of these sports tends to lengthen some muscle groups at the expense of the contralateral group. Extreme flexibility is not recommended for many athletes. Highly flexible knee and shoulder joints are less stable.

FLEXIBILITY TRAINING

Coaches should plan flexibility programs designed to bring about the typical ranges of motion required for each sport. Since pre-event stretching does not seem to prevent injury but may possibly reduce performance, we recommend putting flexibility training more toward the end of practice. Static stretching is the most recommended form of flexibility training. Three stretching sessions a week with four to five repetitions per muscle group for 30 seconds is sufficient (27). Only one stretch per muscle group is necessary even though some athletes like to perform multiple exercises per group. The general areas recommended for stretching are listed in Table 2.4.

Dynamic stretching routines have become much more popular. Because sport is a dynamic activity, muscles should be prepared to move through a range of motion, not to simply maintain one static position. Do not confuse dynamic stretching with ballistic stretching. Dynamic stretching involves controlled body movements such as arm and leg swings and torso twists that gradually increase in intensity. Dynamic stretching is often performed in conjunction with a warm-up but is normally done at the end of the warm up. Ballistic stretching is not recommended as a means of increasing flexibility since the body is often forced beyond a normal range of motion and considerable soreness can occur as a result.

Sprained Ankles

The sprained ankle is the most common joint injury in sport and accounts for huge expense and significant time lost for sport participation (28). Some ankle injuries can even cause long term disability. Most sprained ankles occur when landing from a jump, a possible misstep, or when an athlete loses their balance. Athletes in basketball, soccer, volleyball, and football are particularly vulnerable. About 90% of sprained ankles occur to the lateral, outside, of the foot (29). Athletes with prior ankle injury appear to be at greater risk of getting a subsequent injury. One study on over 10,000 basketball participants indicated that players with a history of ankle injury were almost five times more likely to sustain an additional ankle injury (30). Sex does not appear to be a risk factor as male and female athletes suffer ankle sprains at about the same rate (27).

Because the sprained ankle is so common, literally hundreds of studies have addressed this subject. For example, Fong et al reviewed 227 studies observing the injury pattern of ankle sprains. They concluded that the ankle was the most common injury in 24 of 70 sports (31). Osborne and Rizzo reviewed 40 studies dealing with prevention and treatment of ankle sprains (32). Considerable studies exist on the epidemiology and

TABLE 2.4 **Flexibility Training for Sport**		
Muscle Area	**Primary Sports Involved***	**Comments**
Hamstrings	Any sport involving sprinting or high speed running	Normally use in conjunction with quadricep stretching.
Quadriceps	Similar to sports for hamstring group but also for crew athletes	Also perform quadricep stretches following weight workout such as squats.
Calf and Achilles Tendon	Sports that involve sprinting, jumping, and quick stopping and starting	Important to make sure Achilles tendon is warm and should be actively stretched in addition to static stretching.
Groin and Hip Flexors	Very important for sports involving quick turns, sprinting, and kicking.	
Lower Back	Most athletes need moderate lower back flexibility.	Rowers, high jumpers, gymnasts, and hurdlers are in particular need of good low back flexibility.
Chest	Athletes who throw or hit (e.g., tennis or squash) need good chest ROM. Some swimmers may reduce ROM by training and need to stretch this area.	Athletes who perform strength training for the chest need to stretch this area following a workout.
Upper Back	Swimmers, throwers, and racket sport athletes need good upper back flexibility.	
Neck	Wrestlers and football players need good neck flexibility.	Perform neck stretches at the end or practice or after a neck strengthening workout.

treatment of ankle sprains, but far less on prevention. The most frequently studied prevention technique has addressed ankle bracing. Three basic techniques are currently used to prevent ankle injuries.

- *Bracing* of ankles through tape or various reusable braces has been around for many years. Although the subject of ankle bracing is considered in more depth in Chapter 5, the basic finding is that bracing reduces the incidence of ankle sprain (32). Furthermore, bracing is particularly important for those athletes with recurring ankle injuries.
- *Balance training.* Since so many ankle sprains occur either from improper landing or when an athlete is off balance, recent work has shown the positive effects of improving balance and a subsequent reduction in ankle injury (27,29). Researchers at the University of Wisconsin utilized a randomized controlled trial in which half of the participants participated in a balance training program while the control group participated in their normal training program. The study was conducted on 765 high school basketball and soccer players. Results indicated that a simple balance training program reduced the rate of ankle sprains by 38% in male and female high school soccer and basketball players. This program was particularly effective for those athletes with a history of ankle injury (27).
- *Plyometric and jump training.* Plyometrics has long been touted as a method of improving power. Additionally, plyometric and jump training has been successfully used in prevention programs to reduce anterior cruciate ligament (ACL) injuries (Chapter 3). Sports medicine researchers in Cincinnati conducted plyometric and dynamic balance training with a group of female high school athletes (29). Subjects performed a 7-week plyometric or balance training program. Following the training subjects were filmed while landing from jumps. Both plyometric and balance trained subjects appeared to land with improved ankle movement suggesting a more stable ankle. It remains uncertain whether plyometric training reduces ankle injury but we highly recommend this type of preseason work simply from the standpoint of improving knee stability. Since improved balance and power are very desirable athletic attributes, this is a perfect example of how coaches can design programs to improve performance and reduce injury at the same time.

FOCAL POINT

Balance Training: A Defense Against Ankle Sprains

Balance is one of those performance variables that we often do not bother to train, presuming that balance will naturally improve simply with participation. While this may be true, specific balance training has been shown to reduce ankle injury. Fortunately, such training is easy, inexpensive, and not time consuming. In addition, coaches can adapt balance training to meet the demands of their sport. Researchers associated with the Sports Medicine Center at the University of Wisconsin have utilized balance boards consisting of a wooden disk 16 inches in diameter with a 4-inch half sphere attached to the bottom. These boards typically cost $50 to $60. Subjects in their study participated in a progressive 5 week preseason (five times per week) program with a maintenance program (three times per week) during season. The first 2 weeks of training were conducted without the balance board and consisted of single-leg and double-leg balance activities with eyes open or closed. Subjects then progressed to single- and double-legged balance activities on the board while also performing basketball activities such as dribbling and passing (See Fig. A).

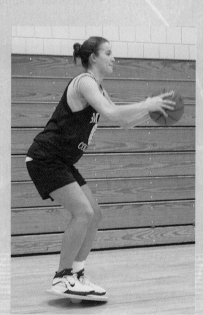

McGuine T, Keene J. The effect of a balance training program on the risk of ankle sprains in high school athletes. *Am J Sports Med* 2006;34:1103–1111.

OVERUSE INJURIES

Overuse injuries are often the result of repetitive submaximal loading resulting in degenerative change. Overuse injuries occur when there is not sufficient recovery, when tissues lose their ability to adapt. The problem is not an acute one, remedied by a couple of days' rest, but much more chronic. Distance running, throwing, swimming, and striking games (e.g., tennis, soccer, squash) are sports that require movements that are very repetitive. Training causes fatigue to specific parts of the body or to the whole body. Sufficient recovery allows athletes to adapt to the demand and to recover to a state that allows for further training without injury.

Data indicate that overuse injuries have increased considerably (30). For example, one study reported that fully 50% of all injuries presented to a sports medicine clinic for youth were classified as overuse (31). Consider that one estimate suggests that approximately 35 million children and young adults in the United States between the ages of 6 and 21 participate in sports and you get an idea how serious overuse injuries are (30). We suspect that there are two primary causes for the increase in overuse injuries. First, the number of girls and women participating in sport has increased dramatically in the past three decades, simply adding many more sport participants. Second, the nature of sport in the U.S. has changed from seasonal participation to more sport-specific, year-round training. As specialization increases so does the risk of overuse. Compounding this problem involves the nature of sport specialization programs; they are frequently not school related. As a result, coaches are usually not required to satisfy academic standards to coach young athletes. But overuse injuries are not specific to children and young adults. There are countless examples of overuse in college and professional sport athletes.

Interestingly, overuse injuries are probably the easiest to avoid yet we are observing an increase in such injuries. Children are particularly susceptible to overuse injuries, but DiFiori suggests that children rarely suffer overuse injuries when they control their own play (30). Multiple factors result in overuse injuries ranging from growth patterns to inappropriate equipment. Some of the basic factors over which coaches have some control include the following:

- Inappropriate practice procedures
- Poor technique
- Parental, coach, and peer pressure
- Uneven or hard surfaces
- Inappropriate equipment

FOCAL POINT

Overuse Injuries are Often Related to Training Errors

Jeff watched with excitement as the city built six new tennis courts in the park across from his house. He had not had the opportunity to play real tennis but he had been hitting balls against his garage wall for the past year. He had gotten pretty good at it. As soon as the courts were finished Jeff started playing with a group of his friends. He was a natural, very quick and agile at age 13. He was still growing. Summer came and the recreation department in his town sponsored lessons and a season ending tournament. Jeff made it to the finals in his age group. His dad decided that professional training would help Jeff and enrolled him in a year-round tennis academy run by a professional player. Jeff started playing tennis daily with long sessions on the weekends. "Repetition is the key to success," his coach said. One hundred forehands were followed by 100 backhands and then 100 serves. Jeff's elbow starting hurting, especially during the backhand drills. He mentioned it to his coach. "You'll adapt to the training, just keep practicing," his coach said. But Jeff's elbow didn't get better, it got worse. What started out as a mild inflammation of the tendon had now become much more serious—there were structural changes to the tendon and bone. Jeff's tennis career ended at age 15.

Reduce High Repetition Training

Since overuse injuries are normally the result of high repetition activities, the first stumbling block is how to organize practice without excess repetition. Clearly, the attainment and improvement in athletic performance requires practice. Athletes must practice to improve skills and to increase or maintain their conditioning. Can motor skills be taught without excessive repetition? The attainment of skilled performance requires extensive deliberate practice, but deliberate practice is not very fun and athletes tend to lose their motivation. But motivation to learn is an important variable for teaching (32). The coach is faced with the task of providing sufficient practice time, yet not so much that the athlete acquires an overuse injury or becomes unmotivated. Is intense repetition the best way to learn a skill? Research in motor learning suggests that endless repletion may not be the best way to learn.

MASS VERSUS DISTRIBUTED PRACTICE

Athletes must practice skills that they intend to utilize in competition. One important variable regarding the organization of practice relates to the distribution of practice time. Let's say that you've planned to devote 40 minutes to skill development during a practice. How are you going to distribute active practice (time spent performing the skill) with rest time? The motor learning literature suggests that this distribution is a question of mass vs distributed practice.

Massing means to run work periods very close together with little or no rest. Distributing practice means to intersperse rest periods between shorter periods of work. Since high repetitions are one cause of overuse injury, rest periods will help prevent overuse injury. Does the distribution of practice affect learning? Research suggests (Schmidt and Lee) that distributed practice is better for performance as well as learning (32). In fact, they even suggest that longer rest periods are better than shorter ones. Continuous practice causes muscular fatigue and reduces performance. In fact, not only do individuals learn better with distributed practice, they tend to retain their skill development longer. Distributing practice by scheduling active practice between rest intervals appears to improve learning and performance. Distributing learning activities by interspersing rest with work is great for learning and injury prevention.

CONTEXTUAL INTERFERENCE: BLOCK VERSUS RANDOM PRACTICE

Another aspect of learning motor skills relates to the actual learning task itself. In the case study of our young tennis player, he was required to hit 100 backhands in a row. He then went on to hit 100 forehands, followed by 100 serves. This is an example of blocked practice, performing the identical task until some level of achievement is reached. Random practice is just the opposite and involves mixing it up, forehand—backhand—volleys—etc. This last example has been called contextual interference, first presented in a study in 1979 (33). Schmidt and Lee (32) use the following example to explain contextual interference. Presume that a golfer has 60 golf balls to hit at a practice range with a driver, 5-iron, and wedge. The golfer can hit 20 balls in a row (blocked) with each club or he can randomly rotate through the 3 clubs (random), until all 60 balls have been hit.

Schmidt and Lee report that the immediate acquisition of performance is better when practice is presented in a blocked fashion. However, retention of the motor task is better with random practice. When asked to repeat the task(s) at a later date, subjects who practiced in a random fashion were superior in performance (32). Randomizing practice reduces joint stress and enhances retention. Since coaches teach athletes motor skills for performance at a later date, random, rather than blocked, practice appears to be a better method of distributing learning activities. Since random practice uses different muscle groups, there is more time for the athlete to recover between repetitions and less risk of overuse.

We recommend the following to enhance learning as well as reduce the risk of overuse injury:

- Create practices in which active practicing of learning tasks is combined with rest periods.
- Create practices in which learning activities are presented in a random approach. Varying the practice tasks improves learning and retention.
- Create practices that are interesting and challenging. Athletes who are motivated will learn more and perform better. Athletes need to deliberately practice but mixing up practice reduces boredom as well as overuse injuries.

Progress Gradually to Reduce Overuse Injury

Coaches should be able to quantify their practices. Volume, intensity, distance, repetitions, and time are all variables that coaches can use to judge how difficult practice is. The concept of Hard-Easy (presented in more detail in Chapter 7) is important. Hard workouts should be followed by easy workouts. Rest must be planned into all practices and between practices. Most athletes cannot adapt to an abrupt change in training. They must be given time to adapt to each phase of training. Slow steady progression is the key to training as well as preventing overuse.

Good Technique Reduces Joint Stress

Athletes with poor technique tend to place undue stress on particular body parts, increasing the incidence of overuse injury. Baseball reporters often said that Nolan Ryan, the great Hall of Fame fastball pitcher, suffered few injuries because of his flawless form (Ryan pitched for 27 years in major league baseball). Ballistic activities such as throwing, kicking, and hitting (tennis forehand, serve, etc.) involve the kinetic chain, a series of movements that normally start on the ground and end with contact or release. The kinetic chain involves the transfer of momentum from the ground through the trunk and onto the extremities in a coordinated accelerating fashion. Proper form results in reduced stress on any one body part. All coaches should be well aware of the proper technique for performance in their individual sport. Time spent teaching proper technique is well spent and should not be relegated only to beginners. Professional athletes practice to improve their technique during their entire careers.

Playing Surface Should be Well Maintained and Stable

Hard uneven playing surfaces present undue lower extremity stress to field players such as soccer, lacrosse, and field hockey. Fields that are very dry tend to increase stress. Training is also very specific to the surface on which it occurs. Athletes can adapt to various surfaces but must be given time to adapt. For instance, if athletes are trained to participate in a specific workout on a grass field, they will find that same workout more stressful on a turf field. Switching fields requires a progressive approach, allowing the athletes to adapt to the new surface.

FROM THE ATHLETIC TRAINING ROOM

Improving Technique: Speed vs. Accuracy

When individuals practice skills there is the normal expectancy that the motion pattern will improve with time. However, the goal of the practice session may affect how the motion pattern actually changes. In a classic study of speed versus accuracy, Southard had subjects perform an arm striking skill (a ballistic task) with the goal of speed or accuracy. Subjects were told to either strike an object as fast as possible or accurately. High speed cameras monitored the development of efficient joint movements (transfer of momentum via the kinetic chain) of the groups. All subjects started out performing this task with constrained, inefficient, movements. The requirement of speed was found to significantly improve the efficiency (reduced joint stress) of the task without sacrificing the attainment of accuracy.

Southard D. Changes in limb striking pattern: effects of speed and accuracy. *Res Q Exerc Sport* 1989;60(4):348–356.

STRESS FRACTURES

Stress fractures are classified as overuse injuries and are normally the result of repeated stress that is insufficient to fracture a bone in a single event. Bones are living tissue and are in a constant state of change. Stress fractures usually occur when there is a negative balance between bone formation and resorption; that is, more bone is being lost than gained resulting in a gradual reduction of bone density until small fractures occur. The site and frequency of stress fractures depends primarily on the activity. Runners develop stress fractures to their lower extremities, throwers to their humerus, and rowers to their ribs. Some athletes are more susceptible to stress fractures and females with irregular menstrual cycles (see Chapter 10) are particularly susceptible (34). The incidence of stress fractures in children is increasing but adult athletes have more stress fractures than children (35).

According to Pecina and Bojanic, training errors are the most common cause of stress fractures (35). In fact, they suggest that training errors account for as many as 22% to 75% of stress fractures and that "mileage mania" (excessive mileage) and too rapid changes in training are the primary training errors. Several factors must be constantly considered regarding overuse and stress fractures:

1. Training must allow rest so that bones can adapt (repair) to the stress of high repetition training.
2. Increased mileage must be gradual.
3. Coaches must constantly balance the possible benefit of increased mileage with the risk of overuse. Will the increased mileage actually result in better performance?
4. Proper footwear (Chapter 5) is critical, especially for athletes involved in long distance training.
5. Fatigue reduces foot stability and the ability of the muscles in the foot and ankle to stabilize and reduce stress on the foot (36).

FATIGUE IS RELATED TO INJURY

Sports medicine personnel have long suspected that fatigue and injury are related. An injury that is frequently associated with fatigue is the muscle strain. For instance, as early as 1971 researchers in Australia provided data suggesting that hamstring injuries were related to fatigue (37). Muscle strains tended to occur very early in practice/games or very late. The explanation was that early strains were caused by inadequate warm-up and later strains were caused by fatigue. Clinical evidence for the relationship between fatigue and muscle strain is supported by laboratory studies on animal muscle. Orthopaedic researchers at Duke University studied the effects of fatigue on the eccentric loading capacity of leg muscles. Muscles that had been fatigued lost some of their ability to absorb energy and tended to tear more easily (38). Since muscle strains tend to occur during eccentric contractions, athletes are more vulnerable to muscle strains when fatigued.

Muscle strains are not the only injury in which fatigue is a factor. Fatigue causes increased joint laxity and decreased neuromuscular control, balance, and coordination (36,39,40). As discussed earlier in this chapter, joint stability is highly related to coordinated muscle contractions. We suspect that fatigued athletes are more susceptible to joint injuries such as ankle, knee, and shoulder sprains. Fatigue inhibits balance and coordination, making an athlete more vulnerable to opponents, especially during collision games like football.

Obviously, the primary way to reduce fatigue is training. Athletes during preseason are particularly susceptible to fatigue. Coaches are anxious to proceed, competition is approaching, athletes are motivated, and there is the urgency to get athletes prepared as soon as possible. As presented in Chapter 7, interval training is a primary strategy, allowing a significant amount of training while reducing excessive fatigue. Athletes are going to get tired during training. In fact, we believe that athletes need to learn to perform while tired, but excessive fatigue is not necessary to develop fit athletes. Balance high quality training with rest periods to get the most out of your athletes.

COLLISION INJURIES

Collisions are natural in many sports but tend to cause many injuries. Knee and shoulder sprains occasionally occur because of collision but most collisions result in bruises, contusions, lacerations, and occasionally concussions. Broken bones are almost always the result of trauma. The best protection for injuries due to collision is protective equipment (see Chapter 5). However, other techniques should be used.

Since athletes spend more time practicing than competing, more injuries tend to occur in practice. Athletes must learn proper hitting techniques such as blocking and tackling during practice. They must become thoroughly familiar with contact. However, excessive use of full-speed contact puts the athletes at risk. Coaches occasionally get angry with players and put them through multiple high-speed full-contact drills. Not only are these drills fatiguing, they put the athlete at significantly more risk of injury. Coaches must weigh the benefits of such training with injury risk. In our opinion, it's normally not worth it.

Good technique is a powerful weapon against collision injuries. All football athletes must be taught the proper, legal way to block and tackle. Rules against the use of the head in blocking and tackling have made huge reductions in head and neck injuries. Illegal play should never be endorsed and coaches must work to schedule opponents of equal size and ability. Every year in American football we see teams that are decidedly inferior playing teams that are superior to them in size and ability. Sports reporters commonly suggest that such events are scheduled to raise more money. Athletes are not expendable; they are not commodities to be used to make money for weak teams. In our view such competitions should not be scheduled.

Maintain a Safe Playing Environment

The playing environment is an important consideration regarding injury prevention. Coaches cannot leave the responsibility of the gymnasium floor or athletic field totally to maintenance personnel. Prior to practice and games the athletic trainers are often totally absorbed with duties in the training room. They do not have time to inspect the playing area. Coaches should inspect the environment, making sure that such things as hoses or sprinklers have not been left in place. Has the field been cut? Is the lawnmower right next to the field of play? Has the field been watered? Is there water on the floor? These are all things that coaches must constantly observe.

Every year athletes are injured because of unpadded goal posts, spectators on the sidelines, and inappropriate gym mats. Many of these injuries are fairly serious such as concussions due to hitting an unpadded wall under the basketball goal. Occasionally funds are available for a new facility but protective equipment is not funded. Everyone is so excited to use the new facility that simple safety rules are compromised. All coaches should be aware of the specific requirements for safe play in their sport. Some of the basics are:

- Padded goal posts
- Wall (or post) padding under the basketball goal (or any wall too close to competition)
- Dry floors
- Ample room on the sidelines
- Fixed bleachers should not be close to the side or endlines
- Even grass fields that are frequently watered (remove sprinkler heads, hoses)

SUMMARY

- Athletic injuries are costly and painful, some even causing lifelong changes in one's health. Athletes who have been previously injured are at greater risk. Injury prevention is not a waste of time.
- Preparing athletes for competition is not dissimilar from preparing athletes for injury prevention.
- Functional strength training helps strengthen joints.
- Eccentric strength training helps prevent hamstring injuries.
- Specific warm-up helps prevent injuries.

- Athletes need to warm up after half-time breaks.
- Pre-event stretching is unproven as a prevention strategy for injuries, but pre-event stretching does tend to reduce power and strength.
- Balance training helps prevent ankle sprains.
- Overuse injuries can be reduced and learning can be improved by teaching motor skills in a distributed, rather than mass, schedule.
- Use contextual interference to teach motor skills to reduce overuse and to improve retention.
- Prevent "Mileage Mania" to reduce overuse injury.
- Use gradual increases in training to reduce overuse and fatigue.
- Athletes who are fatigued are more susceptible to muscle strains and are less coordinated, making them more vulnerable to contact injury.
- Coaches need to supervise the practice and playing environment for safety considerations.

References

1. Powell JW, Barber-Foss KD. Injury patterns in selected high school sports: a review of the 1995–1997 seasons. *J Athl Train* 1999;34(3):277–284.
2. Gelber AC, Hochberg MC, Mead LA, et al. Joint injury in young adults and risk for subsequent knee and hip osteoarthritis. *Ann Intern Med* 2000;133:321–328.
3. Parkkari J, Kujala UM, Kannus P. Is it possible to prevent sports injuries? *Sports Med* 2001;31(14):985–995.
4. Gabbe BJ, Bennell KL, Finch CF, et al. Predictors of hamstring injury at the elite level of Australian football. *Scandinavian J Med Sci Sport* 2006;16:7–13.
5. Orchard JW. Intrinsic and extrinsic risk factors for muscle strains in Australian football. *Am J Sports Med* 2001;29(3):300–303.
6. Petersen J, Holmich P. Evidence based prevention of hamstring injuries in sport. *Br J Sports Med* 2005;39:319-323.
7. Askling C, Karlsson J, Thorstensson A. Hamstring injury occurrence in elite soccer players after preseason strength training with eccentric overload. *Scandinavian J Med Sci Sport* 2003;13(4):244–250.
8. Asmussen E, Boke O. Body temperature and capacity for work. *Acta Physiologica Scandinavica* 1945;10:1.
9. Bishop D. Warm up II. *Sports Med* 2003;33(7):483–498.
10. Safran MR, Garrett WE, Seaber AV, et al. The role of warmup in muscular injury prevention. *Am J Sports Med* 1988;16(2):123–129.
11. Brooks GA, Fahey TD, White TP. *Exercise Physiology: Human Bioenergetics and Its Applications*, 3rd ed. Mountain View: Mayfield Publishing Company, 2000.
12. Bixler B, Jones RL. High-school football injuries: effects of a posthalftime warm-up and stretching routine. *Fam Pract Res J* 1992;12(2):131–139.
13. Shrier I. Stretching before exercise does not reduce the risk of local muscle injury: a critical review of the clinical and basic science literature. *Clin J Sports Med* 1999;9:221–227.
14. Witvrouw E, Mahier N, Danneels L, et al. Stretching and injury prevention: an obscure relationship. *Sports Med* 2004;34(7):443–449.
15. Thacker SB, Gilchrist J, Stroup DF, et al. The impact of stretching on sports injury risk: a systematic review of the literature. *Med Sci Sports Exerc* 2004;36(3):371–378.
16. Nelson AG, Kokkonen J, Arnall DA. Acute muscle stretching inhibits muscle strength endurance performance. *J Strength Cond Res* 2005;19(2):338–343.
17. Nelson AG, Kokkonen J. Acute ballistic muscle stretching inhibits maximal strength performance. *Res Q Exerc Sport* 2001;72:415–419.
18. Behm DG, Button DC, Butt JC. Factors affecting force loss with prolonged stretching. *Can J Appl Physiol* 2001;26:261–272.
19. Evetovich TK, Nauman NJ, Conley DS, et al. Effect of static stretching of the biceps brachii on torque, electromyography, and mechanomyography during concentric isokinetic muscle actions. *J Strength Cond Res* 2003;17:484–488.
20. Wilson GJ, Murphy AJ, Pryor JF. Musculotendinous stiffness: its relationship to eccentric, isometric, and concentric performance. *J Appl Physiol* 1994;76:2714–2719.
21. Avela J, Kyrolainen H, Komi PV. Altered reflex sensitivity after repeated and prolonged passive muscle stretching. *J Appl Physiol* 1999;86:1283–1291.
22. Fowles JR, Sale DG, MacDougall JD. Reduces strength after passive stretch of the human plantarflexors. *J Appl Physiol* 2000;89:1179–1188.
23. Hartig DE, Henderson JM. Increasing hamstring flexibility decreases lower extremity overuse injuries in military basic trainees. *Am J Sports Med* 1999;27(2):173–176.
24. Arnason A, Sigurdsson SB, Gudmundsson A, et al. Risk factors for injuries in football. *Am J Sports Med* 2004;32(No. 1 Supplement):5S–16S.
25. Dadebo B, White J, George KP. A survey of flexibility training protocols and hamstring strains in professional football clubs in England. *Br J Sports Med* 2004;38:388–394.

26. Shrier I. Does stretching help prevent injuries? In: MacAuley D, Best T. *Evidence-Based Sports Medicine*. London: BMJ Publishing Group, 2002.

27. Taylor DC, Dalton JD, Seaber AV, et al. Viscoelastic properties of muscle-tendon units: the biomechanical effects of stretching. *Am J Sports Med* 1990;18:300–309.

28. Beynnon BD, Murphy DF, Alosa DM. Predictive factors for lateral ankle sprains: a literature review. *J Athl Train* 2002;37(4): 376–380.

29. McGuine TA, Keene JS. The effect of a balance training program on the risk of ankle sprains in high school athletes. *Am J Sports Med* 2006;34(7):1103–1111.

30. McKay GD, Goldie PA, Payne WR, et al. Ankle injuries in basketball: injury rate and risk factors. *Br J Sports Med* 2001;35: 103–108.

31. Fong D, Hong Y, Chan L, et al. A systematic review on ankle injury and ankle sprain in sports. *Sports Med* 2007;37(1):73–94.

32. Osborne MD, Rizzo TD. Prevention and treatment of ankle sprain in athletes. *Sports Med* 2003;33(15):1145–1150.

33. Myer GD, Ford KR, McLean SG, et al. The effects of plyometric versus dynamic stabilization and balance training on lower extremity biomechanics. *Am J Sports Med* 2005;34:445–455.

34. DiFiori JP. Overuse injuries in children and adolescents. *Phys Sportsmed* 1999;27:75–89.

35. Watkins J, Peabody P. Sports injuries in children and adolescents treated at a sports injury clinic. *J Sports Med Phys Fitness* 1996;36(1):43–48.

36. Schmidt RA, Lee TD. *Motor Control and Learning*, 3rd ed. Champaign, IL: Human Kinetics, 1999.

37. Shea JB, Morgan RL. Contextual interference effects on the acquisition, retention, and transfer of a motor skill. *J Exp Psychol Learn Mem Cogn* 1979;5:179–187.

38. Arendt EA. Stress fractures and the female athlete. *Clin Orthop Relat Res* 2000;372:131–138.

39. Pecina MM, Bojanic I. *Overuse Injuries of the Musculoskeletal System*, 2nd ed. New York: CRC Press, 2004.

40. Gefen A. Biomechanical analysis of fatigue-related foot injury mechanisms in athletes and recruits during intensive marching. *Med Biol Eng Comput* 2002;40(3):302–310.

41. Dornan P. A report on 140 hamstring injuries. *Au J Sports Med* 1971;4:30–36.

42. Mair SD, Seaver AV, Glisson RR, et al. The role of fatigue in susceptibility to acute muscle strain injury. *Au J Sports Med* 1996; 24(2):137–143.

43. Rozzi SL, Lephard SC, Fu FH. Effects of muscular fatigue on knee joint laxity and neuromuscular characteristics of male and female athletes. *J Athl Train* 1999;34(2):106–114.

44. Johnston RB, Howard ME, Cawley PW, et al. Effect of lower extremity muscular fatigue on motor control performance. *Med Sci Sports Exerc* 1998;30(12):1703–1707.

Noncontact ACL Injuries:
Causes and Prevention

Upon reading this chapter, the coach should be able to:

1. Understand the basic anatomy and function of the anterior cruciate ligament (ACL).

2. Be aware of the basic mechanisms of noncontact ACL injuries.

3. Comprehend rationale for why women athletes tend to injure the ACL more frequently than men.

4. Design and implement an ACL injury prevention program.

5. Assist with the functional rehabilitation of an athlete recovering from ACL injury.

Kelly was looking forward to her senior year as a mid-fielder on the soccer team at her small New England college. She had spent the summer as a lifeguard and had tried to keep in shape by swimming. In addition, her coach had recommended a jogging program that she had participated in on a fairly regular basis. Practice started quite vigorously since the first full scrimmage was only 10 days away. Kelly quickly realized that while jogging may have helped her general endurance, it had not prepared her for the start and stop action of soccer.

It was just the third day of a fairly long practice. Toward the end of practice Kelly was tired and moving a little sluggishly when she jumped up to head the ball. She landed awkwardly, heard a distinct "pop" in her right knee, and collapsed. Considerable swelling started soon after the injury. Magnetic resonance imaging (MRI) results indicated that Kelly had ruptured her anterior cruciate ligament (ACL) and done extensive damage to her medial meniscus and medial collateral ligament. In an instant, Kelly's season was over.

At the suggestion of her physician, Kelly will not have immediate surgery (unless her leg is locking) but will start working to reduce swelling and regain range of motion (ROM). Kelly will then go on to knee reconstruction surgery and a long recovery period. Prognosis for ACL reconstruction is quite good and Kelly should recover full use of her knee. What is more uncertain is the effect of this injury later in life. Will she have early arthritis? Will this injury result in a diminished capacity for activity later in life?

This story is typical of thousands of injuries to young athletes year after year. In general, more males than females sustain a serious ACL injury. This is because there are far more male athletic participants than females. However, NCAA data indicate that in those sports in which women and men compete at the same level, women are two to eight times more likely to suffer an ACL injury than men (1). Griffin estimated that 1 out of every 10 female collegiate basketball players will suffer an ACL injury during her playing career (2). Boden et al have indicated that there are approximately 250,000 ACL injuries a year in the United States (3). Griffin et al indicate that approximately 50,000 ACL reconstructions are done each year, resulting in a financial impact of just under a billion dollars (2). This figure does not take into account the initial cost of ACL injury care or the conservative treatment of individuals who do not undergo ACL reconstruction. Further, the long-term cost of ACL damage during one's youth is unknown.

When Surgery is Necessary

ACL reconstructive surgery has advanced tremendously in the past 20 years. Arthroscopic reconstruction is now the norm and the success rate is quite high. Several short-term studies indicated that 65% to 88% of patients return to sport within the first year of surgery (1–3). Success rate is somewhat variable depending on how success is measured. Upon injury, most surgeons recommend that the athlete spend several weeks working to reduce pain and swelling prior to surgery. Leg strengthening is also part of presurgery.

ACL reconstruction usually involves one of three choices, a choice frequently made by the orthopaedic surgeon. Since every knee is different, the method of reconstruction often depends on the patient. The patella tendon bone graft has been the "gold standard" choice for years. A small section of the patella tendon (along with small bone blocks from each end) is harvested from the injured knee and inserted into the tibia and femur. The patella tendon is very strong and the surgeon only has to fit the blocks of bone into small bone tunnels on each end. Anterior knee pain is one disadvantage of this procedure. Patients who already have anterior knee pain as a result of other problems often receive an alternative graft.

Using hamstring tendons to reconstruct the ACL is also very popular. Surgeons often use multiple tendons to construct this graft. One disadvantage is that soft tissue must now be connected to bone and the initial rehabilitation is slower. A third alternative is to use cadaver tissues (allografts). Since tissues are not removed from the patient, surgical time is quicker and there is less damage and discomfort to the patient. The biggest risk is infection since hepatitis and HIV can be transmitted through these tissues. The process is fairly safe due to recent screening techniques. Cost and availability are also problems. Allografts are frequently utilized when a patient has had prior ACL reconstruction.

Synthetic ligaments have been utilized but with mixed results. Research continues in this promising field. Patellar and hamstring grafts remain the most popular and both grafts seem to provide excellent functional results. At this point, it appears that there is no clear advantage of using patellar or hamstring tissues (2,3).

1. Siegel MG, Barber-Westin SD. Arthroscopic-assisted outpatient anterior cruciate ligament reconstruction using the semitendinosus and gracilis tendons. *Arthroscopy* 1998;14:268–277.
2. Gobbi A, Mahajan S, Zanazzo M, et al. Patellar tendon versus quadrupled bone-semitendinosus anterior cruciate ligament reconstruction: a prospective clinical investigation in athletes. *Arthroscopy* 2003;19(6):592–601.
3. Feller JA, Webster KE. A randomized comparison of patellar tendon and hamstring tendon anterior cruciate ligament reconstruction. *Am J Sports Med* 2003;31:564–573.

Is it possible to prevent any of these injuries? Is there something Kelly and her coach could have done that would have allowed her to play soccer her senior year? Apparently, Kelly was not in top physical condition for the beginning of the soccer season. Students in fall sports like soccer, field hockey, volleyball, and football are often not prepared for the intensity of early season training. Kelly's jogging/running program may have helped her if she planned to run cross-country, but it did not prepare her for soccer. To answer this question of prevention, let us first take a look at the ACL and the various injury mechanisms.

ACL ANATOMY AND FUNCTION

The ACL is a small knee ligament that stretches from the top of the tibia to the back of the femur. Working in conjunction with the posterior cruciate ligament, it is largely responsible for stabilizing the knee during front to back motion (Fig. 3.1). It prevents the tibia from sliding forward on the femur and

FOCAL POINT

Life Without an ACL

In 1960 I jumped off an oilfield platform, landed awkwardly, and heard a loud "pop" in my knee. I immediately went down. One month later a surgeon removed my torn medial meniscus. As an athlete I knew about rehabilitation and went about an intense rehab program, lifting weights and running. Although my collegiate athletic experience was over, I resumed my normal activities, working out regularly and playing a wide variety of sports. Over the years I have played several sports very competitively, competing in USVBA championships, tennis, squash, and rowing. Badminton, a tough sport on the knees, is my primary sport and one in which I have competed nationally. Although none of these things are exceptional, a few years ago I had an MRI on my knee and the physician told me that I didn't even have an ACL! Apparently, I had torn it that summer day in 1960. Obviously, I was able to cope with this loss. My knee has never given out. I do have a little arthritis but was told this was from the lost meniscus. There is life after ACL loss.

—A senior athlete, age 62.

prevents the femur from moving backward. It particularly comes under tension when an individual is decelerating (stopping, landing, and pivoting). It also assists with lateral forces that are the result of fast turning activities such as a quick change of direction. Due to the anatomy of the ACL, it is more strained when the knee is close to full extension, at about 10 to 30 degrees of flexion. In addition to the stress that occurs as a result of body movements, outside forces such as a block or tackle in football also cause ACL stress.

Remember that ligaments are only partly responsible for the stability of the joint. Muscles cross joints and as they contract they tend to stabilize these joints. Almost all muscle contraction results in increased stability of joints. Therefore, muscles that are strong and contract in a correct manner result in stronger and more stable joints. The activities described in this chapter are designed to enhance the ability of muscles to stabilize the knee joint.

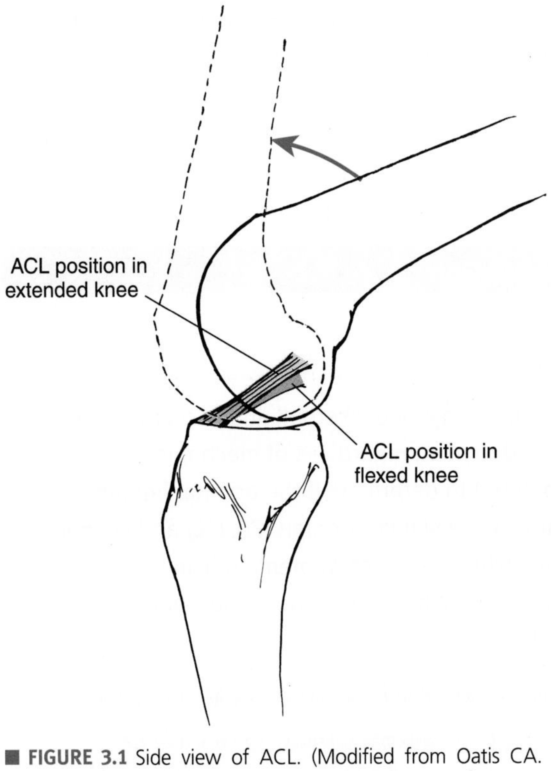

ACL position in
extended knee

ACL position in
flexed knee

■ **FIGURE 3.1** Side view of ACL. (Modified from Oatis CA. *Kinesiology—The Mechanics and Pathomechanics of Human Movement*. Baltimore: Lippincott Williams & Wilkins, 2004.)

INJURY MECHANISMS

Interestingly, approximately 70% of all ACL injuries are not the result of contact but happen as a result of an athlete's movements (2). These noncontact injuries usually occur during the deceleration phase of movement. That is, the athlete is either landing from a jump or pivoting to change direction. Both landing and changing directions require deceleration. The typical scenarios that result in such injuries are: landing with the knees straight or locked, quick planting and cutting, and sudden stopping with straight or hyperextended knees. Another factor is the addition of an opponent or teammate. Two volleyball players may go up to block a spike, collide, and land off balance. A basketball player may react awkwardly to a surprise movement of an opponent. Such activities may not involve direct contact with the knee, but they can cause sufficient knee stress to rupture the ACL. There are thousands of noncontact ACL injuries per year in soccer, basketball, and volleyball. Although there are far fewer participants, the incidence of ACL injury to female gymnasts is also quite troubling.

Although sudden deceleration to stop or change directions is often the type of activity that precedes an ACL injury, athletes need to jump, land, turn, and decelerate quickly and successfully. In fact, the more proficient athlete is one who can stop and start quickly. Are certain individuals more susceptible to ACL injury? Is it possible to weed out those athletes who appear to be vulnerable? Although considerable research is being conducted on this subject, no definitive test is yet able to identify those individuals who are at risk.

THE FEMALE ATHLETE AND ACL INJURIES

The number of girls and women playing competitive sport has risen greatly in the past 20 years. Not only has the number of athletes increased, the style of competition has moved from fairly slow, defense-dominated play to a faster, high-powered game requiring quick stops, starts, turns, and higher jumping. The result has been a significant increase in ACL injury. Several theories have been introduced to suggest why females have such a high incidence of ACL injury (3). Specifically, the primary theories have attempted to explain why women appear to be more susceptible than men. The foremost theories are hormonal, anatomic, muscle imbalance, neuromuscular control, and playing posture.

Hormonal

Since women have a cyclical change in hormones, one hypothesis is related to the fact that estrogen can relax soft tissues and thus predispose female athletes to ACL tears. Since estrogen rises during the mid-cycle of the menstrual period, researchers have suggested that female athletes may be more susceptible during this period. A variety of studies have been designed to determine if female athletes are more frequently injured during this mid-cycle phase. However, the results have been nonconclusive (4). Female athletes may be at more risk during mid-cycle but more research is needed before this relationship is established.

FOCAL POINT

ACL Injuries in NCAA Basketball and Soccer

In 1995, Arendt and Dick reviewed knee injuries among men and women playing basketball and soccer (1). This original report indicated the high rate of female ACL injuries compared to men, regardless of mechanism (contact or noncontact). Agel et al completed a 13 year review (1990 to 2002) to determine if the original findings had changed (2). Results indicated that the rate of noncontact injuries were similar for men (70.1%) and women (75.7%). However, in soccer, only 47.8% of injuries were noncontact, while 58.3% of women's ACL injuries were noncontact. Women continue to encounter significantly more ACL injuries than men whether in soccer or basketball. The rate of ACL injuries for female athletes has not changed.

1. Arendt E, Dick R. Knee injury patterns among men and women in collegiate basketball and soccer: NCAA data and review of literature. *Am J Sports Med* 1995;23:694–701.
2. Agel J, Arendt E, Bershadsky B. Anterior cruciate ligament injury in national collegiate athletic association basketball and soccer: a 13 year review. *Am J Sports Med* 2005;33(4):524–531.

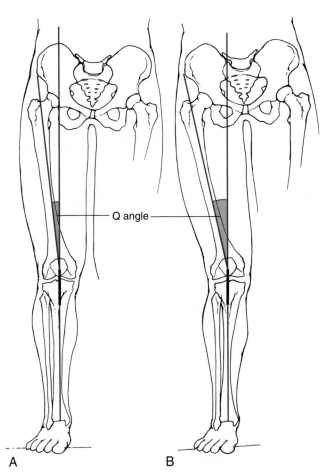

■ **FIGURE 3.2** "Q"-angle. The angle between a line drawn from the anterior superior iliac spine of the pelvis to the center of the patella and another from the center of the patella to the center of the tibial tuberosity. (Modified from Oatis CA. *Kinesiology—The Mechanics and Pathomechanics of Human Movement*. Baltimore: Lippincott Williams & Wilkins, 2004.)

Anatomic

The most common hypothesis regarding anatomic differences is related to the quadriceps angle ("Q"-angle—Fig. 3.2). Women generally have a wider pelvis than men resulting in a greater angle between the upper and lower leg, possibly resulting in an unstable knee. A larger Q-angle is associated with the valgus (knee is inward in relation to hip) orientation of the knee. Women tend to have greater valgus knee motion during landing, suggesting that they are at greater risk of injury (5). For example, Hewett et al found that valgus knee motion was a predictor of increased susceptibility to knee injury (6). Females with increased valgus alignment of the knees during activity appear to be at risk. The extent of this risk is still uncertain since relatively few studies have linked Q-angle to ACL injury.

Neuromuscular Differences

The ACL (along with the muscles around the knee) helps stabilize and restrict the tibia from moving forward during activity. Weak musculature (especially hamstring) in athletes reduces the stability of the knee. During deceleration activities the load on the ACL is very high, and excessively so if the knee musculature is imbalanced (7). The athlete must then rely more on their ligaments for knee stability rather than their muscles, putting the athlete at additional risk. We suspect that fatigue may also reduce the effectiveness of the muscle's ability to stabilize the knee. For example, the incidence of ACL injuries to rugby players is higher at the end of the game (8), and professional women soccer players receive more injuries later in the season (9).

Women, compared with men, land from a jump and pivot with less lower limb stability than men (10). Two factors may be responsible for this occurrence. First, although it is well known that the hamstring muscles are weaker than the quadriceps, some reports have found that women have a higher quadriceps to hamstring ratio than men (11). During deceleration activities (e.g., landing from a jump) the quadriceps contract eccentrically to limit knee flexion. When the quadriceps contracts, there is an additional load on the ACL since *the actions of the quadriceps are antagonistic to the function of the ACL* (Fig. 3.3). Conversely, the hamstrings act in line with the ACL (in opposition to the quadriceps) and tend to keep the tibia from sliding forward. Athletes with hamstring muscles that are insufficient to offset quadriceps activity may be more at risk.

Secondly, muscles have to be strong but they have to contract in an organized, synchronous way in order to support the knee. Neuromuscular control of the knee involves complex unconscious control of the muscles surrounding the knee. This control (or lack thereof) has led some researchers to recommend that females may need to improve their muscular control to protect the ACL (2). Huston and Wojtys found that male athletes tended to recruit their hamstring muscles earlier than females when presented with an activity that stressed the ACL (7). It has also been suggested that women tend to have more aggressive quadriceps activity relative to hamstring activity (12). Therefore, strong hamstring muscles that are also recruited quickly may be a deterrent to ACL injury.

Playing Posture

The late Chuck Henning, a well known orthopedic surgeon in the Kansas City area, was one of the pioneers in ACL injury prevention. Henning suggested that women tend to play sport in a more erect posture, resulting in less knee flexion during maneuvers. Boden et al report that Henning was one of the first to develop a neuromuscular prevention program for ACL injuries (3). He developed drills to teach athletes to increase flexion in the hip and knee during stopping and turning activities. Although unpublished, early results of his program demonstrated a significant reduction in ACL injuries.

Kirkendall and Garrett point out that for the ACL to tear there is either movement of the tibia forward or rotation of the femur on the tibia (13). As described earlier, the tibia tends to move forward during quadriceps activation (especially if not counterbalanced by hamstring contraction). They also point out that if the athlete is more erect during a cutting or stopping procedure, the quadriceps has a mechanical advantage over the hamstring. In laboratory studies, Chappell et al have found that women athletes tend to land with a straighter leg, supporting Henning's original suggestion (14).

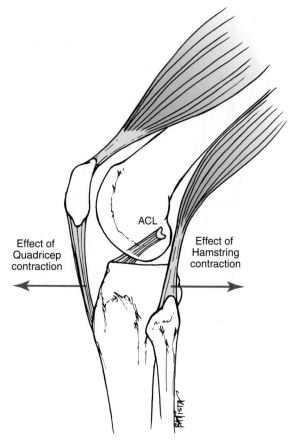

■ **FIGURE 3.3** Quadricep/hamstring tension on ACL.

THE COACH'S ROLE IN ACL PREVENTION

The difference between the ACL injury rate in males and females is probably due to a combination of factors, and the fact is that the coach has little or no control over many of the suggested causes (2). Female athletes will continue to have hormonal changes and a different anatomy. Both male and female athletes

FOCAL POINT

Knee Flexion Reduces ACL Stress

Cedric Bryant, exercise physiologist for the American Council on Exercise, suggests that we should train all female athletes more like tennis players. "If you look at female tennis planers, ACL injuries are relatively rare. Female tennis players learn very early on to flex the knee joint when moving. That's how they're taught to hit good ground strokes. But they also learn to better absorb the stress on the knees because of how they're taught to move on the tennis court."

Wheeler T. Programs help female athletes avoid ligament injuries. *Star-Telegram*, 5 January 2004.

must continue to jump, land, pivot, and stop suddenly. So what can the coach do to help prevent ACL injuries to male and female athletes? Neuromuscular control is one factor that the coach can change. Fortunately, studies have shown that improving neuromuscular control can reduce the incidence of ACL injuries (15–18). Coaches (especially those in the high risk sports) should be well aware of conditioning practices that help reduce the risk of ACL injury to their players.

Neuromuscular training programs have been highly successful, demonstrating as much as an 88% reduction in ACL injuries (15–18). Athletes need strong muscles, but they also need well-balanced muscles that act in a controlled manner. Traditional strength training should be supplemented by functional training. Since noncontact ACL injuries tend to take place during deceleration, prevention programs have been oriented to improving the ability of the athlete to decelerate in a controlled manner and to improve balance and kinesthetic awareness.

An important benefit of neuromuscular training is that power increases while the risk of knee injury decreases. For example, in one neuromuscular training study by Hewett et al, they found that athletes were able to decrease landing forces by about 22% as a result of jump training (19). In addition, the hamstring to quadriceps muscle peak torque improved significantly. Not only did the jump training improve neuromuscular control, the athletes also significantly increased their power. Since the development of power is a common goal of training, coaches can now introduce neuromuscular training into their schedules knowing that they are achieving two goals with the same activity.

Suggested Prevention Plans

Table 3.1 outlines three phases of an ACL injury prevention program. The typical ACL prevention program (Table 3.2) uses a specific training sequence that can be conducted in about 15 to 20 minutes. These are normally performed during the warm-up period (18). Initially, these activities may take a little longer since the athletes are unfamiliar with the exercises. Also, you should know that there is no exact training system for ACL prevention. We believe that the innovative coach can use the recommended principles to blend sport specific activities into their practices to create very interesting and effective training techniques.

We have also developed a 6 week out-of-season plan (Table 3.3) with great success. We often conduct this program for around 90 athletes at a time. Following a dynamic warm-up, we generally have all of the participants pair up and perform the jumping drills we recommend. The athletes then rotate through four to five stations utilizing agility, balance, level plyometrics, and depth jumping plyometrics. Athletes spend about 6 to 8 minutes at each. The emphasis is on high speed activities with enough rest to repeat at high intensity.

FOCAL POINT

Neuromuscular Training Improves Lower Limb Stability in Young Female Athletes

Researchers at the Cincinnati Sportsmedicine Research and Education Foundation measured the lower limb alignment of 325 female athletes ranging in age from 11 to 19 (mean age is 14.1) years during a drop-jump test. Subjects were asked to jump off a 12 inch high box; upon landing they were to immediately perform a vertical jump. Video cameras recorded the lower limb alignment during landing and take-off. The majority (80%) of the females demonstrated a valgus alignment (i.e., the knees tended to move inward possibly placing additional stress to the ACL) upon landing. Following these measurements, 62 of the athletes completed a 6 week neuromuscular training program followed by a retest of the drop-jump test. Results indicated a significant improvement in lower limb alignment upon landing and take-off following neuromuscular training.

Noyes FR, Barber-Westin SD, Fleckenstein C, et al. The drop-jump screening test. *Am J Sports Med* 2005;33(2):197–207.

TABLE 3.1	Seasonal ACL Injury Prevention Programs		
	Out of Season	**Preseason**	**During Season**
Days/week	2–3 nonconsecutive	3	1–2
Time/session	45 minutes	15–20 min	15 min
Description	A progressive program as described in Table 3.3 focusing on jumping drills, agility, balance and power. General strength training should accompany this program on alternate days.	An abbreviated program as described in Table 3.2 focusing on sport specific agility, balance, eccentric hamstring strength, and power.	A maintenance program similar to preseason.*

*Athletes who perform extensive jumping (e.g., volleyball and basketball players) during practice and competition do not need additional jump training during their competitive season.

Training Principles for ACL Prevention

The basic theme of ACL prevention training is to improve the biomechanics of deceleration as well as improving balance and kinesthetic awareness of the lower limbs. The following principles of training should be utilized regardless of season.

1. In order to reduce peak landing forces, encourage athletes to focus on controlled, quiet landings. Landing on your toes while flexing the ankle, knee, and hip reduces the landing force and the stress on the knee. "Knees over feet" should be encouraged repeatedly. Athletes need feedback to achieve the correct alignment and prevent the knees from moving inward or outward. Hewett suggests using such verbal cues as "straight as an arrow, light as a feather, recoil like a spring, be a shock absorber, and on your toes" (20).
2. Recruit fast twitch fibers. High intensity exercises use the fast twitch (FT) fibers. These fibers are only recruited when the athlete performs exercises at high speed. Since FT fibers fatigue quickly, athletes need sufficient rest between jumping repetitions. In general, we recommend that exercises (especially plyometrics) last about 10 to 20 seconds (or less) with about 60 seconds rest between repetitions. Remember that these are not endurance exercises. However, occasionally require repetitions of 30 seconds to replicate specific sport activities.
3. Emphasize quality, not quantity. Since a major focus of this training is neuromuscular control, you must emphasize the proper mechanics. When athletes become fatigued neuromuscular control is compromised. When athletes begin to falter, landing improperly, they should rest until ready to perform additional high-quality activities.
4. Spend as little time on the floor as possible. Athletes need to recoil from a landing as quickly as possible. This type of bounding activity improves power and the neuromuscular coordination necessary for

TABLE 3.2	Suggested 15 to 20 Minute Preseason ACL Injury Prevention Program	
Activity	**Time**	**Description**
Warm-Up	5 min	General warm-up similar to typical sport-specific activities normally used. End this with some side to side running, backward running, and skipping forward and backward.
Jump Drills	3 min	Perform jump drills—20 seconds each—as described in Table 3.4
Russian Hamstring (Figure 2.2)	3 min	Perform 2 sets of 10 repetitions of exercise described in Figure
Agility	4 min	High speed shuttle runs using forward and backward running
Plyometrics	4 min	Level plyometrics

TABLE 3.3 Six Week Prevention Program					
Week 1	**Week 2**	**Week 3**	**Week 4**	**Week 5**	**Week 6**
Jump drills	Jump drills	Jump drills	Jump drills	Jump drills	Jump drills
Agility run	Agility run	Agility run	Agility run	Agility run	Agility run
		Hill runs	Hill runs		
		Level Plyometrics	Level Plyometrics	Level Plyometrics	Level Plyometrics
				High Intensity Plyometrics	High Intensity Plyometrics

success in sport as well as joint stability. Encourage athletes to rebound off the floor quickly without pause.

5. Bend at the knee and hip when turning. As mentioned earlier, the ACL is particularly stressed when the knee is straight. Landing and turning on a bent knee results in less ACL stress. Encourage your athletes to lower their center of gravity, putting less stress on the ACL.

6. Move backwards as well as forward. As mentioned earlier, the hamstring assists the ACL. Strong hamstring muscles tend to aid the ACL with anterior-posterior stability. Running, hopping, bounding, and skipping backward all require extensive hamstring involvement. Athletes who have to move backward quickly (like fencers) have particularly well-developed hamstring muscles. So train your athletes to make quick backward movements.

ACL Prevention Exercises

Clearly, the off-season program we recommend provides time for more repetitions, but the training principles and exercises are essentially the same. Each training session should involve the following:

WARM-UP

Precede each session with a warm-up. A well-organized warm-up can be accomplished in 5 to 10 minutes. Start by slow jogging for a minute or two, and then be creative, using activities that are similar to what your

FOCAL POINT

The PEP Program

One ACL prevention program that has received considerable attention is the PEP Program (Prevent injury, Enhance Performance). The PEP program was started by a group of sports medicine personnel at the Santa Monica Orthopaedic and Sports Medicine Research Foundation. They have conducted a 2 year clinical prevention program with 1,400 Division I female soccer players. Reports indicate that individuals completing the PEP program can substantially reduce (88%) noncontact ACL tears.

The PEP program is specifically designed for soccer, takes about 20 to 25 minutes to complete, and is composed of stretching, balance, strength, agility, and power exercises. All of the activities are designed to be performed on the athletic field without equipment. Information on the PEP program can be found online at www.aclprevent.com.

Mandelbaum B, Silvers H, Watanabe D, et al. Effectiveness of a neuromuscular and proprioceptive training program in preventing anterior cruciate ligament injuries in female athletes. *Am J Sports Med* 2005;33:1003–1010.

athletes will do in practice but at lower intensities. The end of the warm-up should include mild forms of bounding type activities. Forward and backward skipping with increasing intensity, jumping, and hopping are all examples.

JUMPING ACTIVITIES

Jumping exercises should be performed on a soft surface. Typical gym mats or a soft playing field will work. Our suggestion is to pair up all the athletes and have them face each other. One athlete performs the drills while the other athlete watches the alignment of hip, knee, and ankle. The athlete performing the jumps should be encouraged to land in a balanced and controlled position (Fig. 3.4). Figure 3.5 indicates an athlete landing improperly. Upon observation of an improper landing, the observer should stop the athlete and indicate what was wrong. This procedure not only provides feedback for the performer, but impresses upon the observer the possible landing errors. Following a set of jumps, the observer becomes the performer while the partner rests. Utilizing this method, each athlete is continuously observed and also receives the appropriate rest. Table 3.4 describes the seven recommended jumps illustrated in Figures 3.6 to 3.12.

AGILITY DRILLS

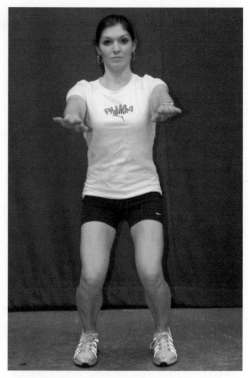

■ **FIGURE 3.4** A good landing from a jump: knees are directly over the feet.

Agility is the ability to change directions quickly. Since pivoting activities are particularly stressful on the knee and athletes need to train for these activities in a controlled setting. Try to perform these on the playing surface athletes will utilize in competition. It is our experience that coaches are already aware of many agility exercises and should be able to design those that replicate the activities in their sport. What are the common required movements in soccer, basketball, or volleyball? Now design some progressively high-speed drills that imitate those movements. Stress the following points during agility drills:

- Stops and turns should be done with bent knees and hips. Teach the athletes to drop down for stops and turns. Focus more on a rounded accelerated turn rather than planting the outside foot and turning.
- Use forward and backward movements. Have athletes make quick movements backwards as well as forward. Athletes need to run forward and backward quickly and to stop in a controlled fashion.
- Have athletes do some agility drills close together to imitate the types of bumping and jarring that occur in their sport.

BALANCE

Start your balance program without commercial balance devices but then increase the difficulty by including such devices as wobble boards, balance discs, and balance pads. Focal Point Box: Overuse Injuries Are Often Related to Training Errors (see Chapter 2) provides a recommended balance progression that also reduces the incidence of ankle injuries.

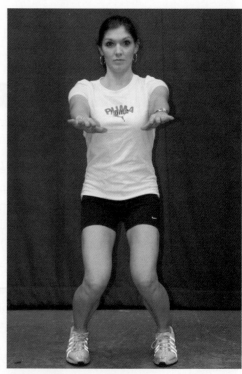

■ **FIGURE 3.5** An improper landing from a jump: knees are not directly over the feet.

TABLE 3.4 Jumping Drills*			
Activity	**Week 1 Time/ Number**	**Week 2 Time/Number**	**Description**
Wall jumps	20 sec	25 sec	Perform repeated vertical jumps landing in the same spot without using arms— soft, controlled landings
Tuck jumps	20 sec	25 sec	Repeated vertical jumps with use of arms and bring knees up to chest and repeat with control
Split jumps	10 reps	12 reps	From the lunge position (one leg forward and one back), jump upward and switch leg positions
One leg jumps	15 reps	20 reps	Stand on one leg—jump straight up and then land on other foot—focus on balanced landing—repeat when stable
Lateral Cone jumps	15 sec	20 sec	Quick jumps from side to side over small cone or collapsible bar. Focus on soft landings.
Single Leg Lateral Cone Jumps**	6 reps	8 reps	Same jump but on one leg. Focus on balance. (Do not use high inflexible cones.)
180 degree jumps**	12 reps	15 reps	Jump into the air and turn a half circle. Stick and control landing, then repeat.

*These drills can all be repeated if time permits and athletes receive the proper rest.
**These jumps should all be performed under control. The athlete should be encouraged to "stick" (without movement on landing) the landing and to do it in a silent fashion. Once balance has been attained, repeat the jump.

PLYOMETRICS

Plyometric exercises (see Chapter 8) are often misunderstood. Many people think of plyometrics as "Depth jumping"—jumping on and off high benches. But plyometrics are any activity that utilizes and trains the "Stretch-Shortening Cycle" (SSC). A muscle that is quickly stretched will subsequently contract with more tension. Plyometric exercises are designed to train this natural elastic characteristic of muscle to apply greater tension. "Depth jumping" (Fig. 3.13) is an advanced form of plyometrics but many common activities can be construed as plyometrics. A simple game like hop-scotch uses the SSC as children bound from one square to the next. Plyometric exercises do not have to be high intensity, placing great stress on muscles and tendons. Gradual progression is one key to a successful plyometrics program as athletes need time to adapt to these fairly stressful exercises.

Start off with *level plyometrics* (athletes start and stop at same elevation). Make sure the surface is appropriate (gym mats, padded runway, and grass or turf fields). Start slowly and gradually increase intensity and repetitions. Look for those athletes who are having trouble and adjust their exercises accordingly. Sufficient rest is required between repetitions for high quality training. Some typical suggestions are:

- Skipping forward and backward (focus on getting height)
- Two legged jumping (focus on soft landing and quick takeoff). We recommend plastic collapsible bars that can be easily adjusted for height.
- One legged bounding focus on getting height while landing on alternate legs
- One legged hopping (Fig. 3.14—land on same leg as you cross mat)
- Backward hopping/jumping on one or two legs
- Cone jumping (there are many varieties of these one can use)

After 3 to 4 weeks, athletes should be able to perform level plyometrics with relative ease. Few directions are needed. We introduce higher intensity plyometrics by using plyometric boxes. We use a padded runway with about 10 platforms ranging in height from 12 to 24 inches. We cycle about 15 to 20 athletes

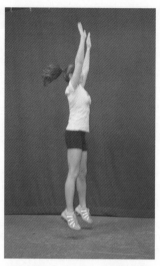

■ **FIGURE 3.6** Wall jump: observer watches and corrects landing

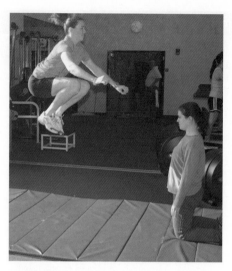

■ **FIGURE 3.7** Tuck jump

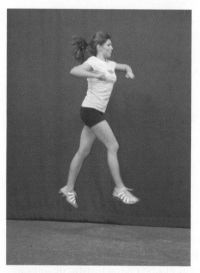

■ **FIGURE 3.8** Split jump

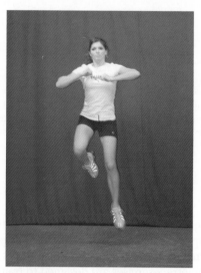

■ **FIGURE 3.9** One leg jumps

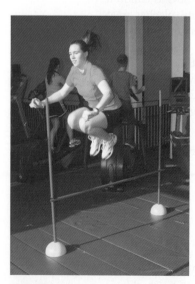

■ **FIGURE 3.10** Two foot jump over collapsible bar

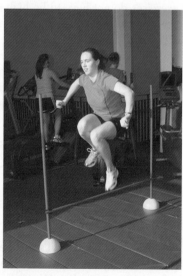

■ **FIGURE 3.11** One foot jump over collapsible bar

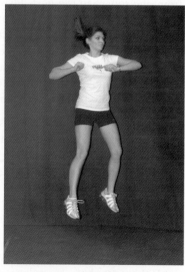

■ **FIGURE 3.12** 180-degree jump

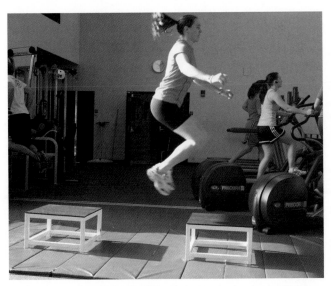

■ **FIGURE 3.13** Plyometrics. Traditional plyometrics involve landing from a height followed by a subsequent jump.

at a time down the runway. Athletes are encouraged to move as quickly as possible, focusing on good landings and quick take-offs. Athletes who still have trouble with the lower intensity exercises should not perform high-intensity plyometrics. Also, be cautious with any athlete who has complained about knee or muscle pain. High-intensity plyometrics require strength and coordination and are not appropriate for all individuals.

HILL AND/OR STAIR RUNNING

We've occasionally used high-speed hill or stair running in our program. This is an excellent way to develop functional leg strength and power. A fairly steep hill about 15 to 20 feet high with good footing is ideal. The hill runs should last anywhere from 3 to 10 seconds and allow athletes to carefully walk back down. If a suitable hill is not available, find a flight of stairs with at least 20 steps. Stair running should be done both from a standing start or a running start of about 20 feet. Athletes should attempt to bound up the stairs as quickly as possible landing on each third step (for the typical 7-inch step) and to walk back down. Repeat anywhere from 5 to 10 times dependent on the height.

Sport Specificity

How much emphasis should each of these forms of training receive? Comparatively speaking, the physical requirements and demands of each sport are quite different. While basketball and volleyball require extensive jumping, basketball may be more problematic since competitors are often jumping simultaneously as they fight for ball control. While soccer athletes jump to head the ball, soccer is more horizontal

FROM THE ATHLETIC TRAINING ROOM

Can Surgery Wait?

An article in *Exercise and Sport Sciences Reviews* discussed the stability of the knee after ACL rupture. The writers discussed the position that some athletes can delay surgery for a *temporary* return to their sport without significant risk of additional damage. About 20% to 30% of individuals with ACL ruptures tend to be able to cope with ACL rupture. Other individuals experience knee instability, or a "full episode of giving way," during vigorous activities. Some even have instability during normal daily activities. The authors discussed a screening examination designed to identify those individuals who can cope with vigorous activity without failure. Additionally, they suggest a rehabilitation protocol designed by Fitzgerald in which athletes are trained to improve their lower extremity muscle activity patterns. The Fitzgerald system involves perturbation training using rocker- and rollerboards. Individuals participating in this program were five times more likely to successfully return to temporary high-level activities than individuals participating in traditional rehabilitation programs.

1. Lewek M, Chmielewski T, Risberg M, et al. Dynamic knee stability after anterior cruciate ligament rupture. *Exerc Sport Sci Rev* 2003;31:195–200.
2. Fitzgerald G, Axe M, Snyder-Mackler L. The efficacy of perturbation training in nonoperative anterior cruciate ligament rehabilitation programs for physically active individuals. *Phys Ther* 2000;80(5):526–527.

than vertical, requiring athletes to stop, start, and turn frequently. Preventive training should reflect the needs of the sport and coaches need to plan accordingly. Basketball and volleyball players should therefore spend more time focusing on landing while soccer players should spend more of their training time on turning and stopping.

Sticky Floors and New Shoes: A Risky Combination

Friction is one factor in ACL injuries. Friction is the resistance to movement between the floor and the shoe of the athlete.

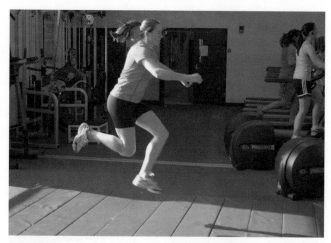

■ **FIGURE 3.14** Level plyometrics. Hopping on one leg is a good plyometric activity.

High friction often improves performance since athletes can stop and start more quickly. However, when athletes stop and/or turn quickly, little give between the floor and the shoe results in increased joint stress. A high level of friction between shoe and floor has been identified as a risk factor for noncontact ACL injury (21). It would seem likely that athletes would be at less risk of joint injury if friction is reduced. As discussed in Chapter 5, athletes should wear athletic shoes designed for the surface on which they play and practice.

One potentially hazardous condition exists in many venues with little consideration for the effects. Many schools redo floors during the summer season. Athletes return to floors that had relatively low friction at the end of the year to floors with increased friction. In addition, many athletes start the season with new shoes. This combination of a new floor and new shoes provides unusually high friction and an increased potential for injury. This is further compounded when athletes enter the preseason in an untrained state. *New shoes, new floors, and an untrained athlete are a recipe for injury.* Coaches can prevent some of these problems by knowing the condition of the floor in advance. Work with the floor crew to make sure the floor is not overly sticky. One additional solution is to have the athletes wear older shoes if possible until they are more conditioned and familiar with the new surface.

The Coach's Role in Rehabilitation

The initial rehabilitation of the athlete from ACL surgery is normally the responsibility of the athletic training staff in consultation with the medical team. Since one goal of rehabilitation is to return the athlete to competition, we believe that the coach should be involved with the functional aspects of rehabilitation. As the athlete recovers strength and ROM the coach should get involved with rehabilitation. Athletes need to relearn how to move on the playing surface. Working in combination with the athletic trainer, the coach should create drills designed to return the athletes to their sport. Obviously, early drills must be simple and progress slowly. As time passes and the athlete gets stronger and more mobile, the activities presented in the preseason workout can be utilized. However, these should be reduced in intensity so that the athlete is comfortable. The goal of this rehabilitation should be to perform those activities we suggested in our preseason program in addition to those activities coaches may develop specific to their sport.

Coaches need to realize that all ACL injuries cannot be prevented. However, the ACL prevention program presented in this text has been shown to effectively reduce the incidence of ACL injuries (15–18). All coaches involved in high risk ACL sports should incorporate a prevention program.

SUMMARY

- Thousands of ACL injuries occur annually, resulting in a loss of participation, significant discomfort and expense, and possible long-term complications.

- The frequency of ACL injuries is greater for female athletes.
- The majority of ACL injuries are noncontact injuries.
- Most noncontact ACL injuries occur during the deceleration phase when landing, stopping, or pivoting.
- Athletes in sports involving considerable pivoting and jumping are at greater risk of ACL injuries.
- Specific neuromuscular training reduces the frequency of ACL injury.
- Neuromuscular training should include jumping and landing drills, agility, balance, and plyometrics.
- Neuromuscular training does not require an extensive time commitment and also increases power.
- Coaches should work with the athletic trainer to assist with specific sport-specific rehabilitation activities.

References

1. Arendt E, Dick R. Knee injury patterns among men and women in collegiate basketball and soccer. *Am J Sports Med* 1995; 23(6):694–701.
2. Griffin L, Agel J, Albohm M, et al. Noncontact anterior cruciate ligament injuries: risk factors and prevention strategies. *Am J Orthop* 2000;8(3):141–150.
3. Boden B. Etiology and prevention of noncontact ACL injury. *Sports Med* 2000;28(4):53–60.
4. Griffin LY, Albohm MJ, Arendy EA, et al. Understanding and preventing noncontact anterior cruciate ligament injuries; a review of the Hunt Valley II meeting, January 2005. *Am J Sports Med* 2006;34(9):1512–1532.
5. Ford KR, Myer GD, Hewett TE. Valgus knee motion during landing in high school female and male basketball players. *Med Sci Sports Exerc* 2003;35(10):1745–1750.
6. Hewett TE, Myer GD, Ford KR, et al. Biomechanical measures of neuromuscular control and valgus loading of the knee predict anterior cruciate ligament injury risk in female athletes: a prospective study. *Am J Sports Med* 2005;33:492–501.
7. Huston LJ, Wojtys EM. Neuromuscular performance characteristics in elite female athletes. *Am J Sports Med* 1996;24(4): 427–436.
8. Dallalana R, Brooks J, Kemp S, et al. The epidemiology of knee injuries in English professional rugby union. *Am J Sports Med* 2007;35(5):818–830.
9. Giza E, Mithofer K, Farrell L, et al. Injuries in women's professional soccer. *Br J Sports Med* 2005;39:212–216.
10. Zeller B, McCrory J, Kibler W, et al. Differences in kinematics and electromyographic activity between men and women during the single-legged squat. *Am J Sports Med* 2003;31(3):449–456.
11. Cabaud H, Rodkey W. Philosophy and rationale for the management of anterior cruciate injuries and the resultant deficiencies. *Sports Med* 1985;4(2):313–324.
12. DeMorat G, Weinhold P, Blackburn T. Aggressive quadriceps loading can induce noncontact anterior cruciate ligament injury. *Am J Sports Med* 2004;32:477–483.
13. Kirkendall D, Garrett W. The anterior cruciate ligament enigma: Injury mechanisms and prevention. *Clin Orthop* 2000;372: 64–68.
14. Chappell B, Kirkendall D, Garrett W. A comparison of knee kinetics between male and female recreational athletes in stop-jump tasks. *Am J Sports Med* 2002;30:261–267.
15. Caraffa A, Cerulli G, Projetti M, et al. Prevention of anterior cruciate ligament injuries in soccer. A prospective controlled study of proprioceptive training. *Knee Surg Sports Traumatol Arthrosc* 1996;4:19–21.
16. Hewett T, Lindenfeld N, Riccobene J, et al. The effect of neuromuscular training on the incidence of knee injury in female athletes: a prospective study. *Am J Sports Med* 1999;27(6):699–706.
17. Myklebust G, Engebretsen L, Braekken IH, et al. Prevention of anterior cruciate ligament injuries in female team handball players: a prospective intervention study over three seasons. *Clin J Sports Med* 2003;13(2):71–78.
18. Mandelbaum, B, Silvers H, Watanabe D, et al. Effectiveness of a neuromuscular and proprioceptive training program in preventing anterior cruciate ligament injuries in female athletes. *Am J Sports Med* 2005;33:1003–1010.
19. Hewett T, Stroupe A, Nance T, et al. Plyometric training in female athletes: decreased impact forces and increased hamstring torques. *Am J Sports Med* 1996;24(6):765–773.
20. Cincinnati Sportsmetrics. *A Jump Training Program Proven to Prevent Knee Injury*. Cincinnati Sportsmedicine Research & Education Foundation, 1998.
21. Heidt R, Dormer S, Cawley P, et al. Differences in friction and torsional resistance in athletic shoe-turf surface interfaces. *Am J Sports Med* 1996;24:834–842.

Environmental Challenges: Heat, Playing Surface, and Thunderstorms

Upon reading this chapter, the coach should be able to:

1. Identify how heat is gained and lost in exercising athletes.

2. Comprehend the relationship between athletic performance and dehydration.

3. Recognize how to treat the various heat illnesses.

4. Understand how to prevent heat illnesses by assessment of the environment, hydration, acclimatization, and the manipulation of exercise clothing.

5. Explain the relationship between playing surface and injury rate.

6. Determine safe and unsafe environments during an electrical storm.

7. Implement the 30:30 rule during thunderstorms.

In 1966 Fox described the deaths of nine young football players from heatstroke. The players were all interior linemen. Seven died during the first 2 days of practice and all were wearing the full football uniform and practicing in conditions that were either hot or humid. Five of the nine were not allowed water during the workout, a common practice in the 1960s (1). One of the players (let's call him Bryan) was 15 years old. Bryan was out of shape and overweight but wanted to play football. Bryan's coach decided that he needed to lose weight and ordered Bryan to put on a rubber suit under his football uniform. He was then told to run laps around the field.

When Bryan started running his heat production increased. Normally, this increased heat might be lost through the air and through the evaporation of his sweat. But this was a hot day and Bryan could only lose heat by the evaporation of his sweat. Bryan sweated heavily but the sweat could not get through the rubber suit, football uniform, and helmet so that it could evaporate. His body temperature began rising and did not stop until he collapsed. Bryan died from exertional heat stroke, hyperthermia.

Such coaching procedures are now quite unusual and there are fewer deaths related to hyperthermia. But athletes still die from excessive heat. Sandor reported that 5 high school athletes died from heatstroke in the United States in 1995 (2). Some may remember Korey Stringer, the popular Pro Bowl offensive tackle for the Minnesota Vikings. Korey started the preseason with a determination to prove himself. From early on, he was taught not to quit, to "suck it up." But on the morning of August 9, 2001, conditioning drills in high heat and humidity took their toll. He lost consciousness and died 15 hours later. His body temperature was 108.8°F!

Coaches must understand the factors involved in temperature regulation. With regard to Bryan, there were some obvious flaws in the coach's procedure. For example:

- Athletes exercising in hot environments will benefit if provided water on a regular basis. Athletes get sick when *not* given water. Athletes do not get sick from consuming water during practice.
- Athletes should never practice with full football equipment in a hot environment until some acclimatization has occurred.
- The rubber suit Bryan had to wear increased his likelihood of heat injury because it did not allow evaporation to occur.
- Losing weight by excessive sweating is not fat loss. You cannot melt fat off the body. Weight lost through sweating is temporary.

HEAT BALANCE

Humans are warm blooded animals and can only live within a relatively narrow temperature range. We have several control mechanisms to maintain body temperature. These range from perspiring in the heat and shivering in the cold, to knowing which clothes to wear. Occasionally, this ability to control our temperature is severely challenged. Hyperthermia is particularly problematic for athletes since exercise produces heat and athletes are often required to practice and compete in hot environments. Various combinations of exercise, temperature, humidity, sunlight, and clothing are all factors that affect our ability to maintain body temperature. Figure 4.1 indicates that some of these factors can be positive or negative. For instance, the air temperature surrounding the body can be hot or cold, adding or taking away heat respectively. The following heat balance equation identifies these factors more specifically:

$$M \pm R \pm C - E = 0$$

Body temperature is determined by a combination of these factors. For a thorough understanding of heat balance, let us examine each factor in this important equation.

M for *Metabolism*

Metabolism is always positive since humans continuously make heat. Increased metabolism, such as exercise, can produce a large amount of heat. Typical athletic events often cause the athlete's metabolic heat production to increase 10 to 15 times. In some sports, like distance running, athletes can raise their metabolic rate 15 to 20 times for extended periods. This explains why athletes are often comfortable on cold days with little extra clothing. Heat production and exercise intensity go hand in hand—the more intense the exercise the higher the heat production. High production of heat tends to quickly raise the temperature of the muscles, blood, and internal organs.

R for R*adiation*

Radiation can be positive or negative. We all know that standing in the shade is cooler than standing in direct sunlight. Although humans give off electromagnetic heat waves, the radiant heat with which we are most familiar comes from the sun. Increased heat from radiation is particularly gained when there are few clouds. Further, between 12:00 p.m. (noon) and 4:00 p.m. radiation from the sun is particularly concentrated.

C for Convection and Conduction

Heat gained or lost is a result of convection and conduction. These two variables can be positive or negative. Convection is the transfer of heat as the result of air currents around the body. If the air temperature is higher than the skin temperature (usually about 33°C or 91°F) then this variable is positive and the individual *gains* heat from the environment. Cooler air results in heat *loss* through convection. Clothing affects the ability of air to cool the body. Wind is also a factor with regard to convective heat exchange. Since the body tends to warm that layer of air just next to the skin, a breeze helps cool the body as the warm air layer is shuttled away from the skin. Conduction is the transfer of heat by touching. For instance, cool water rapidly conducts heat away from the body resulting in a quick drop in body temperature. This is one reason why cold water immersion is a common treatment for hyperthermia.

E for *Evaporation*

Evaporation is always negative. As the athlete sweats the moisture on the skin can evaporate, resulting in heat loss. Evaporation is a powerful mechanism, resulting in approximately 55% of the heat loss in an exercising athlete (3). Evaporation is particularly important when the athlete is exercising in a hot environment and cannot lose heat through convection. Humidity is a powerful predictor of one's ability to cool through evaporation. As humidity increases, the ability to lose heat by evaporation decreases. Exercise clothing also influences the ability to evaporate sweat. While evaporation of sweat is a highly effective method of dispersing heat, excessive sweating can result in dehydration.

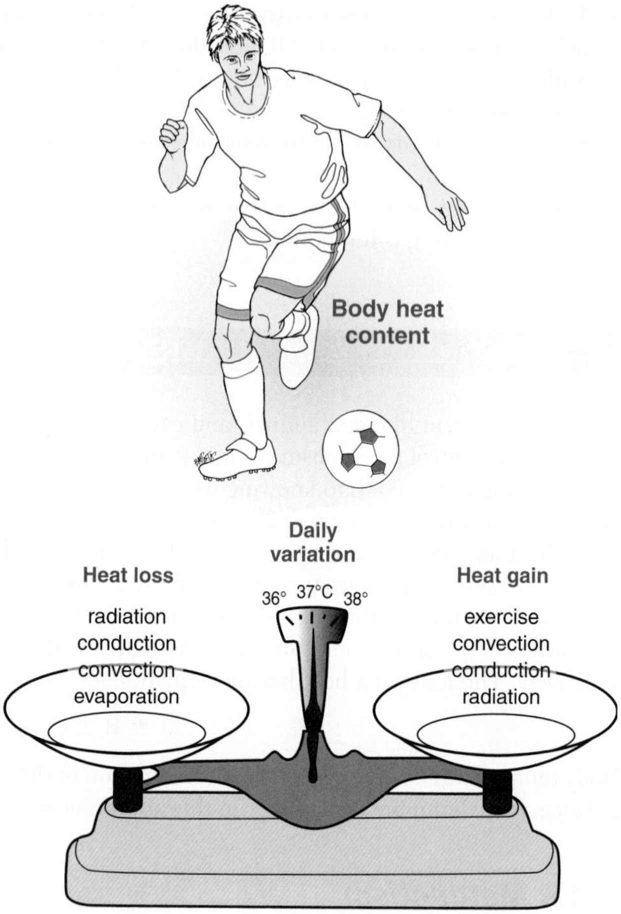

O for *Zero*

Zero represents a body that is in homeostasis (neither gaining nor losing heat). Heat produced is balanced by heat lost, resulting in a constant temperature. This is the normal situation within the body. But the combination of exercise and environmental stress presents sufficient challenge so that body temperature almost always rises slightly during exercise. Fortunately, this usually helps performance and is the typical result of a warm-up. Warmer muscles contract and relax faster, enzymes function better, and a whole host of other physiological events are improved by a slight temperature rise. However, body temperature that is too high results in serious malfunction, injury, and occasionally death.

■ **FIGURE 4.1** Temperature balance factors. (Modified from McArdle W, Katch F, Katch V. *Exercise Physiology-Energy, Nutrition, and Human Performance*, 6th ed. Baltimore: Lippincott Williams & Wilkins, 2006.)

THE CHALLENGE OF HEAT

Exercising in heat and humidity exposes athletes to considerable stress. Such exposure results in an increased susceptibility of heat illness as well as a decline in performance. Heat stress presents three major problems to the athlete.

Dehydration

Athletes lose large quantities of water and salt through sweating. On a warm day a large football player will typically lose 5 pounds of fluids. Since a pint of water is about 1 pound, the athlete will need to drink 5 pints of water to replace this fluid loss. Unfortunately, the thirst mechanism of the athlete is normally satisfied with much less. Even when athletes are provided a steady supply of water, they will not voluntarily drink as much water as they lose. On a hot day, water loss through sweating can be even higher. For instance, it has been reported that athletes have lost as much as 20 pounds of water on a hot humid day (4). This amount of water is equal to $2\frac{1}{2}$ gallons of water! Such a water loss places tremendous stress on the individual.

There is a fairly large range of sweat rates between individuals. For example, the sweat rate of soccer players depends on many factors such as position, playing style, and time on the field (5). Likewise, tolerance of dehydration varies among individuals. However, a fluid deficit of greater than 2% of body weight is a common benchmark for increased physiological strain (6). Dehydration is highly linked to the various heat illnesses. Dehydration of 2% degrades aerobic exercise performance and increases the perceived effort of tasks. Further, dehydration can decrease cognitive/mental function, an important attribute when tactics and strategy are required for success (6).

Cardiovascular Effects

The heat produced in muscles during exercise is typically dissipated through the skin. On a hot day, blood leaves the heart to carry oxygen to the muscles. The blood also picks up excess heat from the increased muscle activity and then travels to the skin to be cooled by air. This results in a significant increase in blood flow to the skin, thereby reducing the return of blood to the heart and lungs. While this mechanism helps the individual lose heat through convection, there is a reduction of blood flow to the muscles. Since muscles need blood to supply oxygen, the reduced blood flow leads to lowered performance. Further, as the athlete perspires, they lose bodily fluids and blood volume decreases slightly. The primary reason for a reduction in performance during heat is reduced oxygen to working muscles. Coaches should not expect athletes to be able to perform as well in the heat.

High Body Temperature

When an athlete begins exercising in the heat there is a fairly rapid increase in the core temperature. Perspiration, and subsequent evaporation, tends to prevent significant increases in temperature. The athlete feels the heat, slows down a bit, rests, and continues working. Maybe they adjust their clothing.

FOCAL POINT

Drink Like a Dog

When dogs are dehydrated in hot weather they will quickly rehydrate themselves when given the opportunity. Humans tend to not totally rehydrate themselves, resulting in what some call voluntary dehydration. This frequently happens even when athletes are given free access to fluids during training and competition. Apparently, the human thirst mechanism seems to be satiated before rehydration. But there are some things that can be done to enhance rehydration.

- Fluids need to be immediately available during exercise. Anecdotal evidence suggests that if fluids are just within an arm's length, the athlete will tend to drink. If the athlete has to walk across the room to drink, they may not.
- Athletes will tend to drink more of cooler beverages than those at room temperature.
- Athletes will tend to drink more of flavored drinks than plain water.
- A final important factor is the beverage delivery system. We often see huge athletes drinking out of a tiny squirt bottle. Some schools have little pump stations on the playing field where athletes stand in line and then pump water into their mouths. Use wide-mouth bottles or cups filled with a cool, good-tasting beverage.

Typically, body temperature rises but stabilizes. Occasionally, the combination of exercise and environment may overwhelm the body's cooling mechanisms. Body temperature does not stabilize, and continues to rise as a result of heat stress. This can be the most devastating challenge of exercise in the heat and must be avoided at all costs.

HEAT ILLNESS

Heat illness can range from mild discomfort to death. Each of these heat illnesses has different outcomes but is the result of similar factors, combinations of environmental stress and exercise.

Muscle Cramps

Involuntary spasmodic muscle contractions have long been associated with heat illnesses. The common belief is that muscle cramps are the result of dehydration and imbalances in electrolyte concentrations. However, recent research on endurance athletes has found no difference between the electrolyte concentration of athletes who tend to cramp and those who do not (7,8). Muscle cramps typically follow long periods of exertion and occur in those muscles utilized during exercise. One might expect that if electrolyte imbalance was the cause, muscle cramping would occur in a more generalized fashion. The fact that muscle cramps tend to be localized suggests that neuromuscular fatigue is the cause. The ability of nerves to contract and relax muscles is compromised by fatigue. As muscles adapt to training, the incidence of cramping appears to diminish. Although this recent line of research needs replication, these findings strongly suggest that muscle cramps are more due to fatigue and not dehydration or electrolyte loss.

Heat Exhaustion

Heat exhaustion is fairly common in athletes but is a poorly defined syndrome. Typical symptoms include fatigue, weakness, dizziness, nausea, muscle cramps, and mild confusion. Unlike the more serious exertional heat stroke (EHS), athletes do not suffer changes in their mental status other than mild confusion (2). Heat exhaustion is primarily the result of excessive fluid loss along with fatigue which leads to inadequate blood flow to muscle and skin (9). Although heat exhaustion is not generally considered dangerous, this is a good indication that the athlete's ability to control their body temperature is seriously reduced.

Heat Syncope

Heat syncope is also fairly common, resulting in lightheadedness and occasional fainting. The condition is temporary and usually related to reduced blood flow to the brain. Blood may tend to pool in the peripheral veins resulting in reduced blood flow to heart and subsequently to the brain. Reduced blood flow to the brain affects control.

Exertional Heat Stroke

Exertional heat stroke (EHS) is the most serious of the heat illnesses and can lead to death. Research indicates that current heatstroke survival is 90% to 100%—a considerable improvement over the 20% survival rate early in the 20th Century (10). As mentioned earlier, the primary cause of EHS is overloading of the thermoregulatory system. The result is an excessive body temperature ($>40.5°C$ or 104 to105°F) possibly leading to cardiac, liver, and kidney damage, as well as death. Other than a very high temperature, a common symptom of EHS is a change in mental status. There is often confusion, disorientation, and possibly psychotic behavior (6). Athletes with EHS most often physically collapse. Contrary to popular belief, athletes with EHS may continue to sweat (10).

TREATMENT FOR HEAT ILLNESSES

The three typical heat illnesses are normally the responsibility of the athletic trainer. However, in the event that the athletic trainer is not available, coaches should have a basic understanding of heat illness treatment.

- Muscle Cramps: Passively stretching the cramped muscle usually releases the tension but a return to play or practice will likely result in continued cramping. Since local muscular fatigue is probably the cause of muscle cramping, rest is probably the best treatment. Maintenance of fluid and electrolyte levels is still important and athletes who have undergone sufficient exertion to cause cramping will normally require rehydration and replenishment of electrolytes.
- Heat Exhaustion: The temporary treatment for heat exhaustion is fluid replacement and cooling. Remove any clothing that prevents cooling, place the athlete in a shaded or air conditioned space and have the athlete lie comfortably with legs propped above heart. The recovery with such treatment is normally rapid.
- Heat Syncope: Similar to heat exhaustion, move the athlete to a cool location and have them lie down. Place feet above their heart if lightheadedness continues.
- Exertional Heat Stroke: EHS is the most serious of the heat illnesses and requires the most drastic measure. Early recognition of EHS is the overriding key to survival (11). Symptoms often include signs of central nervous system dysfunction including confusion, disorientation, poor balance, and unusual or irrational behavior. Upon observing such behaviors, EHS should be suspected. Since athletes with EHS have high temperatures, it is necessary to cool them immediately (see Focal Point: Cooling Methods for Heat Stroke). If possible, the best treatment is cold water immersion. If immersion is not available, remove clothing/equipment and spray with cold water, apply ice packs, use fans, place in air conditioning, and apply cold towels. If it is not possible to cool the athlete on site, transport to a hospital.

FOCAL POINT

Cooling Methods for Heat Stroke

The primary difficulty with exertional heat stroke (EHS) is the dangerously high temperature of the body. Immediate and aggressive cooling of the body is the preferred treatment in order to reduce the core (internal) temperature of the body. A study of the literature reveals three typical methods of cooling that are also practical in the athletic arena. Water immersion in cold water has been studied at length using various water temperatures. Since very cold water tends to cause restricted blood flow to the skin, some research has suggested combining cold water immersion with massage. However, immersion in cold water has been found to be very effective. A second technique utilizes evaporation to cool the body. This technique involves spraying finely misted water over an individual while a fan blows warm air over them. A third technique involves placing ice packs over the large vessels in the neck, groin, and underarm. Hadad et al reviewed 77 studies on cooling techniques and indicated that all three techniques are effective. In general ice packs are not as effective as immersion or evaporative cooling techniques.

Hadad E, Rav-Acha M, Heled Y, et al. Heat stroke: a review of cooling methods. *Sports Med* 2004;34(8):501–511.

THE COACH'S ROLE IN HEAT ILLNESS PREVENTION

The treatment of heat illness is normally the responsibility of the athletic trainer, but the prevention of heat illness is the responsibility of the coach. Coaches plan practice, determine rest periods, and are generally in charge. Fortunately, there are a number of procedures coaches can utilize to prevent heat illness. First, you should understand the heat balance equation and the factors that result in heat illness. Second, you should be fully aware of how to implement prevention techniques. Coaches are usually very good observers and close to the action. Your observation of players, especially on those days when environmental heat stress is challenging, is critical. Athletes are often highly motivated to work hard. Peer pressure may push an athlete beyond a safe body temperature. Do not wait for the athletes to quit or pass out, as it may be too late. Coaches have the responsibility to take charge, educate their athletes, and make good decisions.

We continue to stress in this text that healthy athletes are the best performers. Working athletes until they are sick should be avoided. Plainly stated, athletes can train more effectively when the best heat prevention procedures are utilized. In addition to the prevention procedures we recommend below, we believe it is important to educate your athletes about the deteriorating effects of heat. Athletes need to be aware of the best measures to prevent heat illness; how to dress, what to drink, and what to eat are important behaviors and largely controlled by the athlete. Athletes need to recognize the symptoms of heat illness and to be able to communicate that information to the coach without penalty. Education is one key to prevention. The basic prevention procedures utilized by the coach include:

- Assessment of the environment
- Planning practice according to environmental heat stress
- Hydration of athletes
- Clothing
- Acclimatization
- Monitor Body Weight Changes

Assessment

The coach needs to determine whether heat illnesses have a high probability of occurring. Assessment procedures are very simple and inexpensive and the informed coach can make better decisions. But you need to realize that none of the following procedures to assess the environment is perfect and to be cautious. In our experience, the observant and educated coach is the best weapon against heat illness.

Following assessment, you can modify your practice and/or game to suit the conditions. A challenging heat environment should lead to frequent breaks in practice, more water, and multiple substitutions in games. There should be an increased awareness on your part. You need to be flexible to be able to modify practice to meet the demands of the environment. You may need to change the time of practice so that athletes can work to their capacity without undue heat fatigue. Some coaches schedule practice at night to reduce the debilitating effects of solar radiation. Football coaches can modify the uniform, possibly only working part time (if at all) with full uniforms. Accurate assessment involves multiple variables:

The Ambient ("Dry") temperature is simply the temperature on *the field or playing surface*. Some playing surfaces (such as synthetic surfaces) may be hotter than the temperature announced from the weather station. Ambient temperature measures the ability to either gain or lose heat through convection and conduction. The presence or absence of wind also affects convection. Ambient temperature does not take into account the ability of the athlete to evaporate sweat or the effect of solar radiation. While it is the easiest method to use, it provides the least amount of information and is not a valid procedure for assessing heat stress. In fact, it may even be deceiving to those who do not understand heat balance. For example, when Fox and his coworkers made observations on football deaths from heat stroke, one of the deaths occurred when the temperature was only 64°F. However, the relative humidity was 100% (1). Simply knowing the temperature of the day was insufficient. The combination of the football uniform and high humidity resulted in a deadly combination.

FROM THE ATHLETIC TRAINING ROOM

Uniform Effects

Kulka and Kenney conducted a very interesting experiment on how different football uniforms affect the heat balance equation. Subjects performed exercise designed to replicate the energy demands of a football game while wearing:

1. Shorts only
2. Practice uniform: helmet, undershirt, shoulder pads, jersey, shorts
3. Full uniform: helmet, undershirt, shoulder pads, jersey, game pants with thigh and knee pads.

The experiment was designed to determine the environmental combination of temperature and humidity at which the athlete could not control their body temperature. As expected, they found significant uniform effects. As an example, if the temperature was a constant 90°F, the critical humidity for the full uniform was 45%, while it was 55% for the practice uniform and 90% for shorts only. Similarly, if humidity was a constant 50%, the critical temperature for full uniform was about 85°F, practice uniform—94°F, and shorts 101°F. Simply having athletes wear a reduced football uniform has profound effects on their ability to cool themselves.

Kulka T, Kenney W. Heat balance limits in football uniforms. *Phys Sportsmed* 2002;30(7):29–39.

The Heat Stress Index (HSI), compiled by the National Weather Service, is a more sophisticated procedure for assessing environmental heat stress and takes into consideration the dry temperature as well as relative humidity (Fig. 4.2). Relative humidity indicates the amount of moisture already in the air. For instance, if the relative humidity is 60% then the surrounding air is already more than half full of the moisture it can hold. A relative humidity of 40% will result in faster evaporation (and therefore faster cooling) than humidity of 80%. Relative humidity of 100% will not result in any evaporative heat loss. You should know that even though athletes will continue to sweat profusely in this environment (high humidity), the perspiration that drops onto the ground or is trapped in the clothing does not evaporate and therefore does not cool. The HSI requires the dry bulb temperature and a measure of relative humidity. If you do not have a gauge to measure relative humidity, the local weather station (or radio station) will usually provide such information. (Note: a sling psychrometer accurately measures relative humidity and can be purchased for about $55.)

The Wet Bulb Globe Temperature (WBGT) adds the variable of radiation to the assessment of heat stress. Three different temperatures are required to determine the WBGT; the dry bulb temperature, the wet bulb temperature, and the globe temperature. While you are already familiar with dry bulb temperature, the wet bulb and globe temperature are less familiar. The wet bulb temperature is obtained by first wetting a wick that is wrapped around a dry bulb thermometer. As water evaporates from the wick the temperature is lowered; the lower the relative humidity, the greater the difference between the dry bulb temperature and the wet bulb temperature. If the two numbers are the same, either the wick is dry or the relative humidity is 100%! The globe temperature is measured by placing an ordinary thermometer into a black globe (such as the copper float in a toilet). The WBGT provides good evidence of anticipated environmental heat stress since it takes into account convection, evaporation, and radiation.

Bowers and Fox describe an apparatus that is very easy to build. Simply place the device on the field of play for about 30 minutes and record the values (4). Fortunately, commercial WBGT measuring devices are now available. For instance, Quest Technologies (www.quest-technologies.com) sells a WBGT thermometer (Fig. 4.3) that is reasonably priced and very easy to use.

The standards for the Heat Stress Index as well as the WBGT (Table 4.1) pertain to lightly clothed individuals. It is important to be aware that these estimates of environmental stress do not take into account

General Heat Stress Index		
Danger Category	**Apparent Temp. (°F) (Humiture)**	**Heat Syndrome**
IV. Extreme Danger	**>130°**	**Heatstroke or sunstroke imminent**
III. Danger	105°–130°	Sunstroke, heat cramps, or heat exhaustion likely. Heatsroke possible with prolonged exposure and physical activity.
II. Extreme Caution	90°–105°	Sunstroke, heat cramps, or heat exhaustion possible with prolonged exposure and physical activity.
I. Caution	80°–90°	Fatigue possible with prolonged exposure and physical activity.

* Note: Degree of heat stress may vary with age, health, and body characteristics

Relative Humidity										
		10%	**20%**	**30%**	**40%**	**50%**	**60%**	**70%**	**80%**	**90%**
Temp °F	**104**	98	104	110	120	>130	>130	>130	>130	>130
	102	97	101	108	117	125	>130	>130	>130	>130
	100	95	99	105	110	120	>130	>130	>130	>130
	98	93	97	101	106	110	125	>130	>130	>130
	96	91	95	98	104	108	120	128	>130	>130
	94	89	93	95	100	105	111	122	128	>130
	92	87	90	92	96	100	106	115	122	128
	90	85	88	90	92	96	100	106	114	122
	88	82	86	87	89	93	95	100	106	115
	86	80	84	85	87	90	92	96	100	109
	84	78	81	83	85	86	89	91	95	99
	82	77	79	80	81	84	86	89	91	95
	80	75	77	78	79	81	83	85	86	89
	78	72	75	77	78	79	80	81	83	85
	76	70	72	75	76	77	77	77	78	79
	74	68	70	73	74	75	75	75	76	77

■ **FIGURE 4.2** Heat stress index. (Modified from McArdle W, Katch F, Katch V. *Exercise Physiology-Energy, Nutrition, and Human Performance*, 6th ed. Baltimore: Lippincott Williams & Wilkins, 2006.)

clothing. For example, an HSI of less than 80°F presents little or no danger of heat illness, but protective clothing such as a football uniform may add another 10°F. Since the HSI does not take radiation into account, it is suggested that if the athlete is in direct sunlight, 10°F should be added to the index.

Hydration

McArdle et al suggest that "adequate hydration provides the most effective defense against heat stress" (12). Further, hydrated athletes can perform at their potential. Some dehydration is unavoidable because athletes sometimes cannot replenish fluids at the rate they are lost. Mild dehydration (<2% of body weight) is common and hinders performance, but is probably not that serious (13). Severe dehydration can be prevented by establishing a hydration protocol based upon environmental factors, work intensity and duration, and individual differences. The American College of Sports Medicine has issued a position stand on exercise and fluid replacement with the following general guidelines (6):

1. *Prehydration*: One goal is to start practice or competition with normal body water content (euhydration). About 4 hours before activity the athlete should slowly drink the amount of beverage recommended in Table 4.2. During the 4 hours prior to activity if the individual does not produce urine or if the urine is dark s/he should slowly drink more liquid.

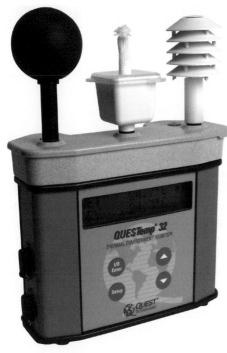

■ **FIGURE 4.3** WBGT measuring device. (Courtesy of Quest Technologies, Inc.)

2. *During Practice:* Make sure replacement beverages are easily accessible, cool, and palatable to the athlete. Individual containers permit easy monitoring. Frequent drinking should be encouraged. The goal of hydration during practice is to prevent excessive dehydration (>2% of body weight). The exact amount needed for replacement is highly individual.

3. *Postexercise:* Following exercise, the goal is to correct for fluid and electrolyte loss. Normally, rehydration is accomplished by the consumption of meals and snacks (some high in sodium) and plain water. However, if rehydration must happen quickly (e.g., twice daily practices), more aggressive rehydration methods should be used. Fluid intake should be based upon the amount of body weight lost during practice. For instance, athletes should be encouraged to drink about 6.5 cups of liquid for every 2.5 pounds of lost weight. Replacement drinks should be consumed over time and should include water, carbohydrates (CHO), and electrolytes. The CHO percentage in the replacement drink should be fairly low.

The question of what to drink has been a source of considerable research. While water is the most important ingredient lost through sweating, electrolytes such as sodium

FROM THE ATHLETIC TRAINING ROOM

Can You Drink Yourself to Death?

Chris was a triathlete who had trained all year to compete in the Ironman Triathlon in Hawaii. His goal was simply to complete the race. Training in New England, he was worried about handling the Hawaiian heat. He was in the best shape of his life but afraid of the heat. He started drinking water as soon as he arrived and for the 2 days prior to the race. He felt a little bloated prior to the race but figured he would sweat it off. Sure enough, it was a hot day and Chris started sweating as soon as he completed the swim. But he had ample water bottles for the bike ride and started drinking again. Soon thereafter, he started having a severe headache, became listless, and somewhat delusional. He was forced to drop out of the race before he completed the bike ride. Upon examination in the medical tent, Chris's rectal temperature was normal and fluids were not administered—he had too much fluid already!

Chris was suffering from hyponatremia, or what is sometimes called "water intoxication." This condition arises primarily in ultraendurance events (greater than 4 hours) and is the result of *excessive* fluid intake. The athlete sweats and loses electrolytes and replaces this with copious amounts of water. Such a combination results in very low serum sodium levels. Hyponatremia is a disorder in fluid-electrolyte balance that results in an abnormally low plasma sodium concentration. The decreased plasma sodium concentration disrupts the osmotic balance across the blood-brain barrier, resulting in a rapid influx of water into the brain. Hyponatremia can be fatal and excessive water intake should be avoided. How common is hyponatremia? Slower athletes who sweat profusely are at greater risk. Speedy et al followed 330 triathletes in New Zealand and found that 58 (18%) had symptoms of hyponatremia. About one-third of these sought and received medical attention.

Speedy D, Noakes T, Rogers I, et al. Hyponatremia in ultradistance triathletes. *Med Sci Sports Exerc* 1999;31(6):809–815.

TABLE 4.1 Wet Bulb Globe Temperature and the Risk of Heat Illness		
°F	**°C**	**Risk Level**
<64	<18	Low
64–73	18–23	Moderate
73–82	23–28	High
>82	>28	Hazardous

and potassium are also lost. Considerable research on exercise in the heat has been conducted in Australia, and Sports Medicine Australia recommends that plain (cool) water is an adequate replacement for activities lasting up to 1 hour. For activities lasting longer than 1 hour they recommend some form of sports drink containing carbohydrates and electrolytes lost during prolonged activity (14). During the competition, it is important that fluids be easily available so that athletes do not have to expend extra energy to obtain fluids. Athletes will normally replace only about one-half of fluid loss if plain water is used for rehydration, so the flavoring of a sports drink may enhance voluntary rehydration. Drinks with a bit of sodium also stimulate thirst. Beverage temperature is very important and cool drinks are more palatable and will rehydrate athletes faster than warm drinks.

Acclimatization

Acclimatizing athletes to the heat is a highly effective method of combating heat illness and improving performance. Athletes who are acclimatized to exercising in the heat will perform far better in practice and games. Table 4.3 indicates the typical physiological effects of acclimatization. A lack of acclimation to the heat as well as poor fitness is double jeopardy for heat illness and inferior performance. Heavier athletes make more heat and may be more susceptible to low fitness and heat illness. Fall sports such as football, soccer, and field hockey appear to be the most problematic. Athletes often report in late summer after an extended period of reduced physical activity. Athletes who are less fit take longer to acclimatize (15).

The most desirable situation is for the athlete to start preseason already acclimated to the heat. Athletes should be strongly encouraged to achieve heat acclimatization and cardiovascular fitness prior to the start of the season. This is easily accomplished if the athletes jog in the heat for about 30 to 45 minutes per day. Athletes need to pay attention to hydration during this acclimatization period. Athletes living in cooler environments can wear additional clothing to imitate hotter climates (16). The acclimatization process is rea-

TABLE 4.2 Recommended Fluid Intake for Prehydration	
Body Weight (lbs)	**Fluid (ounces)**
110	8.5–12
132	10–14
154	12–16.5
176	13.5–19
198	15–21
220	17–24
242	18.5–26
264	20–28.5
286	22–31
308	24–33
330	25–36

TABLE 4.3 Effects of Heat Acclimatization	
System	**Acclimatization Effect**
Heart Rate	Decreased
Skin Blood Flow	Decreased
Muscle Blood Flow	Increased
Sweat Production	Increased
Evaporation Cooling	Increased
Electrolytes in Sweat	Decreased
Central Nervous System	Less discomfort, nausea, dizziness
Body Temperature	Decreased

sonably effective after 7 to 14 days but diminishes significantly after 6 days of no heat stress (15,17). Remember that the athletes must *exercise* in the heat to achieve acclimatization, not just be in the heat. Sitting by the pool on a hot day will not result in heat acclimation. Unfortunately, athletes will report to the fall season in a deconditioned and unacclimatized state. Improving the state of acclimation should be one of the primary goals for the first 3 to 5 days of practice. *But remember that the best way to achieve optimal heat acclimation is to make sure that the athletes are properly hydrated and well fed.*

Clothing

The type of clothing that an athlete wears affects the ability to lose heat through convection and evaporation. All clothing interferes with the ability of moisture from the skin to evaporate; the best clothing provides the least resistance from skin to air. Clothing should be loose fitting to allow the surrounding air to circulate. Although sunburn can be a problem, bare skin allows for the best heat loss through evaporation and convection. Natural fibers, such as cotton, are quite suitable and allow evaporation. Some composite fabrics have high wicking properties but many nylon-like materials actually reduce evaporation. Fabric construction is also important. For example, fishnet construction allows more effective ventilation than tightly woven cloth (18). Exercise clothing should also be light in color as dark colors absorb more radiation.

Headgear is of particular importance. Since a significant amount of sweating and evaporation occur in the head region, players should be encouraged to remove their helmets during all rest periods. Light colored caps or visors (preferably mesh or cotton) can be helpful if it is sunny. On cloudy days when there is little to no radiation, hats actually reduce evaporation.

FOCAL POINT

Rest and Shade May Not be Enough

In Fox's study of high school football deaths, he tells the story of a 16-year-old boy who reports for football for the first time. On his first day he is required to wear the complete football uniform. During practice the boy begins to feel ill and the coach places him in the shade (but without water). Practice continues for approximately 2 hours after which the boy is approached and discovered to be unconscious. Efforts to revive him failed and he died there that day sitting in the shade. Apparently, sitting in the shade was not enough to cool him since the day was hot and his uniform significantly reduced evaporative cooling. The original illness probably caused high body temperature and dehydration. The combination of the football uniform and absence of water overwhelmed this boy's cooling mechanisms.

Body-Weight Chart

Since the human thirst mechanism is not always adequate for replacing fluid loss, athletes occasionally lose too much weight through fluid loss. One way for coaches and athletic trainers to track these changes is the daily measurement of weight before and after practice. An accurate scale should be readily available in the dressing area alongside the body-weight chart. Athletes should not wear their uniforms during weighing since moisture in the clothing will overestimate body weight. Preferably, athletes should wear their underwear when weighing.

Daily monitoring of the body-weight chart is normally conducted by the athletic trainer (or manager) but some routine should be in place. In general, weight lost during practice should be replenished in 24 hours. Athletes who have losses greater than 2% should be monitored carefully.

WOMEN, CHILDREN, AND HEAT

Two basic factors have led many to believe that women do not tolerate exercise in the heat as well as men. Since women perspire less than men, many believed that women could not cool themselves as well as men. Second, early studies suggested that women suffered more heat strain than men when working in a hot environment. But these early studies did not control for aerobic fitness and the women were working at a higher exercise intensity. Since body temperature and exercise intensity are highly related, the difference in body temperature was related to aerobic fitness and not heat control. More recent studies matching males and females for aerobic fitness have determined few differences in the ability to regulate heat (19). Women do tend to sweat less than men but are also better able to lose heat through convection than men.

Children are less tolerable to heat than adults and are at a disadvantage in the heat (20). For instance, children have a lower cardiac output which is problematic since cardiovascular stress is significant in the heat. Children also have a lower plasma volume and a reduced sweating capacity (20). Also, children tend to start sweating at a higher threshold resulting in higher body temperatures. Rowland suggests that children need a longer and more gradual acclimatization period (21). Additionally, children tend to feel acclimatized prematurely and thus tend to do too much too soon.

PLAYING SURFACE

There was a time when all outdoor fields were grass and all indoor surfaces were wood. The relationship between playing surface and injury risk was not a commonly studied phenomenon. In 1965, the Astrodome was constructed and an attempt was made to grow natural grass inside the dome. Interestingly, there was even speculation that clouds could form inside the dome, causing rain! But the grass was difficult to maintain and a huge synthetic carpet (originally called Chemgrass) was installed. Astroturf® (patented by Monsanto in 1965) was born. It was not long before synthetic surfaces were installed in outdoor venues. Since the advent of Astroturf, additional synthetic surfaces have been created including Tartan Turf, Super Turf, Stadia Turf, Momentum Turf, and Field Turf.

As a result of the increased variety of playing surfaces (both indoors and out), a common question is whether athletes are more at risk on some surfaces. The question is not an easy one to answer since so many variables are involved. For instance, one surface may be more problematic for one type of injury and less risky for others. The type of shoe worn on the various surfaces is a very important and often uncontrolled variable in research studies. Weather is an important variable regarding injury rate and playing surface. Temperature and moisture affect sport surfaces. One important consideration is whether injuries occurred in early or late season (22). For example, despite the negative outcry by traditionalists, the Baltimore Ravens removed their natural grass playing field and installed Momentum Turf into their football stadium in 2003. Their grass field deteriorated so significantly toward the end of the season the owners and coaches felt that players were at additional risk of injury. Irregular playing surfaces are inherently dangerous and synthetic surfaces may help to reduce injury toward the end of the season (24).

Playing Surface Factors and Injury Risk

Coaches often have little control over the playing surface. This is particularly true for away contests. However, coaches are often involved with field maintenance and when new playing surfaces are being selected. Important factors include the following:

FIELD REGULARITY

There is no question that a well maintained field is far safer than one filled with potholes and irregularities (23). A surface that is predictable for the athlete reduces awkward movements or uncertain foot placements that often lead to lower leg injury. Maintaining the field in the best shape throughout the season helps to reduce irregularities. Coaches need to recommend regular watering and mowing of fields. Also, coaches should reduce practice time on the game field. Use alternate fields whenever possible to reduce wear and tear and maintain the integrity of the game field. Since many injuries occur during the game, saving the game field for competition helps reduce injury (24).

FRICTION

Traction between shoe and surface is important for athletes who need to stop, start, and turn quickly (see Chapter 5). However, increased friction results in greater stress on muscles and joints (especially ankle, knee, and hip) possibly increasing injury rate (25). Powell and Schootman examined the relationship between knee injuries and playing surface (natural grass versus Astroturf) and found an increased incidence of anterior cruciate ligament (ACL) injury during football games on the synthetic surface (26). Likewise, Hagel et al found increased injury rates for head and neck as well as lower leg injuries for football players on synthetic surfaces (27). FieldTurf is a more recent synthetic surface that manufacturers claim is safer and similar to natural grass. Meyers and Barnhill compared the injury rate of high school football players on FieldTurf and natural grass for 5 years. Results were unclear since both surfaces exhibited unique injury patterns. For instance, there were more noncontact and muscle-related traumas on FieldTurf but more head and ligament injuries on natural grass. The authors recommended further investigation.

Another aspect of friction to consider is the weather. In a very interesting study, Orchard and coworkers followed all players in the Australian Football League for 6 years during which they competed in 2,280 football matches (29). Their interest specifically concerned the relationship between noncontact ACL injuries and the condition of the grass field. They found that higher rainfall and/or low evaporation significantly reduced the risk of noncontact ACL injuries. They recommended that consistent extra watering would likely lower the rate of such devastating injuries.

CUSHIONING

A common complaint of artificial surfaces is that they are harder than natural grass. Since impact with a hard surface is a common cause of head injury, a hard playing surface should be more problematic. Although severe head injuries are relatively rare, they have the potential to dramatically change an athlete's life (30). In addition, research has shown that mild traumatic brain injury (MTBI) has cumulative effects. Athletes who had suffered an MTBI are more prone to subsequent brain injury (31). The most compelling evidence that synthetic surfaces increase the risk of brain injury was in a study by Guskeiwicz and coworkers in 2000 (32). They tracked the injury rates among 17,549 high school and college football players and documented 1,003 cases of MTBI of which 10% were due to contact between the athlete's head and playing surface. The rate of head injury for the synthetic surface was about double the grass surface. Perhaps more importantly, head injuries on the synthetic surface tended to be more serious resulting in loss of consciousness.

All synthetic surfaces are not the same, but neither are grass surfaces. For instance, Naunheim et al studied three different playing fields in St. Louis. They found that the artificial surface of the domed stadium was harder than an outdoor grass practice field. However, the grass practice field was harder than a nearby indoor artificial turf (33). Grass surfaces, especially dry ones that are sparsely planted, can be very hard.

The relationship between injury risk and playing surface remains a question. Manufacturers and researchers continue to study this important relationship. The numerous types of synthetic surfaces as well as the wide range of conditions on grass surfaces make such study quite difficult. Unfortunately, unequivocal recommendations regarding the best surface for injury prevention are not available. Both grass and synthetic surfaces have advantages with regard to injury rate and performance.

ELECTRICAL STORMS

Lightning strikes the ground in the U.S. every summer day and most days of the rest of the year (34). Lightning strikes are seemingly random and prediction is difficult. As a result of the unpredictable nature and power of lightning, it is the second leading cause of storm-related deaths (second only to flooding) and greater than tornadoes and hurricanes. About 100 people a year are killed by lightning and more than 500 are injured (35). Since many athletic events and practices are conducted in environments that are often listed as unsafe, it is important that coaches are aware of such dangers and to work with the training staff to incorporate safe practices.

The National Athletic Trainers' Association (NATA) has issued a position statement regarding lightning safety for athletics and recreation (36). Recommendations include the following:

- A lightning safety policy should be in place including an established chain of command (who makes the call to remove individuals and teams to a safe location).
- A designated weather watcher (athletic trainer or manager).
- A means of monitoring the local weather.
- A designated safe location should be listed for each practice setting.
- Adhere to the 30:30 rule. Compute the time between viewing lightning (flash) and hearing thunder (bang). Seek a safe shelter when the "Flash to bang" count approaches 30 seconds. Wait at least 30 minutes after the last sound of thunder before resuming activity.

Safe and Unsafe Locations

According to the American Meteorological Society (AMS), no place is absolutely safe from lightning threat (34). Most of us think of avoiding a direct lightning strike, but individuals may be injured in other ways. For instance, individuals may be injured by touching an object that is struck by lightning or even when lightning strikes objects near someone. Lightning can also create a ground current in which voltage radiates outward from a point of contact. So what are the safe locations? According to the AMS:

- Large enclosed structures with plumbing and electricity are normally safe.
- Large enclosed structures are much safer than smaller open structures.
- Fully enclosed metal vehicles such as cars, truck, buses, and vans normally offer good protection.

Places to avoid during a lightning storm include:

- Being in or near high places such as open fields.
- Avoid rain or picnic shelters, baseball/softball dugouts, metal fences, bleachers, golf carts, flag and light poles.
- Indoor swimming pools and locker rooms.
- Open water.

Bennett has recommended that if there is no safe structure you should crouch in a thick grove of small trees surrounded by tall trees or in a dry ditch. Crouch down with only your feet touching the ground and do not lie down. Try to make yourself as small as possible (37).

Risky Situations

The 30:30 rules recommended by several knowledgeable groups are applicable for most situations, but remember that lightning strikes are still not predictable. A conservative approach is best. Lightning is always generated and connected to a thundercloud. The precursor to lightning normally includes high winds, rainfall, and cloud cover allowing persons in charge to take early and appropriate action.

Golf and crew athletes are particularly susceptible to lightning. These athletes compete and train in very open conditions and often at a considerable distance from a safe environment. We recommend that golf and crew coaches adopt a very conservative plan. Transportation may be the primary issue for crew athletes since they may be many miles from a safe environment. For instance, a flash-to-bang count of 30 seconds equates to about 6 miles (9.7 km). A thunderstorm traveling 12 miles per hour will cover that distance in 30 minutes.

SUMMARY

Heat

- Thermal balance is a function of metabolism, convection, radiation, and evaporation.
- Exercise in high heat and humidity makes athletes highly susceptible to heat illnesses.
- The coach is responsible for the prevention of heat illness.
- Coaches need to observe their athletes at all times to look for symptoms of heat illness. Coaches should not overexert athletes into heat illness.
- Athletes who are hydrated and acclimatized will be able to train and compete better.
- Unfit athletes are more susceptible to heat illness.
- Educate your players about the need for hydration and electrolyte replacement.
- Make acclimatization a priority during the early season.
- Assess the environment prior to practice to determine risk of heat illness.
- Adjust practice and clothing accordingly in difficult situations.
- Practice during the coolest part of the day.
- Provide cool water in convenient receptacles at all times.
- Provide sport drinks for practices over 1 hour.
- Encourage athletes to drink liberally and salt food following practice.
- Weigh players before and after practice and counsel those who lose more than 2% of their weight to increase fluid intake.
- Women tend to experience heat illnesses at the same rate as men.
- Children handle heat less effectively than adults and need a longer acclimatization period prior to intense practice and competition.

Playing Surface

- Well maintained playing fields prevent injury.
- Fields that are regularly watered provide less friction and decreased incidence of lower leg injuries.
- Artificial surfaces provide a uniform playing surface but often increase shoe-surface friction resulting in increased lower leg injuries.
- Some artificial surfaces are harder than natural grass resulting in an increased incidence of head injuries.
- Unequivocal recommendations regarding injury risk are difficult because of the numerous variables involved.

Electrical Storms

- Approximately 100 people a year die from lightning strikes.
- Athletic teams that play outdoors should have a warning system in place.

- Coaches need to observe the 30:30 rule suggesting that when the flash to bang count approaches 30 seconds the players should be in a safe place. Resume play 30 minutes after last lightning strike.
- Golf and crew athletes need a more conservative electrical storm plan to remove them from danger.
- A safe place is a large building with plumbing and/or electricity, bus, or van.
- Unsafe facilities are bleachers, open water, open fields, under trees or light poles, or dugouts.

References

1. Fox E, Mathews D, Kaufman W, et al. Effects of football equipment on thermal balance and energy cost during exercise. *Res Q* 1966;37:332–339.
2. Sandor R. Heat illness: on-site diagnosis and cooling. *Phys Sportsmed* 1997;25(6):35–40.
3. Gisolfi CV, Wenger CB. Temperature regulation during exercise; old concepts, new ideas. *Exerc Sport Sci Rev* 1984;12:339–372.
4. Bowers R, Fox E. *Sports Physiology*, 3rd ed. Dubuque: Wm. C. Brown Publishers, 1988.
5. Shirreffs S, Ragon-Vargas L, Chamorro M, et al. The sweating response of elite professional soccer players to training in the heat. *Int J Sports Med* 2005;26:90–95.
6. American College of Sports Medicine. Position stand: exercise and fluid replacement. *Med Sci Sports Exerc* 2007;39:377–390.
7. Schwellnus M, Nicol J, Laubscher R. Serum electrolyte concentrations and hydration status are not associated with exercise associated muscle cramping (EAMC) in distance runners. *Br J Sports Med* 2004;38:488–492.
8. Sulzer N, Schwellnus M, Noakes T. Serum electrolytes in ironman triathletes with exercise-associated muscle cramping. *Med Sci Sports Exerc* 2005;37(7):1081–1085.
9. Plowman S, Smith D. *Exercise Physiology for Health, Fitness, and Performance*, 2nd ed. New York: Benjamin Cummings, 2003.
10. Shapiro Y, Seidman D. Field and clinical observations of exertional heat stroke patients. *Med Sci Sports Exerc* 1990;22:6–14.
11. Heled Y, Ray-Acha M, Shani Y, et al. The "golden hour" for heatstroke treatment. *Mil Med* 2004;169:184–186.
12. McArdle W, Katch F, Katch V. *Exercise Physiology, Energy, Nutrition, and Human Performance*, 6th ed. Baltimore: Lippincott Williams & Wilkins.
13. Noakes R. Hyponatremia in distance athletes. *Phys Sportsmed* 2000;28(9):71–76.
14. Sports Medicine Australia. *Policy: Preventing Heat Illness in Sport*. Sports Medicine Australia, 2001.
15. Armstrong LE, Maresh CM. The induction and decay of heat acclimatisation in trained athletes. *Sports Med* 1991;12:302–312
16. Dawson B. Training in sweat clothing in cool conditions to improve heat tolerance. *Sports Med* 1994;17(4):233–244.
17. Binkley H, Beckett J, Casa D, et al. National Athletic Trainers' Association position statement: exertional heat illnesses. *J Athl Train* 2002;37(3):329–343.
18. Gavin T. Clothing and thermoregulation during exercise. *Sports Med* 2003;33(13):941–947.
19. Drinkwater B. Women and exercise: Physiological aspects. *Exerc Sport Sci Rev* 1984;12:21–52.
20. Bar-Or O. Children's responses to exercise in hot climates: Implications for performance and health. *Sports Sci Exch* 1994;7(2):1–4.
21. Rowland T. *Exercise and Children's Health*. Champaign: Human Kinetics, 1990.
22. Orchard J. Is there a relationship between ground and climatic conditions and injuries in football? *Sports Med* 2002;32(7):419–432.
23. Irvin R, Iversen D, Roy S. *Sports Medicine*, 2nd ed. Boston: Allyn & Bacon, 1998.
24. Soderman K, Alfredson H, Pietila T, et al. Risk factors for leg injuries in female soccer players: a prospective investigation during one out-door season. *Knee Surg Sports Traumatol Arthrosc* 2001;9:313–321.
25. Torg J, Quedenfeld T, Landau S. The shoe-surface interface and its relationship to football knee injuries. *Am J Sports Med* 1974;2:261–269.
26. Powell J, Schootman M. A multivariate risk analysis of selected playing surfaces in the National Football League: 1980 to 1989. An epidemiologic study of knee injuries. *Am J Sports Med* 1992;20:686–694.
27. Hagel B, Fick G, Meeuwisse W. Injury risk in men's Canada west university football. *Am J Epidemiol* 2003;157:825–833.
28. Meyers M, Barnhill B. Incidence, causes, and severity of high school football injuries on FieldTurf versus natural grass. *Am J Sports Med* 2004;32:1626–1638.
29. Orchard J, Seward H, McGivern J, et al. Rainfall, evaporation and the risk of non-contact anterior cruciate ligament injury in the Australian Football League. *MJA* 1999;170:304–306.
30. Shorten M, Himmelsbach J. Sports surfaces and the risk of traumatic brain injury. In: Nigg B, Cole G, Stefanyshyn D. *Sports Surfaces*. Calgary: University of Calgary, 2003.
31. Collina M, Lovell M, Iverson G, et al. Cumulative effects of concussion in high school athletes. *Neurosurgery* 2002;51(5):1175–1181.
32. Guskiewicz K, Weaver N, Padua D, et al. Epidemiology of concussion in collegiate and high school football players. *Am J Sports Med* 2000;28(5):643–650.
33. Naunheim R, McGurren M, Standeven J, et al. Does the use of artificial turf contribute to head injuries? *J Trauma* 2002;53(4):691–694.
34. Holle R, Lopez R, Zimmermann C. Updated recommendations for lightning safety, 1998. *Bulletin of the American Meteorological Society* 1999; 80(10):2035–2041.

35. Lopez R, Holle R. The distance between successive lightning flashes. *NOAA Technical Memorandum ERL NSSL-1XX.* Norman, OK: National Severe Storms Lab, 1999.
36. Walsh K, Bennett B, Cooper M, et al. National Athletic Trainers' position statement: lightning safety for athletics and recreation. *J Athl Train* 2000;35(4):471–477.
37. Bennett B. A model lightning safety policy for athletics. *J Athl Train* 1997;32(3):251–253.

Protective Equipment

Upon reading this chapter, the coach should be able to:

1. Understand the principles of protective equipment.
2. Determine procedures for correct fitting of protective equipment.
3. Develop a plan to select and maintain protective equipment.
4. Recognize the importance of wearing safety equipment during practice as well as competition.
5. List the equipment requirements of various sports.
6. List the advantages and disadvantages of prophylactic bracing.
7. Explain the risks of footwear designed for playing fields and courts.
8. Describe favorable characteristics of a good running shoe and the possible consequences of ill-fitted or improperly designed shoes.

Lacrosse was the family game in Jenny's family. Her mother had been a star player in college and both of her brothers were currently playing collegiate lacrosse. Jenny had spent countless hours in her youth tossing the ball around with her mother and brothers. In high school, Jenny led her team to the district championship and was the lead scorer. She was highly recruited to college and ended up at a small school in New England. Jenny was a powerhouse. She was quick, strong, and her lacrosse skills were well developed. At 5'10" and 150 pounds, she was the ideal athlete.

Jenny was also a free spirit and made fun of all the equipment her brothers wore to play lacrosse. Jenny wore her mouthpiece for practice and games but this was her only protective equipment. During her years of play she had seen players hit in the face with the ball, but she just did not think it would happen to her. Jenny's college team was good, but not great; but in 2001 the team finally came together in her senior year to make the playoff finals. The winner would go to the NCAA tournament. Jenny's team was leading toward the end of the second half when a thrown ball hit Jenny in her left eye, breaking one of the orbital bones and her nose. The pain was intense. Fortunately, her eye did not suffer any permanent damage but she did have a huge black eye. She had double vision for 4 days. The orbital bones did not require surgery but the broken nose was very painful. Jenny's team went on to play in the NCAA tournament, losing in the first round. Jenny watched from the sidelines.

Fortunately, what happened to Jenny is extraordinary today since lacrosse players are not allowed to play without eye protection. Athletes in schools normally participate under the auspices of various governing bodies. Organizations such as the National Collegiate Athletic Association (NCAA) and the National Federation of State High Schools (NFHS) mandate specific protective equipment. The NCAA's Committee on Competitive Safeguards and Medical Aspects of Sports mandates guidelines and maintains a website with safety suggestions (1). Coaches should be thoroughly familiar with the protective equipment required for their specific sport. These same governing bodies also publish lists of equipment that are considered illegal and/or dangerous to opponents.

Equipment standards have also been specified for some pieces of safety equipment such as the helmet. The American Society for Testing and Materials (ASTM) established the Committee on Sports Equipment and Facilities in 1969 and has supported important improvements in athletic safety equipment. The standardization of helmets is controlled by the National Operating Committee on Standards for Athletic Equipment (NOCSAE) and the Hockey Equipment Certification council (HECC). Although protective equipment is required for many sports, stringent standards (such as with helmets) do not exist with other types of protective equipment. For example, shoulder pads are required for footballers but the pads do not have to pass a standardized test. Further, many pads are under athletic jerseys and not observed by the officials. For this reason, coaches must be well aware of the principles and practices of safety equipment. New safety gear is constantly being created and tested, but coaches must be very diligent regarding protective equipment innovations. Advertising can be deceptive and all coaches should be thoroughly familiar with the principles of protection. For example, Robbins and Waked suggested that deceptive advertising of protective devices may represent a public health hazard and pointed out that individuals may be less cautious when using new devices of unknown benefit (2).

PRINCIPLES OF PROTECTION

Protective equipment can work to cushion blows, reducing the impact forces from balls thrown at high velocities, the force of hitting one's head against the ground, or absorbing forces due to collisions with other players. Safety gear can protect vulnerable areas. Joints can be stabilized with bracing and footwear can help absorb the force of thousands of footsteps of the endurance runner. Although protective equipment has improved significantly with the advent of new, lighter materials for protection, the basic principles of protection remain the same.

Protective equipment works in several ways to reduce injury:

- Reduces the shock (force) of impact
- Protects vulnerable areas (such as the eyes and mouth) from contact
- Increases joint stability
- Increases friction (traction) between the feet and the playing surface
- Provides cushioning and support for the foot and ankle

Shock Absorption

Most protective equipment is designed to absorb forces from direct contact. Figure 5.1 illustrates how a single force can be reduced to a smaller dispersed force when a protective pad is worn. The basic principle of shock absorption is to increase the distance and area over which a force is applied. As a result, the eventual stopping force applied to an area such as the head, shoulder, and shin is reduced. Figure 5.2 illustrates how shoulder pads might reduce injury to the shoulder joint by reducing and dispersing the blow to surrounding tissues. Although thicker pads might be more effective in reducing impact forces, there is a tradeoff between protection and mobility. You can wear gigantic pads all over your body but you will not be able to move very quickly. An athlete that is over protected might actually be more vulnerable.

Bracing

Prophylactic bracing has been utilized in athletics for centuries. The stability of various joints may be increased by applying athletic tape or wearing braces. Athletes without any injury, or even a history of injury, often wear protective devices. Many athletic trainers routinely tape the ankles of all football players prior to a contest, as well as participants in many other sports such as volleyball and lacrosse. Ankle braces have become increasingly popular. Due to the nature of their position, football linemen are under significant stress and frequently wear prophylactic knee braces designed to increase knee stability. Yet, prophylactic bracing continues to be a controversial subject. Part of the controversy is rooted in the concern that bracing one joint may increase the stress on other (and possibly weaker) joints. For instance, recent design of ski boots has changed the pattern of ski injuries from the area immediately above the ankle to the shin and knee area (3). Therefore, coaches must view the body as a complete system and not as a series of isolated joints.

Footwear

One of the most important equipment decisions coaches and athletes make is the type of shoe to be worn. This decision used to be a simple one because there were only a few types of athletic shoes as well as playing surfaces. Now, not only is there a wider variety of footwear, but numerous playing surfaces exist as well. *Simply stated, the selection of footwear must be related to the specific playing surface.* By knowing the playing surface, the coach can determine the most appropriate shoe to be worn. Shoes are often specifically designed for one particular surface. The interface between shoe surface and playing surface is what determines friction, not just shoe surface alone. Athletes need sufficient friction between shoe and playing surface to stop and turn, but too much friction results in increased torque on the lower extremities as well as the lower back and even the neck (4). Shoes must also provide sufficient support and padding for the heel, toe, and arch. Finally, if the shoe is not stylish, the athletes might not wear it. Footwear decisions are often complex.

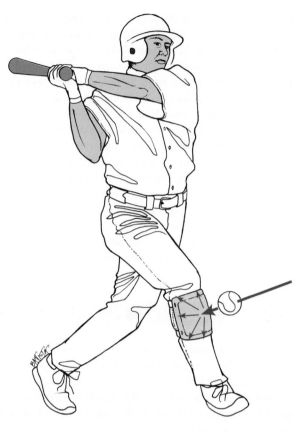

■ **FIGURE 5.1** A large force can be absorbed by a pad resulting in smaller more dispersed forces.

Recommended Equipment Procedures

Coaches should be very involved in the purchase, as well as regulating the use of safety equipment. In addition, coaches must insure that protective equipment is maintained. Several factors determine the effectiveness of protective equipment:

- *The equipment has to fit.* Protective equipment has to be individualized. In fact, poorly fitted protection may be more harmful than no equipment at all. Since all athletes should be considered equally important, the practice of handing down old and outdated equipment should be avoided. Beware of companies that suggest "one size fits all." A piece of equipment that fits one athlete will often not be appropriate for another. Coaches

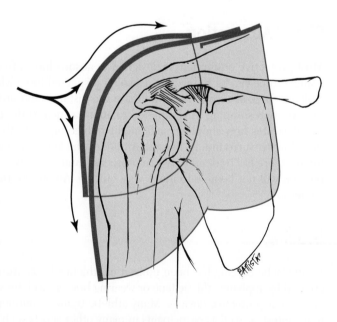

■ **FIGURE 5.2** Shock absorption. Shoulder pads work by dispersing the energy from a blow to a wider area.

of growing athletes must also be aware that the proper fit may not last the entire season. Adolescent boys and girls can grow several inches and gain significant weight during a competitive season.

■ *Protection during practice is just as important as game protection.* With the exception of a few sports, more injuries occur in practice than in games (5). Athletes spend much more time practicing than competing. *Saving protective equipment solely for game use jeopardizes the athlete.* Athletes must be comfortable with their protective equipment. Protective equipment should not hamper an athlete's ability to move and perform and practice is the best environment to determine performance. Do not wait until game time to determine that a piece of equipment restricts a player, making the athlete less effective and immobile. Athletes can adapt to many situations but they must be allowed to adapt—they have to practice with whatever protective equipment they intend to wear in competition.

■ *Protective equipment should not put the athlete at risk.* The use of protective equipment might make the athlete more vulnerable. For example, one might take a quick look at prophylactic knee braces and think that they are great. Maybe the athlete cannot turn as quickly, but now s/he is more susceptible to side impact forces. Wearing a brace on one joint may just place additional stress on other joints. A large face mask may help reduce facial injuries but such masks place increased torque on the neck upon impact. In fact, protective equipment may give the athletes the false impression that they are invulnerable.

■ *Protective equipment must be maintained.* Procedures for cleaning and checking equipment must be established. Athletes often finish a practice with sweat soaked equipment, possibly with spots of blood and saliva. Routine hygienic cleaning is necessary. Also, pads wear out and need to be changed. Simply handing out equipment at the beginning of the season is not enough. A routine must be put into effect for maintaining, storing, and replacing equipment.

■ *Safety equipment is not a weapon.* Athletes can wear the best equipment, but technique also plays a factor. For instance, anecdotal evidence suggests that some athletes feel invulnerable to injury when wearing equipment. Using the helmet as a weapon was once routine but rule makers initiated changes in 1976 to prohibit leading with the head during blocking and tackling. Prior to 1976 there were approximately 20 permanent quadriplegia cases a year. These devastating injuries were significantly reduced after this rule change (6). All of the NOCSAE helmets have a warning label informing the athlete that no helmet can prevent all injuries and that they are not to strike opponents with their helmets. It is the coach's responsibility to teach their athletes the proper use of safety equipment. Further, coaches must continue to advocate for the enforcement of "spearing" rules by game officials.

FROM THE ATHLETIC TRAINING ROOM

What Not to Wear

Any piece of equipment that is deemed dangerous by the game official is disallowed in competition. Coaches should follow that same rule in practice since some protective equipment may harm other players. NCAA guidelines prohibit specific items for certain sports according to the following table (5):

Sport	Item
Basketball	Casts or braces made of fiberglass, plaster, metal, or any nonpliable substance is prohibited. This does not apply to the upper arm, sholder, thigh, or lower leg if the material is padded.
Field Hockey	Players may wear soft headgear but only with official approval.
Football	Hard substances may be worn on the hand, wrist, forearm or elbow but must be completely covered by ½-inch closed-cell foam padding.
Football	Hard thigh guards unless covered with thick foam
Ice Hockey	Metal pads or protectors. No jewelry.
Women's lacrosse	Players may wear soft headgear if necessitated on medical grounds.

(continues)

What Not to Wear *(continued)*

Men's lacrosse	May only wear standard goalkeeper equipment.
Soccer	Knee braces are permissible but only if metal is not exposed. Casts may be worn if covered. No jewelry.
Softball	Casts may be worn but covered with neutral color. Casts worn by pitcher must not be distracting.
Track and Field	Taping of hand, thumb, or fingers of discus and javelin throwers is disallowed unless covering an open wound.
Volleyball	No jewelry is allowed. Hard splints or hand or arm must be safely covered.
Wrestling	May not wear anything that prevents normal movement or prevents an opponent from applying a hold. Hard or abrasive material must be covered and no jewelry is allowed.

TYPES OF PROTECTIVE EQUIPMENT

Game officials normally have the final ruling regarding the legality of protective equipment. Players shall not be allowed to wear items of equipment that may be dangerous to others. Athletic trainers and athletes may occasionally design special padding or braces for competition. Such protective equipment must meet the approval of the officials. In addition to protective equipment, regulations also exist regarding items that may endanger another player. For instance, jewelry is not allowed (or recommended) in most sports with the exception of religious medals. In such cases, these need to be taped to the body. Soccer players are prohibited from wearing "piercings" in NCAA competitions.

Headgear

Table 5.1 indicates headgear requirements for NCAA competition. High school and club sport organizations have similar requirements but these differ by state and organization. Helmets differ by sport because of the specific potential danger related to each sport. Helmets in sports like baseball, lacrosse, and field hockey must withstand high velocity impacts from relatively small objects. Football helmets need to withstand relatively low velocity impact such as hitting the ground or an opponent.

Buying a NOCSAE approved football helmet is just the beginning of proper head protection. Fitting and maintaining helmets are equally important and The American Equipment Managers Association provides excellent instructions (7). General fitting and maintenance guidelines should include the following:

- Fit helmets when player's hair is the same length to be worn during the season. Hair should also be slightly damp.
- The helmet should fit snugly with the cheek pads firmly against the sides of the face.
- Secure the chinstrap and pad, starting with the front straps, adjusting the chin pad an equal distance from each side of the helmet.
- The helmet should be one inch above the eyebrows and the face mask should extend two to three finger widths from the nose.
- The face mask should not obscure vision.
- Check the crown by locking your fingers on the top of the helmet and firmly pull straight down. The athlete should feel evenly distributed pressure. If the athlete feels pressure mainly in front or back the helmet needs adjustment.
- Check vertical helmet movement by placing your hands on each side of the helmet and force the helmet up and down. The skin on the forehead should move. However, the helmet may move a bit with continued force but it should catch on the eyebrows without coming down on the nose.

TABLE 5.1 NCAA Headgear Requirements in Various Intercollegiate Competitions	
Sport	**Specific Requirements**
Baseball/Softball	Baseball and softball can use interchangeable helmets. Helmets must have the NOCSAE seal and double ear-flaps. Helmets must be worn on deck, when batting and running bases.
Baseball/Softball Catchers	Catchers are required to wear a protective helmet with face guard plus a built-in or attachable throat guard on the facemask.
Fencing	Facemask with maximum mesh space of 2.1mm with a minimum gauge wire of 1mm.
Field Hockey Goalie	A helmet incorporating fixed full-face mask. In addition the goalie must wear a separate wrap-around throat protector.
Football	Helmets must have the NOCSAE seal and a face mask. The helmet must also have a four or six-point chinstrap and carry a warning label indicating the risk of injury.
Ice Hockey	Helmet and face mask that meets the HECC standards. Chin strap must be securely fastened.
Women's Lacrosse Goalkeeper	Goalkeeper must wear a complete helmet with face mask and a separate throat protector.
Men's Lacrosse	All players must wear a NOCSAE approved helmet including a face mask and chin pad with a cupped four-point chin strap. In addition, the goalie must wear a throat protector.
Skiing	Ski racers must wear a helmet designed for ski racing.
Water Polo	Swimmers must wear a cap with protective ear guards.
Wrestlers	Must wear protective ear guards.

- The back of the helmet should cover the base of the skull and ear holes should match the ear canal.
- After proper fitting the helmet must be regularly checked for cracks in any part of the interior or exterior, pads, rivets, screws, Velcro, and snaps.
- All helmets have a shelf life and should be retired according to the recommendations of the manufacturer.

FROM THE ATHLETIC TRAINING ROOM

Who is NOCSAE and What Do They Do?

In 1968 there were 32 football fatalities in organized sport. Since head injuries were the cause of many of these injuries, NOCSAE (pronounced "noxey") was formed the next year in response to a need to standardize football helmets. The first NOCSAE helmet standards were developed in 1973, and the first helmet was tested in 1974. The baseball standard followed in 1983 (since designated the baseball/softball standard), lacrosse helmets and face masks in 1986, and finally football facemasks in 1987. Football helmets' testing involves mounting the helmet on a synthetic head and dropping it from a height of 60 inches onto a firm pad. Repeated drops are made on different locations and in different temperatures. The 60-inch drop is equivalent to an athlete running into a flat surface at 12.2 mph which stopped the athlete in less than an inch. Baseball/softball helmets are tested by shooting balls directly at the helmet at 60 mph. Similar measurements are made on lacrosse helmets, all at different temperatures. Impact accelerations are measured and all helmets must meet the Severity Index established by NOCSAE.

Mouth and Eye Protection

Injuries to the mouth and eyes can be devastating, resulting in long lasting problems. The loss of teeth to an adolescent may result in problems that last a lifetime. Such injuries are easily preventable but the coach must initiate and supervise such prevention. Ice hockey players report that they will often skip wearing mouthpieces during practice but wear them only in games. While the officials oversee games, the coach oversees practice.

MOUTHPIECES

NCAA sports that require a mouthpiece include field hockey, football, ice hockey, and lacrosse. Although not required for soccer, baseball, or softball by the NCAA, many high school and youth sport organizations require participants to wear a mouthpiece. In a recent review of dental trauma, basketball players were found to be at significant risk of orofacial injury. In fact, injury rates in basketball surpass those in football and ice hockey (8). Kumamoto and Yoshinobu also reported a relatively high incidence of dental injuries in baseball and softball. In general, younger athletes appear to be more susceptible to dental injuries (8).

Fitted mouthguards come in the "boil and bite" generic kind and the custom made mouthguard. There are also stock mouthguards that come in sizes but we recommend a fitted mouthpiece. In relation to other safety equipment, the mouthpiece is quite inexpensive and very effective. A properly fitted mouthpiece prevents dental as well as soft tissue injuries to the mouth. Because the mouthpiece absorbs and cushions impact forces, there is some protection for jaw fractures and concussions. There appears to be no difference between the two types of fitted mouthguards regarding concussions (9). In addition to being properly fit, the mouthguard should be durable, odorless and clearly visible to the official. Mouthguards should not be altered or customized to cover only the front teeth. Reducing the size of the mouthpiece makes it easier to swallow and lodge in the throat.

EYE PROTECTION

The development of standardized face masks has been an excellent trend in protective equipment. Further, when governing bodies require eye protection, the decision to wear such protection is no longer a burden on the coach. For example, about one in ten basketball players suffer an eye injury each year but you will rarely see a basketball player with an eye guard unless there are extenuating circumstances (10). The social climate of basketball is such that athletes prefer not to wear eye protection. Although it has been suggested that about 90% of eye injuries are preventable, there are more that 40,000 sports and

FOCAL POINT

Mouthguard History

Reed reported that the first mouthguard was made in 1892 by Woolf Krause. Almost a quarter century went by until the next report in 1915 when professional boxer Ted "Kid" Lewis is reported to have used a mouthpiece during a championship bout. Lewis fought Jack Britton for the title on February 7, 1921. Britton's supporters protested Lewis' mouthpiece and boxing officials declared mouthpieces illegal. Several dental societies started making mouthguards for football players in the early 1950's. Prior to that date about 50% of all football injuries were dental. Mandatory mouthpieces for high school and junior high football players were adopted in 1962 and the NCAA waited until 1973 to list mouthpieces as mandatory equipment for football players.

Reed RV. Origin and early history of the dental mouthpiece. *Br Dent J* 1994;76:478–480.

recreation-related eye injuries each year in the United States (11). Sports that are played with a stick, a ball, or both are the most problematic. Table 5.2 ranks the risk of eye injury by sport.

Since the advent of helmet and face mask regulations by NOCSAE, there have been additional changes aimed toward eye protection. Governing bodies for some sports have responded to the incidence of eye injuries by instituting regulations for eyewear. For example, the NCAA mandated protective eyewear for all women's lacrosse players as of January 1, 2005 (Focal Point: Mouthguard History). Various high school and youth sport leagues require batting helmets with eye protection and intercollegiate squash players must wear eye guards. Standardized eye guards have been established by the American Society for Testing and Materials (ASTM). The ASTM has mandated specific performance standards (ASTM F803-01) for racket sports, baseball, basketball, women's lacrosse, field hockey, and alpine skiing. NCAA sports that require eye protection include fencing, football, ice hockey, lacrosse, and squash. Many state and local organizations require protection in other sports.

About one-third of persons participating in sport require corrective lenses (5). Standard eyeglasses provide little protection and athletes who need corrective lenses should wear safety lenses. Lenses made from polycarbonate plastic are the standard. Many athletes wear contact lenses but these do not protect the eye from direct blows. Additional eyewear protection is needed.

Occasionally a coach will have to meet the needs of an athlete who is functionally one-eyed (whose best corrected vision in their weaker eye is 20/40 or worse), or monocular. Such cases have to be treated conservatively and coaches must go beyond normal sport requirements and insist that the monocular athlete wear ASTM certified eye protection even in those sports with less risk.

Shoulder and Rib Protection

Shoulder injuries are difficult to treat and often take a long time to heal. Many of these injuries can be prevented by wearing the appropriate well-fitted shoulder pad. Sports that require shoulder padding by

FOCAL POINT

Women's Lacrosse Mandates Eye Protection

In the 1990s parents of injured athletes began questioning the absence of eye protection for women's lacrosse players. After all, the men were wearing helmets and face masks! But the only eye protection available was a helmet with face mask. Women's lacrosse has a tradition of noncontact, especially around the head. In fact, there was an unofficial rule by lacrosse participants referring to the six inch "bubble" around the head—no stick should enter that space. But the ball could still enter that space, causing damage to the eye as well as the bones about the eye and nose. In fact, most eye injuries are caused by the ball and not the stick (1).

Serious consideration was given to protective eyewear but there were many concerns. Many traditionalists suggested that eyewear would change the game, that athletes would have a limited field of view. Some indicated that it was a manufacturer's ploy to sell equipment. But a prototype was created in conjunction with the American Society of Testing Materials (ASTM) and the Protective Eyewear Certification Council (PECC). A test season was conducted during the fall nonchampionship season of 2002. Four of the top ten teams wore protective eyewear donated by a manufacturer. Results indicated that the general consensus was positive. It was also recommended that the eyewear be modified to allow a wider view. Some athletes reported more confidence with protective eyewear. In May 2003 the Board of Governor's of U.S. Lacrosse Women's Association rewrote the rules mandating protective eyewear for the 2005 season. In 2004 the NCAA mandated protective eyewear for the 2005 season. The result in NCAA competition was an approximate 400% drop in nose fractures and a 40% drop in eye injuries.

TABLE 5.2	Risk Categories for Eye Injury
High Risk	Baseball/Softball Basketball Fencing Field Hockey Lacrosse Squash
Moderate Risk	Football Soccer Volleyball Tennis Badminton Water Polo
Low Risk	Skiing Swimming Wrestling
Safe	Track and Field Gymnastics

the NCAA include football, men's lacrosse, and ice hockey. Shoulder padding should cushion the ball and socket shoulder joint while allowing for ample movement. Shoulder pads are now designed for a wider range of uses, resulting in multiple types of pads for football alone. Figure 5.3 is an illustration of shoulder pads for an interior lineman and a wide receiver. The interior lineman needs much more shoulder padding while the wide receiver needs padding plus shoulder mobility.

The American Equipment Managers Association's guidelines for football shoulder pad fitting include the following (7):

- Athlete should be fit without a shirt or with only a T-shirt.
- Match the pad with the position.
- Pad should extend approximately one-half inch over the deltoid.
- Athlete should be able to raise their arms without pinching the neck.
- Pads should provide adequate covering of the trapezius and pectoralis major.
- Make sure the acromioclavicular (AC joint) is covered.
- Have the athlete take a football stance and check to see that pads do not choke or pinch the athlete.
- Generally check to determine that pads are secure when straps are engaged.

Some coaches and athletes have elected to add protection for those athletes more vulnerable to rib and lower back injury. Rib protection (Fig. 5.4) is now available for susceptible athletes such as football quarterbacks and wide receivers. Likewise, lower back protection (Fig. 5.5) also exists. These additional devices are usually sold as attachments to shoulder pads. Figure 5.6 illustrates a device known as a channel-

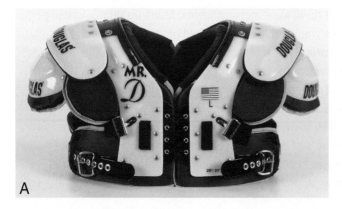
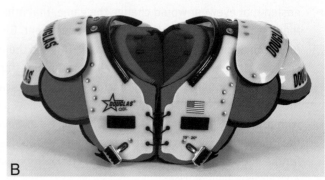

■ **FIGURE 5.3** Shoulder protection by position. **A.** Interior lineman. **B.** Wide receiver or quarterback. (Courtesy of Douglas Pads and Sports, Inc.)

FOCAL POINT

Ice Hockey Protection

Due to the nature of ice hockey, excellent protective equipment is mandatory. The possibility of being hit with a hard puck traveling at a high speed is very high. Additionally, numerous collisions occur between players and the wall. Hockey goalies are particularly susceptible to serious injury from the puck. As with all ice hockey helmets, the goalies helmet should meet HECC certification. Particular care must be given to fitting the goalie's helmet. The upper perimeter of the frontal component should be approximately $\frac{1}{4}$-inch above the eyebrow. All straps should fit snugly with the chin cup snugly against the chin. Goalies must have a neckguard. The chest pad is a vital piece of equipment and must be the right length. Test the length when the goalkeeper is in the crouched, defensive, position. The bottom of the chest pad should meet or slightly overlap the top of the protective cup.

Above all, it is vital that the equipment fit comfortably and to cover vital areas. A recent trend to find the correct size is web-based sizing. Several ice hockey companies maintain interactive websites (such as Hockeygiant.com) to assist with sizing. Participants can enter their measurements and obtain an immediate sizing recommendation.

ing system. This is a removable system, allowing one to create a void over certain areas. Many companies make special pads for specific injuries using this procedure.

Knee Braces

Knee bracing for the injured or rehabilitating athlete is the responsibility of the medical personnel with support from the athletic trainer. The American Academy of Orthopaedic Surgeons indicate that knee braces fit into three categories (12):

1. Prophylactic—braces intended to reduce or prevent knee injury. These braces are normally worn by susceptible athletes such as interior linemen in football.
2. Functional—braces designed to increase the stability of players with unstable knees.
3. Rehabilitative—braces to be worn during rehabilitation to protect and control motion.

The increased attention to knee injuries of high profile athletes along with aggressive marketing of prophylactic braces has generated significant pressure to prevent the debilitating effects of knee injury.

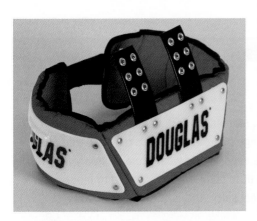

■ FIGURE 5.4 Rib protection. (Courtesy of Douglas Pads and Sports, Inc.)

Coaches are frequently asked whether football players (and occasionally other athletes) should wear prophylactic braces. It is not unusual to see all of the interior football linemen wearing braces. Football coaches often recommend or require athletes with no history of knee injury to wear prophylactic knee braces as a preventive measure. However, the effectiveness of this practice remains controversial.

How did all this get started? In 1979 nine NFL football players were given a single-sided, double-hinged knee brace, the Anderson Knee Stabler. The players had previous medial collateral ligament (MCL) damage and wore the brace to prevent further injury. The players wore the braces for a total of 29 games (around three games per player) during which time they were injury free. As a result, the creators of the brace (Anderson Knee Stabler) indicated the protective effects of their brace (13). Subsequently, other manufacturers have produced prophylactic braces, some with bracing on both sides of the knee. These braces are generally readily available (off-the-shelf) but some companies now produce custom made braces at significant expense.

Following this first report in 1979, a number of studies have been conducted (almost exclusively with football athletes) regarding the effectiveness of prophylactic braces (14–19). Unfortunately, there is still no conclusive evidence regarding the efficacy of prophylactic braces. The primary problem is a lack of control in the studies. Studies have been conducted in which the parents and/or the athletes decided who should wear braces (14,15). A well-controlled study was conducted at West Point but the athletes were intramural football participants and not college athletes (16). Such studies often conclude that further investigation

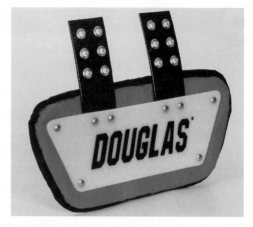

■ **FIGURE 5.5** Lower back protection. (Courtesy of Douglas Pads and Sports, Inc.)

is warranted. Research has shown positive and negative effects. For example, an excellent study recently completed explored the use of protective equipment in athletes at 100 North Carolina high schools over a 3 year period (17). They found that the use of prophylactic knee braces was associated with an increased incidence of knee injury, but that serious (>3 weeks lost) knee injuries were reduced. Conclusion: further study is warranted.

While the protective effect of prophylactic knee braces is still in doubt, one must also question the effect on performance as well as the expense. Purchasing prophylactic knee braces may require teams to compromise on other equipment. Research has also shown that prophylactic knee braces reduce speed and possibly agility (18). Does the athlete feel more secure? Paluska and McKeag have suggested that athletes may have a false sense of security and that the brace may injure other players. Some athletes have suggested that they feel safer (19). The current situation regarding prophylactic knee braces is one of confusion. As a result, we recommend that the utilization of prophylactic knee braces be made on an individual basis in consultation with medical personnel.

Ankle Bracing

The ankle is the most common location of injury in most sports. Since the typical etiology of ankle injury results from forced plantar flexion accompanied by ankle inversion, support systems have been developed to reduce the range of motion of the foot and ankle (20). Adhesive taping and various prophylactic ankle stabilizers are the most common methods of stabilizing the ankle. A wide variety of ankle braces are now available, each offering different levels of support.

FOCAL POINT

To Brace or Not

"After 10 years of organized football I've seen my share of knee injuries. I guess I'm fortunate that my knees are still in good shape. I didn't wear a knee brace until I started playing college ball but our coach required that all interior linemen wear them. If I wanted to play I had to wear a brace. We even had to wear them on noncontact days in practice. I didn't like the brace at all when I first tried it. It was a little cumbersome, tended to move around, and I know I was slower. I finally got used to it and it made be feel safer. Did it help? I don't know."

—A Division 1 offensive tackle.

FOCAL POINT

Ankle Bracing and Agility

Braces are commonly used for prevention of ankle injuries, but does the wearing of ankle braces affect athletic ability? Is performance compromised by the wearing of braces? A recent study addressed this question. Researchers had 34 subjects complete a series of performance measurements involving power and agility while wearing various ankle braces—one rigid, five semirigid, and four soft models. Only the rigid model compromised sport performance while the other nine braces had no effect on ability. However, the subjects did not feel equally comfortable in all of the braces. Subjective evaluation of the braces revealed significant differences with regard to comfort and support. The researchers suggested that athletes choose their own brace, since a comfortable brace might be more conducive to wear.

Rosenbaum D, Kamps N, Bosch K, et al. The influence of external ankle braces on subjective and objective parameters of performance in a sports-related agility course. *Knee Surg Sports Traumatol Arthrosc* 2005;13(5):419–425.

Do ankle braces reduce the incidence of ankle injury? Verhagen et al critically reviewed studies over a 20 year period concerning the efficacy of ankle taping and bracing as a preventive measure to reduce ankle injury (21). They concluded that studies reported a significant decrease in the incidence of ankle sprains using either tape or braces. Thacker et al reviewed 113 studies and found similar results (22). Gross and Liu have also reported that semirigid and laced ankle braces reduce the incidence of ankle injury (23). Even though research tends to support ankle bracing as a method of reducing ankle injury, many athletic trainers and coaches question routine bracing of asymptomatic athletes. The concern is that athletes will rely too heavily on supplemental support and will not develop the strength and balance necessary to prevent ankle injury. Since the most common risk factor for ankle sprain is a history of previous sprain (22) we support the routine administration of taping or bracing of those athletes with a history of ankle sprains. The efficacy of bracing all athletes is still questionable.

Footwear

Athletic footwear can be protective but injuries may result from inappropriate footwear selected for training and competition. Due to the fairly complicated biomechanics of individuals as well as the wide variety of competitive surfaces, specific footwear recommendations are not available. Additionally, coaches must contend with style, color, brand, and general popularity of shoes. Young athletes are susceptible to vigorous advertisements by the various shoe companies. Interestingly, there appears to be no relationship between the expense of a shoe and its effectiveness (2). Expensive shoes are not necessarily the best. We recommend that coaches follow the general guidelines presented below:

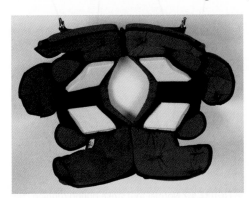

■ **FIGURE 5.6** Channeling protection system (as seen from inside).

- The shoe *must* fit. Since feet tend to swell during the day, fitting of shoes should occur in the afternoon while wearing the same socks to be worn while practicing and competing.
- Fit the shoe to the longest toe and the widest part of the shoe should coincide with the widest part of the foot.
- Athletes must be given ample time to practice in the shoe in which they compete.
- When breaking in new shoes, allow athletes to bring in their older shoes to wear during part of practice. Repeat this until the new shoe has molded to the foot.
- Humans are so unique that the perfect shoe for one athlete may be unsuitable for another. One shoe does not fit all.

- Athletes with special needs, such as orthotics, need to be evaluated by the athletic trainer.
- Since shoes tend to lose cushioning and support over time, athletes should not wear their athletic shoes except during practice and competition.

Athletic shoes come in several categories:

- *Running Shoes*—shoes that are primarily designed for cushioning and support while traveling in a straight line. Running shoes are inappropriate for sports in which the athlete must stop, turn, or decelerate quickly.
- *Game/Court Shoes*—shoes that are primarily designed for cushioning and support while starting, stopping, turning, and landing. Game shoes may or may not have cleats but will have sufficient friction to support the athlete when accelerating or decelerating.
- *Specialized Shoes*—specific shoes have been designed for particular sports. For instance, special shoes have been designed for track and field athletes including javelin and discus throwers, high jumpers, and shot putters.

RUNNING SHOES

The impact between the foot and ground during running has a peak force greater than twice the body weight of the athlete. These highly repetitive forces applied to the foot, knee, and hip are the primary risk factor for numerous running injuries. Of the 10,000 injuries reported in one sports medicine clinic, 37% (more than any other activity) were related to running (24). As the popularity of running increased in the early 1970s the first technical running shoes were manufactured. Early running shoes were rated by *Runner's World Magazine* for price, weight, shock absorption, flexibility, and durability. At this point, little attention had been placed on stability and motion control of the foot and ankle. Recently, Shorten has indicated that the four most common overuse injuries (knee pain, tibial stress syndrome, Achilles tendonitis, and plantar fasciitis) are all associated with misalignment (25).

During running the foot is naturally placed directly under the center of gravity of the runner. This insures the balance of the runner. As a result, the foot makes initial ground contact in a slightly supinated position (slight inversion and adduction of foot) and then rolls into pronation (eversion and abduction of the foot). Figure 5.7 illustrates this natural heel to toe running form. Some runners have inherent pronation of the foot and must undergo a greater range of pronation, possibly leading to additional stress on the lower extremity. To correct this problem, shoe manufacturers now include anti-pronation control features. Since there is a range of pronation problems, shoe manufacturers now make shoes with varying degrees of control, allowing the athlete to choose the shoe that works best. Coaches, athletes, and athletic trainers must work together to find the shoe that works best. Goss and coworkers have suggested the use of shoe clinics as a method of improving shoe selection. These clinics often include a team of sports medicine professionals knowledgeable in foot mechanics.

Cushioning has long been considered an important component of the running shoe. Repetitive loading is a risk factor and cushioning can reduce the stress on the foot. Fortunately, there is a wide variety of cushioning materials available that are effective. During running the peak forces are generally focused on the heel, the metatarsal heads and the big toe; but, improved cushioning can distribute impact forces more widely. Runners often have a shoe for training and a less cushioned (lighter) shoe for competition. Since running kinematics are slightly changed when utilizing a different shoe, athletes must be given time to practice in both.

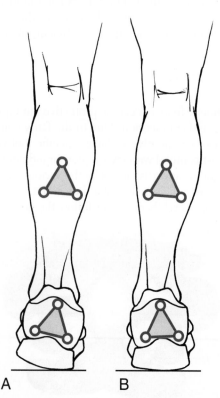

■ **FIGURE 5.7** Normal foot strike during running. The runner's foot rolls from the lateral to the medial side of the foot during each stride.

In general, the selection of running shoes should include:

- A comfortable upper that provides good perspiration absorption and a comfortable feel. A structure composed of various materials is common.
- Cushioning that feels neither too hard nor too soft.
- An outsole of polyurethane rubber for durability and abrasion resistance.
- An insole usually made from polyethylene foam to provide shock absorption and help prevent sliding (26).

GAME/COURT SHOES

Games present a different challenge to the foot and lower body as they involve abrupt changes in direction and velocity. Since the shoe-surface interface determines friction, game shoes must be designed for the specific surface on which the game is played. A shoe designed for a natural grass surface is probably not going to be safe for play on an artificial surface. A common cause of injury is insufficient rotational freedom between the playing surface and footwear (27). The shoe remains fixed to the playing surface while the trunk rotates. An example of this is demonstrated in a study by Wilkinson in which the application of resin on basketball shoes increased the incidence of ankle sprains (28). Since the basketball shoe was designed for court participation (without resin) the addition of resin increased friction beyond safe limits, resulting in less rotational freedom and increased stress on the ankle. The fixation of the foot has been systematically linked to knee injury (4). Increased friction may allow for faster stopping and turning but also results in significantly more stress on the joints of the lower body.

As Shorten suggests, it is desirable for the traction between a shoe and a playing surface to lie in an optimum range, providing adequate resistance to slipping without excessive stress (4). We suggest finding the shoe that results in minimal slippage while maintaining performance. Shoe manufacturers now design shoes for specific surfaces. For instance, in one study of 15 different football shoes made by three different manufacturers, it was found that shoes tested in conditions for which they were not designed exhibited excessive friction characteristics (29). Coaches need to continue to encourage shoe manufactures to label the appropriate use of their athletic footwear. The risk of any shoe on a specific surface is quite variable and specific recommendations are not available. Ultimately, the coach needs to be aware of the factors that determine risk, to involve the athlete in the choice of shoe and to monitor recent innovations in footwear.

SUMMARY

- The basic principles of protection involve cushioning, protection from blows, the increased stability of joints by bracing, and the selection of appropriate footwear to provide cushioning, stability, and appropriate friction between shoe and playing surface.
- Protective equipment must fit, be worn during practice and competition, and needs routine maintenance and updating.
- Various organizations such as the NCAA and the NFHS mandate specific requirements for protective equipment.
- Game officials are the final judge of safety equipment.
- The effectiveness of prophylactic knee bracing continues to be equivocal and has not proven effective.
- Ankle taping and bracing improve ankle stability. Athletic trainers often do not routinely apply taping so that athletes can develop stability without bracing.
- Athletes with a history of ankle injury should wear an ankle brace (or tape) during practice and competition.
- Footwear for running is very different from shoes designed for ball games. Athletes should wear shoes designed for the sport in which they participate.
- Running shoes require cushioning as well as support for excessive pronation. Some runners will require more control than others.
- Game/court shoes should not provide too much friction since foot fixation is the cause of many lower extremity injuries. Shoes with aggressive cleating is normally not recommended.

References

1. NCAA Committee on Competitive Safeguards and Medical Aspects of Sports. http://www.ncaa.org/health-safety. Accessed August 11, 2007.
2. Robbins S, Waked E. Hazard of deceptive advertising of athletic footwear. *Br J Sports Med* 1997;31(4): 299–303.
3. Peterson L, Renstrom P. *Sports Injuries: Their Prevention and Treatment*, 3rd ed. London: Martin Dunitz, Ltd, 2001.
4. Shorten M, Hudson B, and Himmelsback J. Shoe-Surface traction of conventional and in-filled synthetic turf football surfaces. In: Milburn P. *Proceedings XIX International Congress of Biomechanics.* University of Otago, New Zealand, 2003.
5. National Collegiate Athletic Association. *Sports Medicine Handbook.* 2005–2006, 18th ed. Indianapolis. Also found at: http://www.ncaa.org/health-safety.
6. Cantu RC, Mueller F. Fatalities and catastrophic injuries in high school and college sports, 1982–1997. *Phys Sportsmed* 1999; 27(8):35–40.
7. American Equipment Managers Association. http://www.aemal.com. Accessed August 11, 2007.
8. Kumamoto DP, Yoshinobu M. A literature review of sports-related orofacial trauma. *Gen Dent* 2004;52(3):270–280.
9. Wisniewski JF, Guskiewicz K, Trope M, et al. Incidence of cerebral concussions associated with type of mouthguard used in college football. *Dent Traumatol* 2004;20(3): 143–149.
10. Vinger PF. A practical guide for sports eye protection. *Phys Sportsmed* 2000;28(6):49–70.
11. Committee on Sports Medicine and Fitness. Policy Statement: protective eyewear for young athletes. *Pediatrics* 2004;113(3): 619–622.
12. American Academy of Pediatrics Committee on Sports Medicine. Knee brace use by athletes. *Pediatrics* 1990;85:228.
13. Anderson GS, Seman SC, Rosenfeld RT. The Anderson knee stabler. *Phys Sportsmed* 1979;7:125–127.
14. Grace TFG, Skipper BJ, Newberry JC, Nelson MA, Sweetser ER, Rothman ML. Prophylactic knee braces and injury to the lower extremity. *J Bone Joint Surg Am* 1988;70:422–427.
15. Hansen BL, Ward JC, Diel RC. The preventive use of the Anderson knee stabler in football. *Phys Sportsmed* 1985;13:75–81.
16. Sitler M, Ryan J, Hopkinson W, et al. The efficacy of a prophylactic knee brace to reduce knee injuries in football: a prospective, randomized study at West Point. *Am J Sports Med* 1990;18:310–315.
17. Yang J, Marshall SW, Bowling JM, et al. Use of discretionary protective equipment and rate of lower extremity injury in high school athletes. *Am J Epidemiol* 2005;161(6):511–519.
18. Greene DL, Hamson KR, Bay RC, et al. Effects of protective knee bracing on speed and agility. *Am J Sports Med* 2000;28: 453–459.
19. Paluska SA, Mckeag DB. Knee braces: current evidence and clinical recommendations for their use. *Am Fam Physician* 2000; 61(2):411–418, 423–424.
20. Verhagen EA, van der Beek AJ. The effect of tape, braces and shoes on ankle range of motion. *Sports Med* 2001;31(9):667–677.
21. Verhagen EA, van Mechelen W, de Vente W. The effect of preventive measures on the incidence of ankle sprains. *Clin J Sport Med* 2000;10(4):291–296.
22. Thacker SB, Stroup DF, Branche CM, et al. The prevention of ankle sprains in sports; a systematic review of the literature. *Am J Sports Med* 1999;27:753–760.
23. Gross MT, Liu HY. The role of ankle bracing for prevention of ankle sprain injuries. *J Orthop Sports Phys Ther* 2003;33(10): 572–577.
24. Garrick JG. Characterization of the patient population in a sports medicine facility. *Phys Sportsmed* 1985;13:73–76.
25. Shorten MR. Running shoe design: protection and performance. In Tunstall-Pedoe D. *Marathon Med.* Portland: BioMechanica, LLC.
26. Goss D, Tortorelli J, Saylor M. Fitting efficacy: shoe clinics add miles for runners. *Biomechanics* 2005;12(8):21–29.
27. Bartlett R. *Sports Biomechanics: Reducing Injury and Improving Performance.* London: E & FN SPON, 1999.
28. Wilkinson WHG. Dangers and demands of basketball. In: Reilly T. *Sports Fitness and Sports Injuries.* London: Wolfe, 1992.
29. Heidt RS, Dormer SG, Cawley PW, et al. Differences in friction and torsional resistance in athletic shoe-turf surface interfaces. *Am J Sports Med* 1996;24(6):834–842.

Overtraining and Underrecovery in Athletes

Upon reading this chapter, the coach should be able to:

1. Understand the causes of overtraining syndrome.
2. Be aware of the symptoms of overtraining and overreaching.
3. Realize that decreased performance may be caused by excessive training and nontraining stress.
4. Appreciate the interaction of nontraining and training stressors.
5. Understand the importance of recovery when planning training.
6. Develop a system of monitoring their athletes.
7. Comprehend how to develop a periodized training program.

Tim joined the Barracuda Swim Team at age 7. At first it was a neat way to be with his buddies during the summer. The pool was located just down the street from his house and the practices were not too hard. It was fun. Tim thrived in the pool and quickly became one of the age-group stars. Summer ended and Tim started training (sometimes twice a day) and racing all year. He quit his other sports to concentrate on swimming. He was very successful. But things started to change. As Tim said, "Swimming used to be a joy for me. I could not wait to get in the pool. Training was actually fun and I loved the competitions. But the stress of swimming thousands of yards a day caught up with me my first year in college. We'd get up at 6:00 a.m. and put in a good hour of swimming. I'd hurry back for a quick breakfast, eating alone as the other students were already gone. I'm in a small liberal arts college and academics here are very competitive, no breaks for athletes. As a chemistry major, I often have afternoon labs, requiring me to train over the dinner hour. There are countless papers, lab reports, books, and exams. I don't have a social life. Afternoon swim practice is now close to 3 hours with 2 hours in the water and another hour in the weight room. I drag back to my dorm, eat alone, try to study but I'm just so tired. Training isn't fun anymore and I'm not getting any faster. If I get sick I've had it. Is this why I came to college?"

Tim's story is not that unique. Athletics in the United States has changed significantly in the last 30 years (1). Not only is the competitive season longer, there are more competitions. It is not unusual for college athletes to fly cross-country for competitions, and return home for another event only a few days later. College football games are scheduled in August, before school even begins. International travel is commonplace. Even in Division III collegiate athletics, athletes who used to participate in more than one sport now tend to specialize in one sport and train for that sport all year. In many schools, when the competitive season ends, athletes enter out-of-season training programs run by strength and conditioning coaches.

The trend of longer and more intense training is not limited to college athletics. Sport specialization has become common in communities across the country. Hill and Simons have defined sport specialization as students who limit their participation to one sport on a year-round basis (2). Many communities now support travel squads with children traveling several hundred miles to compete. Pam Belluck reported on a small town in Minnesota where the basketball coach wanted to start a "traveling squad" for second graders (3). A *New York Times* article reported that parents of Little League players were paying $70 per hour for batting coaches (4). The parents believed that improved batting makes their children better applicants for college. Bill Pennington of the *New York Times* recently reported on the problems many children face with regard to specialization (5). The prevailing thought is that if children do not specialize by the eighth grade, they will not be prepared for higher level competition. There are literally thousands of club teams playing far too many competitions a year. In San Diego alone there are more than 125 baseball teams for ages 10 and under, many playing 80 games a year (5). When the head coach of a youth baseball team (composed mostly of 9 year olds) in San Diego was asked to described the length of the team's season, he said, "Labor Day to Labor Day"(5).

There is little question that specialization is on the rise, but the number of young people specializing is not known. There are advantages to specialization, including the possibility of enhanced performance and motor skill development, but disadvantages also exist. Excessive sport training may lead to overuse injuries. Young athletes may lose the opportunity to develop skills in other sports. Frequently, their natural talent may exist in other activities. Wiersma has indicated that 98% of athletes who specialize will never reach the highest levels of competition (6). Many agree that to accomplish expertise in sport, specialization is necessary (7). The important question is at what age specialization should begin if an athlete wishes to do so. The American Academy of Pediatrics has recommended that specialization should not begin before adolescence (8). The answer to these questions is still a subject of debate.

Since the latter half of the 20th Century considerable progress has been made to improve the quality of training (9). Coaches and athletes have devised numerous, creative ways to train. Schools compete to provide the best athletic facilities, filled with state of the art equipment. Numerous summer training camps attempt to attract student athletes with high profile athletes and coaches. Access to school and community training facilities is at an all time high. The prevailing thought seems to be "more is better." As a result, we now frequently read about overtraining, staleness, fatigue, overuse injuries, and burnout. Burnout, a frequently used term in today's society, is often used to describe someone who has dropped out of an activity. Athletic burnout has become an increasing problem since, more often than not, the ending result is that the athlete quits the sport completely. The early description by Smith of burnout has withstood the test of time. Smith described burnout to be "a psychological, emotional, and sometimes a physical withdrawal from an activity in response to excessive stress or dissatisfaction" (10). Many researchers have proposed burnout theories where overtraining is a common and prevalent theme (11–13). Athletic burnout is related to overtraining.

FOCAL POINT

Athletes Have Little Discretionary Time

Athletes continue to express frustration at their lack of discretionary time. An interview of a collegiate basketball player by Wrisberg et al is an example:

"At this level, the season is so long. And then there's the traveling and schoolwork and everything. It's really hard balancing basketball with your personal time . . . which basically you don't have any of."

Wrisberg C, Johnson M, Brooks G. Assessing the quality of life of NCAA Division I collegiate athletes: A qualitative investigation. Unpublished data. In: Kellmann M. *Enhancing Recovery*. Champaign, IL: Human Kinetics, 2002.

OVERTRAINING

Lehmann et al report a story about a well known German gymnast competing in the 1996 European Championships (14). As he was preparing to compete, he shook his head, briefly closed his eyes, and left the arena without looking up. "Suddenly, I just couldn't do any more. I just wanted to rest." The fatigue in his body was evident. While this particular occurrence may be a little extreme, Lehmann recounts a number of stories of athletes who credit their success with *less* (rather than more) training. Oddly enough, some stories even relate to events where the imposed rest, due to an injury, actually helped an athlete. As Lehmann reported on an ATP tennis professional, "My recent successes are due to less tennis, more regeneration, and the enforced break (due to injuries); I am less exhausted and burnt out than the other players." Unfortunately, these stories are not unique; the athletes are talking, but few are listening. As a result, overtraining is prevalent.

- Lehmann, et al reported on a group of soccer players during a 4 month season in which 50% were overtrained (15).
- Morgan and co-workers found that 60% of females and 64% of males have been stale (overtrained) at least once during their running careers (16,17).
- Raglin and Morgan found that 91% of swimmers who were stale during their freshman year in college experienced staleness in the following years (18).
- Kentta et al surveyed 272 age-group athletes from 16 sports and found that 37% had experienced overtraining (19).

Overtraining does not just happen to elite level athletes who train year-round; athletes at all levels of competition are susceptible to overtraining (20). Since the most common result of overtraining is reduced performance, coaches must be aware of this phenomenon. For example, if an athlete experiences a decrement in performance due to overtraining, a coach might decide that the athlete needs more training. Increased training, rather than rest, is the opposite of what the athlete may need. In addition to performance, Table 6.1 indicates the most common symptoms of overtraining (21).

The formalized study of overtraining is relatively new. The original evidence of overtraining was mostly anecdotal, but as this information became more common, concern grew. As evidence of this concern, an International Conference on Overtraining in Sport was held at the University of Memphis preceding the 1996 Olympic Games in Atlanta. The edited work *Overtraining in Sport* was the outcome of this symposium (22). Two subsequent publications have addressed this concept (23,24). Overtraining has been described as "an imbalance between training and recovery," (25). Lehmann and colleagues go further and

TABLE 6.1 Symptoms of Overtraining
Reduced Performance
Severe Fatigue
Muscle Soreness
Feelings of Depression
General Apathy
Decreased self esteem
Irritability
Restlessness
Loss of Appetite
Disturbed Sleep
Concentration Difficulties

describe overtraining as the result of an imbalance between stress and recovery (21). Overtraining is not simply the result of too much physical exertion; overtraining is the result of training, competition, and nontraining stressors. Too much stress combined with too little regeneration results in overtraining.

Kellmann suggests that problems at school, time management problems, and arguments with friends or partners, in addition to the requirements of athletics, present a single package load of stress to the individual (24). "Often, individuals can easily handle those situations, but when a heavy training load is added to an already high 'personal package load,' the total impact on the systems simply gets too high." Nontraining stressors are almost always present for student athletes. Students are faced with considerable stress as they compete for grades, entrance to college, entrance to graduate school, boyfriend/girlfriend issues, and simply trying to cope with the rigors of school. The response to this imbalance is overtraining.

Overtraining syndrome (OTS) is the term now commonly used to describe the physiological and psychological symptoms related to excess training and nontraining stressors (26–28). As explained by Meeusen et al, adding the term "syndrome" acknowledges that exercise training is not necessarily the sole cause of overtraining. The problem is multi-factorial (28). Therefore, overtraining syndrome (Fig. 6.1) is an accumulation of training and/or nontraining stress resulting in long-term decrement in performance capacity. Overtraining syndrome may or may not be accompanied by related physiological and psychological signs and symptoms of overtraining. Overtrained athletes cannot be positively influenced by short amounts of rest. Restoration of performance capacity may take several weeks or months (28).

Overtraining or Overreaching?

Successful training involves an overload. But when the overload is not matched with an appropriate recovery, performance often drops. This condition is quite common in athletics and athletes frequently experience this phenomenon during preseason and often during training camps. Due to the nature of the college calendar, many swim coaches regularly schedule a mid-season training camp in late December and early January during which athletes undergo a marked increase in training. Such training often results in a performance decrement. Kreider et al have labeled this state, overreaching (OR), an accumulation of training and nontraining stress resulting in a short-term decrement in performance capacity (22). Recovery usually takes a matter of days. One suggestion is that if an athlete does not recover in 72 hours they have worked too hard and can be considered overreached (29).

Some authors have used the term functional overreaching (or short-term OR). Functional OR should lead to an improvement in performance after recovery. However, when the balance between training and recovery is not respected, performance does not improve and the athlete begins showing signs of psychological disturbance such as decreased vigor and increased fatigue. Functional OR is not that serious unless the coach does not recognize it. Reduced performance by athletes is not uncommon and overreaching is one cause. Unfortunately, a common reaction by coaches to poor performance is to increase training stress. In such cases, overreaching can transition into long term problems.

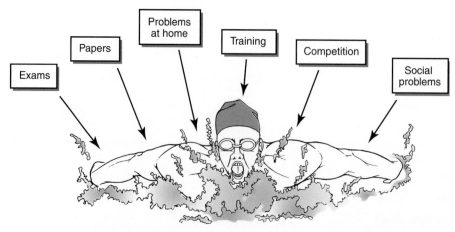

■ **FIGURE 6.1** Training and nontraining stressors on an athlete.

UNDERRECOVERY

Exercise physiology texts contain a full range of training methods. Continuous versus interval training, free weights versus machine weights, circuit training, and power training are endlessly covered. Likewise, training manuals for sport are jam-packed with drills and illustrations of training techniques. Recovery from all of these training methods is given superficial treatment at best. The athlete who is allowed sufficient recovery is better able to withstand the rigors of training. Recovery helps prevent overtraining. An awareness of the importance of the recovery process often marks the difference between a mediocre and an excellent athlete. Certainly, athletes must train hard but they must also recover. What is the purpose of intense training if it results in an athlete who is tired and sore, an athlete who does not recover, or an athlete who underperforms? A heavier or more intense training load without adequate recovery is not the key for success. As McCann writes, "Focusing on optimal recovery shifts from the problem to the solution" (30).

While numerous methods of measuring training exist, measuring recovery is very problematic. How do we know when an athlete has recovered? We do not. A definitive way of measuring recovery has yet to be found. The restoration of the specific energy systems is fairly well known. Classic work conducted in Sweden determined that restoring phosphagens (ATP-PC—Chapter 7) is a very quick process, taking only 3 to 6 minutes (31), while the removal of lactic acid from the blood stream takes about an hour (32). It is generally accepted that resynthesis of muscle glycogen can take as long as 48 hours (33). Table 6.2 summarizes energy system restoration.

But recovery from exercise is much more than restoring muscle glycogen or removing blood lactate. Bompa has also suggested that fatigue is located in the central nervous system (CNS) (34). As the CNS system fatigues, athletes lose their ability to concentrate, coordinate complex movements, and react quickly and powerfully, possibly making them more vulnerable to injury. Because both physical and psychological stress have been found to affect performance, coaches should plan physical and psychological forms of recovery (34).

Causes and Problems of Overtraining Syndrome

As suggested, overtraining syndrome (as well as overreaching) is probably not caused by one single factor, but a combination of many variables. The literature in overtraining commonly lists the following causes:

- Excessive practice and/or physical training
- Too little recovery
- A combination of excess practice and underrecovery
- Too many nontraining stressors
- Malnourishment
- Physical exhaustion and unremitting muscle soreness
- Boredom caused by too much repetition

FOCAL POINT

Athletes Need to be Taught to Slow Down and Recover

Individuals who are highly motivated are frequently victims of overtraining. In an interview by Wrisberg et al, a college tennis player describes a teammate:

"One guy on the team doesn't know when to stop with his training. He's a great guy but he works too hard and now he has a stress fracture in his back. Last year he broke a foot. He goes too much. He wants it too bad."

Wrisberg C, Johnson M, Brooks G. Assessing the quality of life of NCAA Division I collegiate athletes: A qualitative investigation. Unpublished data. In: Kellmann M, ed. *Enhancing Recovery*. Champaign, IL: Human Kinetics, 2002.

TABLE 6.2 Energy System Recovery	
Energy System	**Restoration Duration**
ATP-PC	Complete restoration of ATP takes 3–6 minutes—50%–70% of the phosphagens are restored in the first 20–30 seconds. Phosphocreatine restoration takes a bit longer—up to 10 minutes if all of the PC was exhausted.
Lactic Acid System	Complete removal of lactate takes about 60 minutes providing the athlete continues to perform mild exercise. If the athlete completely rests then lactate removal takes 90–120 minutes.
Aerobic System	About 60% of muscle glycogen is restored in the first 10 hours following prolonged, nonstop activity providing the athlete is given a high carbohydrate meal shortly after exercise. Complete glycogen restoration takes about 48 hours.

Overtrained athletes often suffer declines in performance and/or no improvement despite continued training. Overtrained athletes also tend to burn out, occasionally dropping out of sport completely. Moreover, from the point of view of sports medicine, overtrained athletes suffer:

- Increased risk of injury (35)
- Decreased immune response (overtrained athletes are more prone to infection and illness) (36)

THE COACH AND OVERTRAINING

It is much easier to prevent overtraining than treat it (20). Since coaches are responsible for training their athletes, they may be directly, or at least indirectly, responsible for overtraining as well. As overtraining has been shown to result in poor performance and increased susceptibility to injury, every effort must be made to prevent such a state. Therefore, it is the coach's responsibility to plan for both training and recovery. Coaches also need to be aware of other stressors that may affect their athletes. Student athletes are faced with far more stress than that produced by training and competition. Nontraining stressors may also take a toll on athletes. Boyfriend/girlfriend problems, disturbing news from home, and financial worries may affect sleep. Poor performance on an exam or an all night study session disrupts body rhythms.

Interaction of Nontraining and Training Stressors

The coach normally sees the athlete through a relatively narrow window during practice and competition. If an athlete is not performing well in practice, it could be that he/she has just received a bad grade on an exam or disturbing news from home. The athlete may have stayed up all night studying. Such unpredicted

FOCAL POINT

Is This Meeting Necessary?

Coaches and/or administrators occasionally make decisions without considering the time cost for their athletes. As an example,

"They're (athletic officials) talking about implementing more programs for athletes—more seminars that take about 2 hours each. So I speak up and say 'Hey guys, we don't have any more time!' And they're like 'Well wait, you need to know about this and you need to know about that.' So I say, 'That's great but there comes a point in time when you are putting too much on athletes. I mean we reach a point where we don't even care anymore.' We just have to have some time for ourselves and I'm afraid they don't understand that."

Wrisberg C, Johnson M, Brooks G. Assessing the quality of life of NCAA Division I collegiate athletes: A qualitative investigation. Unpublished data. In: Kellmann M. *Enhancing Recovery*. Champaign, IL: Human Kinetics, 2002.

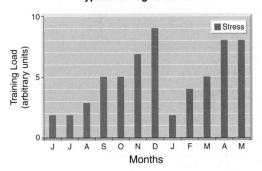

Annual Non-Training Stressors for a Typical College Student

■ **FIGURE 6.2** Annual nontraining stressors for a college student.

stressors are difficult for the coach to recognize but students often experience a series of nontraining stressors related to academic demand. As a result of interviews with college health counselors, we developed a scale of nontraining stress for a typical college student. A timeline of nontraining stressors might look something like Figure 6.2. As expected, the end of a semester is a peak period for nontraining stress. Another factor related to school stressors is the year in school. Sher et al found that individuals reported a clear, steady decline in distress across the 4 years (37). The authors suggested that this appeared to be a function of adaptation to school as well as adjusting to young adult life. As a result of this information, coaches should be more aware of first-year students.

Similarly, we conducted a series of interviews with soccer coaches to develop a scale of performance stressors during a typical collegiate season. As shown in Figure 6.3, the peak periods are October and November, toward the end of the competitive season. Figures 6.4 and 6.5 demonstrate the combination of training and nontraining stressors. Fortunately, as the training stress tends to reduce, nontraining stressors start to increase. However, several soccer coaches indicated that the stress of mid-term exams, coupled with more important soccer events, was problematic for some students.

Every sport has a unique sequence of training stressors. In general, preseason is a time of fairly high stress as athletes experience a relatively sharp increase in physical activity. Then as the season progresses, competitions become more serious, possibly leading to postseason play, conference, and even national championships. Likewise, the nontraining stressors presented by academics follow a fairly predictable path. Some sports are more problematic than others, especially when postseason play coincides with high academic pressure. Further, acute daily stressors related to the unique personal nature and the history of each athlete are often unpredictable. When coaches are aware of such pressures, they can adjust training accordingly.

STRATEGIES FOR PREVENTING OVERTRAINING

There is no one best way to prevent overtraining. Since overtraining is the result of multiple factors, the coach must develop various tactics to help prevent OTS. Diagnosing and preventing OTS is not simple, but we believe that one powerful tool is attentiveness by the coach. The awareness that underperforming athletes may actually be overtrained is critical to prevention. When coaches observe an athlete who is underperforming they need to consider the possibility of too much training and/or too little recovery. Some strategies that we suggest to prevent the overtraining syndrome include:

- Establish two-way, open communication with your athletes. Establish opportunities to debrief athletes to help with recovery.
- Avoid monotonous training.
- Monitor your athletes.
- Periodize training.
- Plan recovery.

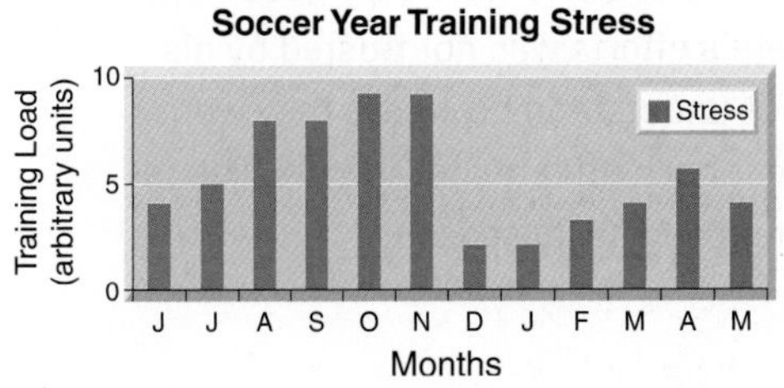

Soccer Year Training Stress

■ **FIGURE 6.3** Annual training stress on a collegiate soccer player.

Two-Way Communication

It is important that coaches develop an environment of openness. Kellmann suggests that coaches should provide a nonthreatening, comfortable and trusting atmosphere in which athletes can discuss personal situations (24). For instance, sometimes an athlete may need to take care of personal issues—problems that when left unresolved may develop to an unhealthy state. Kellmann recommends that it is better to miss a few days of practice to solve a problem than to allow such stress to become magnified (24). Academic pressures on students can be considerable. As one of the coaches we interviewed said, "I recruit a student to achieve both athletically and academically. I have a responsibility to that student to help them achieve in both areas."

Coaches need to be good observers, to be able to evaluate their athletes and to monitor their performance. Johnson and Flamino found that swim coaches were quite good at predicting the effort of their swimmers (38). But swim coaches have the advantage of quantifying each practice and have significant control over intensity and volume. Coaches of other sports may have more difficulty predicting effort. But athletes need reassurance that they are being treated as individuals, that the coach understands their effort as problems may arise if their perception is different. Bompa suggests that coaches need to be aware of the physiological and psychological characteristics of their athletes (34). Remember that no two athletes will respond to the same stimulus identically. The perfect workout for one athlete may be excessive for another athlete.

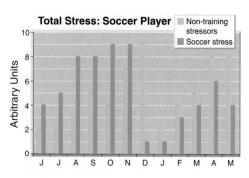

■ **FIGURE 6.4** Training and nontraining stressors on a collegiate soccer player.

DEBRIEFING

Two-way communication should also include debriefing to facilitate recovery. Hogg suggests debriefing as aid to reduce stress (39). Debriefing has received little examination in sport psychology, but Hogg suggests that debriefing is essential for complete mental and emotional recovery from a significant competitive event. Athletes need to reflect seriously on their performance following major competitions (39). Debriefing helps the athlete recover from the mental stress of performance and to move forward. One goal of debriefing is to empower the athlete by enhancing self awareness and the ability to acknowledge strengths and weaknesses. Debriefing provides the necessary information by which the athlete may devise a plan for future performance. Coaches should not attempt to debrief an athlete if they are not able to provide insight toward the future, to give the athlete direction. Hogg suggests the following steps (39):

1. Select the best time and place to meet with the athlete soon after performance.
2. Encourage the athlete toward meaningful self-analysis.
3. Open the environment for healthy interaction—share experiences—do not focus too much on the past.
4. Determine if there is a need for change.
5. Set new goals that are challenging, measurable, and meaningful.
6. Self-monitor for improved performance.

FOCAL POINT

Coaches' Versus Athlete's Perception of Effort

Johnson and Flamino studied several Division III swim coaches for 2 years to determine if coaches could predict the perceived effort of their swimmers during training (32). They found that the coaches were very good at predicting effort. Interestingly, the coach who was best at predicting the athlete's efforts was not trusted by his swimmers. For various reasons, the athletes believed that the coach did not understand how hard they were working. After the coach was informed of this he incorporated a plan to treat each athlete individually. The result was a 31% improvement in the athletes' trust of their coach and an improved swim season.

Johnson J, Flamino Y. Can coaches predict the exertion of swimmers? *Am Swim* 2002;2:21–24.

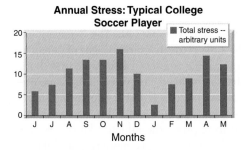

■ FIGURE 6.5 Combination of training and non-training stressors on a collegiate soccer player.

Avoid Monotonous Training

Boredom is frequently mentioned as one of the causes of overtraining as well as burnout (18). Athletes get tired of repeating the same training program day after day. Interestingly, Kentta et al found that overtraining is much more prevalent in individual rather than team sports (29). This might be expected since athletes participating in individual sports spend so much time alone. As suggested in Chapter 2, repetitive drilling is probably not the best way to teach motor skills. Endless drilling may also make athletes more susceptible to overtraining.

We encourage coaches to be creative, to frequently change procedures to make training interesting. This goes for the entire practice from warm-up to cool-down. Play games, have small competitions, but keep it interesting. We observed a swim practice one day in January when the coach stopped practice and had everyone go off the three meter platform. All of a sudden, there was laughter, smiles, and a rejuvenated mood by the swimmers. The coach told us later that he just sensed that a change was necessary. He had not planned this but simply observed that something different was necessary.

Monitor Your Athletes

Considerable attention has been aimed at finding a simple diagnostic to determine overtraining, but such efforts have been unsuccessful (26). This is not surprising since overtraining is a complicated condition. While underperformance is the common sign of overtraining, it is also important to rule out the presence of organic disease or malnourishment as possible causes. Diagnosing overtraining involves physiological as well as psychological symptoms. Overtrained athletes not only suffer a sport-specific decrease in performance, they also experience disturbances in mood. Overtrained athletes experience "heavy legs" and sleep disturbances (26). Overtrained athletes have an increased perception of effort during training (29).

Coaches will always need to systematically monitor each of their athletes. Daily note taking, observations, casual conversations, and the continuous monitoring of performance are common techniques that all coaches should develop. In the absence of a simple diagnostic test, we believe that good observational skills are one key to preventing overtraining. Coaches may also wish to monitor mood state. Some coaches have recommended the use of performance tests as a way of monitoring athletes.

FROM THE ATHLETIC TRAINING ROOM

A Simple Way of Monitoring Staleness

Researchers at the University of Queensland in Australia identified a simple method of predicting staleness (overtraining). They followed a group of swimmers during a 6 month competitive season. Upon arising each morning the swimmers kept a daily log of sleep quality, fatigue, stress, and muscle soreness on a scale of 1 to 7. A rating of "1" was good while a rating of "7" meant the athlete did not sleep or was extremely sore. A normal score for nonstale swimmers was around 3 to 4, but scores of 5 or 6 were related to poor performance. Interestingly, daily log scores were also related to several blood chemistry markers of stress. The researchers suggested that an increased feeling of fatigue coupled with poor sleep were valid markers of impending overtraining.

Hooper S, Mackinnon L, Howard A, et al. Markers for monitoring overtraining and recovery. *Med Sci Sports Exerc* 1995;27:106–112.

THE RECOVERY-CUE

One diagnostic test that is relatively easy to use is the Recovery-Cue (see page 93) (40). The Recovery-Cue was developed to monitor early warning signs of overtraining. The scale measures various signs of perceived exertion and recovery as well as sleep and life quality. The Recovery-Cue is a seven item scale that should be administered on a weekly basis. Kellmann et al recommend that the scale be completed at the same time and day from week to week (40). Completing this weekly scale allows the coach and/or supporting staff to graph the results and to monitor individual trends throughout a season. The best use of this assessment tool is in conjunction with the athlete, since the scale was designed to improve the athlete's knowledge and awareness of recovery. Increased knowledge and awareness allow the athlete to take more responsibility toward being a more integral part of the training and recovery process. Our suggestion (especially in the collegiate setting) is to create a web-based version of the scale in which the results are easily downloaded onto a spreadsheet and graphed. Coaches can then observe each athlete's mood over a season.

PERFORMANCE TESTS

The quantification of performance in some sports is relatively easy. Swim and track coaches can measure the time it takes an athlete to complete a specific distance. Performance in sports like football, soccer, and basketball is more difficult to quantify. For this reason, coaches occasionally develop performance tests that are specific to the sport. As suggested by Meeusen et al, the inability to sustain intense exercise is a prime feature of OTS (28). Athletes suffering from OTS can often start a training sequence or race at the usual speed but then cannot complete the task. Time to fatigue tests probably show more changes in exercise capacity than less strenuous tests (41).

Performance tests should be specific to the sport. For instance, the 1.5 mile run was often used to measure fitness for football even though it is well known that continuous running is not part of football. If performance tests are to be used, they should represent the specific training in which the athlete engages. Performance tests are tough on athletes and should only be administered if the results are utilized for better planning. Performance tests can also indicate to athletes that they are improving, giving them more self confidence.

Use Periodized Training

Athletes cannot possibly stay in top condition year round. Intense periods of training and competition must be followed by periods of reduced activity in order for the athlete to recover. Following an adequate period of recovery, the athlete is renewed and ready to train and compete again. Athletes occasionally cycle through preparation, competition, and recovery several times per year without becoming overtrained. This method of training is typically called "periodization," a deliberate strategy of exposing athletes to intense training followed by a lower training load (34). Since periodized training involves planned recovery, this system of training is frequently recommended as a strategy to prevent overtraining (34,35,42).

The formalized approach to periodized training has been around since the 1960s. The Russians were probably the first to systematize this form of training (43). According to Norris and Smith, Americans have been reluctant to adopt Russian methods of training, presuming that their success was more related to pharmacological enhancement than superior training methods (44). Although originally used for weight lifters and track and field athletes, periodized training can be adapted for all forms of athletic training and is now quite popular in North America.

A comprehensive treatment of the Periodized Model can be found in the periodization literature (34,44,45,46). Although the periodization terminology utilized by authors varies, the concepts are quite similar. These include the following:

- The training of athletes involves a specific plan.
- The plan is flexible.
- Athletic training is conducted in cycles.
- Each cycle has a goal.
- The volume and intensity of training are manipulated to bring about the desired goal.
- The training phases follow a logical sequence.

- Recovery and regeneration are part of the training program.
- Each phase of the program builds upon the preceding plan.

THE ANNUAL PLAN

Creating and following an annual plan is critical to periodized training. Coaches often use various templates to plan out a year or a season. Figure 6.6 is one example of a template that can be utilized to plan

	Pre-Season		Competitive Season		Rest
	General Preparation	Specific Preparation	Early (less important?) Competitions	Late Season Competition (Playoffs)	
Dates					
Priority					
Volume					
Intensity					
Skill Training					
Tactics/ Strategy					
Strength Training					
Macrocycles					
Microcycles					
Academic Stress					

Use H, M, L, or O to score in first 5 rows.
H = High
M = Medium
L = Low
O = None

■ FIGURE 6.6 A competitive season.

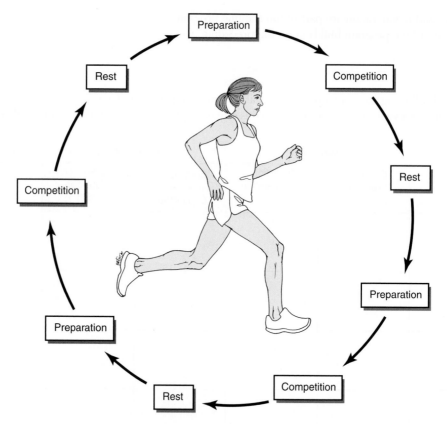

■ **FIGURE 6.7** An annual cycle involving three competitive periods.

one competitive season. Coaches may wish to modify this template for their specific sport, adding or taking away rows or columns. In general, the first step in creating an annual plan is to use a calendar to mark the following:

- The competitive events
- The important competitive events

This establishes when you want athletes to be in peak condition. These dates will vary by sport. For instance, swimmers may compete over a 3 month period, often scheduling less important competitions early in the season. Most importantly, swim coaches want their athletes to peak at the end of the season when conference championships are held. As shown in Figure 6.7, a distance runner may cycle through preparation, competition, and rest several times a year. Many team sports like basketball and soccer schedule conference games later in the season. Athletes will need to be in top competitive condition for several weeks to possibly compete in conference championships.

Once the competitive dates are set, you can answer some basic questions. At what point should athletes be at their peak condition? When should the athletes work hard and when will they need to rest? Once these basic questions have been answered, work backward to prepare your athletes for competition. Fleck and Kraemer recommend that coaches manipulate volume, intensity, and skill training according to a periodized schedule (46). As the season progresses, the volume of training is reduced as the intensity increases (Fig. 6.8). Prior to the most important competitions, intensity is also reduced,

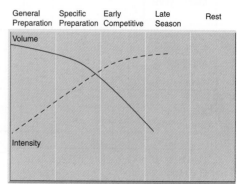

Training Phases Through One Season of Competition

■ **FIGURE 6.8** Training phases through one season of competition.

allowing athletes to perform at their best. Figure 6.9 illustrates a completed template (minus the macro- and microcycles) for a football season, and Figure 6.10 illustrates anticipated changes in fitness over a year. To prevent overtraining, high level training and competition is followed by rest and recovery.

	Pre-Season		Competitive Season		Rest
	General Preparation	Specific Preparation	Early (less important?) Competitions	Late Season Competition (Playoffs)	
Dates	June 3– July 15	July 16– Sept 9	Sept 10– Oct 7	Oct 14– Nov 26	Nov 27– Jan 3
Priority			L M H M	H M H H H	
Volume	M → H	M	L	L	
Intensity	L	M	H	M – H	
Skill Training	L	M	H	M	
Tactics/ Strategy	O	L	M	H	
Strength Training	H	H	M	L	
Macrocycles					
Microcycles					
Academic Stress	L	L	M	M	H

Use H, M, L, or O to score in first 5 rows.
H = High
M = Medium
L = Low
O = None

■ FIGURE 6.9 A competitive season for football.

As shown in Figure 6.6, the preparatory and competitive phases are divided into sub-sections. Each phase of the period should have specific goals. Ideally, athletes should spend as much time during the preparatory phase as the competitive period (20). Unfortunately, due to the constraints of NCAA and state high school regulations, this plan is probably unrealistic for the scholastic athlete. Nevertheless, the athlete should still go through all of

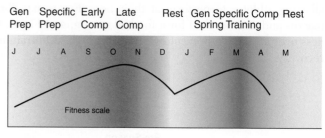

■ **FIGURE 6.10** Annual fitness plan for football.

these phases, transitioning from the general to the specific to the competitive phase. Active rest must follow. In general, the goals of the various periods might look something like the following:

GENERAL PREPARATION

This phase is very important toward the success of the athlete. Athletes should work hard during this phase to improve their general fitness with a high volume of training. Training during this period is tough, starting with medium volume of training and then progressing to high volume. Specific goals are to:

- Improve general physical training
- Improve motor abilities
- Improve technique
- Educate athletes regarding training

SPECIFIC PREPARATION

During this phase athletes are transitioning toward the competitive season. The objectives are similar but much more specific to the sport. Emphasis on fitness continues with an increased accent on technique, strategy, and knowledge. The volume of activity should drop as the precompetitive cycle begins. Reduce general (activities not specific to the sport) activities, as training should involve almost exclusively sport specific activities.

Ideally, the preparatory phase should last at least 2 months. Since many sports such as soccer and football start their competitive seasons early in the fall, it is imperative that athletes train independently during the preseason.

COMPETITIVE SEASON

By the time the competitive season starts, athletes should be fit for competition. Training is highly sport specific and designed to maintain fitness. Coaches are well aware that athletes need some competitive experiences to reach high performance levels. As a result, many coaches treat the first few competitions as less important, as a precompetitive season. Gandelsman and Smirnov claim that it takes 7 to 10 competitions to achieve high performance (47). Although such claims may be somewhat speculative and dependent on many variables, the training goals of the competitive cycle are consistent and include:

- Continued improvement of sport skills and technique
- Continued improvement of competitive strategy and tactics
- Gaining competitive experience
- Maintenance of competitive fitness

THE TRANSITION/REST PHASE

The transition/rest phase does not mean that the athlete stops all activity. The central theme of active rest is change. The second theme is that the athletes continue to be active, but to a lesser extent than during preparation and competition. Encourage your ath-

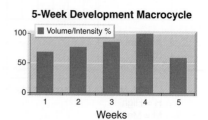

■ **FIGURE 6.11** A 5-week developmental macrocycle.

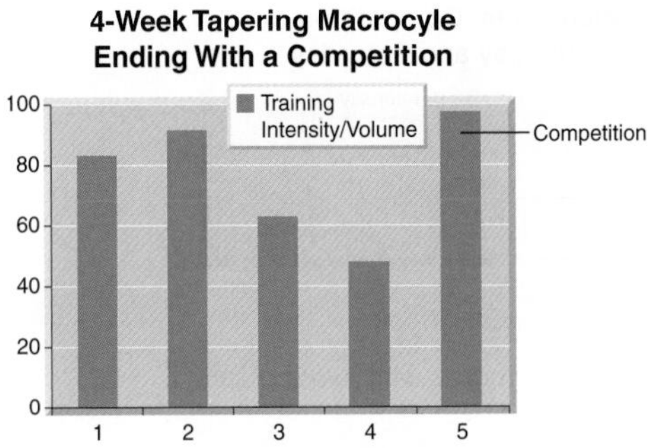

**4-Week Tapering Macrocycle
Ending With a Competition**

■ **FIGURE 6.12** Macrocycle ending with an important competition.

letes to engage in another activity while maintaining a reasonable degree of fitness. This phase ends when the next general preparation cycle resumes.

Planning Cyclic Training

The basic units of cyclic training are the macrocycle and the microcycle. Microcycles might be thought of as short periods (like a week). A group of microcycles make up a macrocycle. One unique aspect of these cycles is that they are goal oriented. The coach decides what is to be accomplished during each cycle and then plans accordingly. Goal setting is inherent throughout the cycles and athletes must be aware of the plan and should play a part in such goal setting. The time frames must be manageable and allow for the overall goal to be accomplished.

THE MACROCYCLE

A macrocycle often lasts about 4 to 6 weeks. The seasonal plan illustrated in Figure 6.6 is composed of four macrocycles. An annual plan is composed of many macrocycles. Each of the macrocycles has a goal and the coach designs training to achieve that goal. For example, during the preseason, preparatory macrocycle, the main goal is adaptation. Such an adaptive (developmental) macrocycle might look like the one shown in Figure 6.11. Each week (microcycle) is a little more difficult with a tapering (reduced activity week) at the end.

A typical macrocycle (Fig. 6.12) that might happen toward the end of a competitive season is the tapering macrocycle. Tapering is used in many sports to bring about top level performance. Approximately 2 weeks of tapering are scheduled for this macrocycle so that athletes are well rested prior to an intense competition.

THE MICROCYCLE

Bompa suggests that the microcycle (usually 1 week of training) is the most important functional tool of planning (34). The structure and content of each microcycle will differ throughout the year as each is designed to achieve the goal of that microcycle. For instance, one microcycle might be oriented toward developing specific skills while another ends with a weekend tournament. The organized coach should use long-term planning to design the microcycle, specifying the dominant training factors for each cycle. But the coach should not plan more than 2 to 3 microcycles at a time, maintaining the flexibility necessary to adapt to individual and team needs.

Microcycles are usually designed with one or two training peaks followed by days of reduced activity. This is one way to reduce susceptibility to overtraining. A microcycle composed of three training peaks may be appropriate during the preparatory period but should not be the normal cycle. A typical training microcycle with Sunday off might look like something similar to Figure 6.13, whereas, a microcycle that ends with a competition on Sunday is illustrated in Figure 6.14.

Remember that there are many examples of microcycles appropriate to the needs of the athletes. However, more than 2 hard days in succession is not recommended. During the competitive season it is not unusual to have one or more competitions a week. Such a microcycle might look like that illustrated in Figure 6.15.

Athletes will need at least 1 to 2 days of regeneration following competition. Occasionally, there are 2 days of competition in a row such as a tournament or big track meet. Athletes will usually need 2 days of lower level work prior to a 2-day competition. Occasionally, the schedule can be altered if you know you are

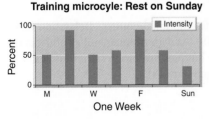

■ **FIGURE 6.13** A 1-week microcycle with Sunday rest.

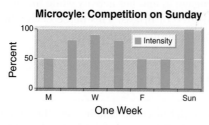

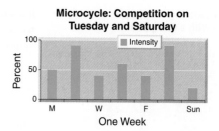

■ **FIGURE 6.14** Microcycle with competition on Sunday

■ **FIGURE 6.15** Microcycle with two competitions in a week.

playing a weak opponent or if it is a competition that is less important. In this manner, more training days with more intense training can be utilized.

The Active Rest Microcycle. Plan these just as you would a practice. Do not simply perform the same old activities at a slower pace. Bompa suggests starting a session with a good, long warm-up of about 30 minutes followed by 30 to 45 minutes of work that is completely different from the specifics of the sport (34). In addition, a number of regeneration ideas (such as the following) should be utilized to revitalize your athletes.

COMPLETE (PASSIVE) REST

Complete rest is the primary method of recovery. Because physically active individuals regularly require 9 to 10 hours of sleep every 24 hours, coaches need to encourage athletes to put themselves into a situation that promotes relaxed sleep. Techniques such as a warm bath, hot tub, herbal tea, and massage may be helpful. Athletes should avoid caffeine, large fatty meals, and alcohol prior to bedtime and be encouraged to regulate sleep patterns by going to bed and rising at specified times.

NUTRITION

Physical activity places greater nutritional needs on athletes (see Chapter 9). Nutrition is particularly important shortly after intense training and/or competition.

HEAT THERAPY

Saunas, hot tubs, moist steam packs, and steam baths are all examples of heat treatments that stimulate the flow of warm blood. Heat treatments immediately after training are contraindicated. External heat robs the deep muscle of the blood needed for recovery and places an increased load on the heart.

COLD THERAPY

Cold therapy presents an analgesic effect on sore and inflamed muscles. Cold is best applied shortly after the cessation of exercise for 20 to 30 minutes. Ice bags can be applied directly to the skin. Individuals occasionally worry that their skin will freeze but skin freezes at 25°F while ice bags are only 32°F. When ice is directly applied there is an immediate sensation of cold followed by some burning. Analgesia follows.

RELAXATION TECHNIQUES

Relaxation lowers the heart rate, reduces muscle tension and aids emotional control. Relaxation techniques have been well documented but are also highly individual (48). As with training, not all athletes respond the same to relaxation techniques. Examples of standard techniques are progressive muscle relaxation, guided imagery, meditation, breath control, and time management (48).

The Recovery-Cue

The Recovery-Cue

1. How much effort was required to complete my workouts last week?

Hardly	6	6	6	6	6	6	6	6
any effort	5	5	5	5	5	5	5	5
	4	4	4	4	4	4	4	4
	3	3	3	3	3	3	3	3
	2	2	2	2	2	2	2	2
excessive	1	1	1	1	1	1	1	1
effort	0	0	0	0	0	0	0	0
Week	1	2	3	4	5	6	7	8

2. How recovered did I feel before my workouts last week?

Energized	6	6	6	6	6	6	6	6
And recharged	5	5	5	5	5	5	5	5
	4	4	4	4	4	4	4	4
	3	3	3	3	3	3	3	3
	2	2	2	2	2	2	2	2
still not	1	1	1	1	1	1	1	1
recovered	0	0	0	0	0	0	0	0
Week	1	2	3	4	5	6	7	8

3. How successful was I at rest and recovery activities last week?

Successful	6	6	6	6	6	6	6	6
	5	5	5	5	5	5	5	5
	4	4	4	4	4	4	4	4
	3	3	3	3	3	3	3	3
	2	2	2	2	2	2	2	2
not	1	1	1	1	1	1	1	1
successful	0	0	0	0	0	0	0	0
Week	1	2	3	4	5	6	7	8

4. How well did I recover physically last week?

always	6	6	6	6	6	6	6	6
	5	5	5	5	5	5	5	5
	4	4	4	4	4	4	4	4
	3	3	3	3	3	3	3	3
	2	2	2	2	2	2	2	2
	1	1	1	1	1	1	1	1
never	0	0	0	0	0	0	0	0
Week	1	2	3	4	5	6	7	8

(continues)

The Recovery-Cue *(continued)*

5. How satisfied and relaxed was I as I feel asleep in the last week?

always	6	6	6	6	6	6	6	6
	5	5	5	5	5	5	5	5
	4	4	4	4	4	4	4	4
	3	3	3	3	3	3	3	3
	2	2	2	2	2	2	2	2
	1	1	1	1	1	1	1	1
never	0	0	0	0	0	0	0	0
Week	1	2	3	4	5	6	7	8

6. How much fun did I have last week?

always	6	6	6	6	6	6	6	6
	5	5	5	5	5	5	5	5
	4	4	4	4	4	4	4	4
	3	3	3	3	3	3	3	3
	2	2	2	2	2	2	2	2
	1	1	1	1	1	1	1	1
never	0	0	0	0	0	0	0	0
Week	1	2	3	4	5	6	7	8

7. How convinced was I that I could achieve my goals during performance last week?

always	6	6	6	6	6	6	6	6
	5	5	5	5	5	5	5	5
	4	4	4	4	4	4	4	4
	3	3	3	3	3	3	3	3
	2	2	2	2	2	2	2	2
	1	1	1	1	1	1	1	1
never	0	0	0	0	0	0	0	0
Week	1	2	3	4	5	6	7	8

Kellmann M, Patrick T, Botterill C, et al. The Recovery-Cue and its use in applied settings: Practical suggestions regarding assessment and monitoring of recovery. In: *Enhancing Recovery: Preventing Underperformance in Athletes*. Kellmann M, ED. Champaign, IL: Human Kinetics, 2002.

Recovery, like stress, is a multidimensional process. Recovery needs to be planned and individualized (see Focal Point: The Recovery-Cue). In addition, athletes younger than 18 require longer periods of recovery (49,50). Athletes who are more experienced tend to recuperate sooner (51). Some authors have suggested that gender may be a factor, indicating that females tend to recover more slowly than males (49,52). Environmental factors, such as temperature and altitude require more recovery. Because negative feelings increase stress which slows recovery, Bompa suggests that coaches should not express fear or indecisiveness (34).

SUMMARY

- Overtraining is more prevalent as a result of increased sport specialization, increased training, and increased athletic competition.

- Overtraining syndrome is caused by a combination of elevated training and nontraining stressors coupled with too little recovery.
- Overtraining syndrome results in increased susceptibility to injury, illness, and poor performance.
- Overtraining syndrome can lead to burnout, a condition in which the athlete gives up a sport.
- Excess training can lead to functional overreaching, normally a short-term condition of reduced performance that can be treated by short term rest.
- Overtraining syndrome is a serious condition, requiring an extensive period of recovery, before an athlete can return to a healthy state.
- Coaches should develop some system of monitoring their athletes for overtraining symptoms.
- Student athletes will have periods when nontraining stressors are higher as well as unpredictable stresses due to personal situations.
- Coaches can prevent overtraining by establishing good communication with athletes and developing a periodized annual plan that includes rest periods.
- Recovery should be planned by the coach and should involve multiple recovery techniques.

References

1. Shulman J, Bowen W. *The Game of Life*. Princeton, NJ: Princeton University Press, 2001.
2. Hill GM, Simons J. A study of the sport specialization in high school athletes. *J Soc Issues* 1989;13:1–13.
3. Belluck P. Parents try to reclaim their children's time. *New York Times*, June 13, p. A18.
4. Johnson D. Seeking little league skills at $70 an hour. *New York Times*, June 24, p. A1.
5. Pennington B. As team sports conflict, some parents rebel. *New York Times*, November 12, p. A1.
6. Wiersma LD. Risks and benefits of youth sport specialization: Perspectives and recommendations. *Pediatr Exerc Sci* 2000;12: 13–22.
7. Ericsson KA. *The Road to Excellence: The Acquisition of Expert Performance in the Arts, Sciences, Sports, and Games*. Mahwah, NJ: Erlbaum, 1996.
8. Committee on Sports Medicine and Fitness, American Academy of Pediatrics. Intensive training and sports specialization in young athletes. *Pediatrics* 2000;106(1):154–157.
9. McCann S. The role of a sport psychologist when addressing overtraining in elite athletes. *Abstracts of the 14th Conference of the Association for the Advancement of Applied Sport Psychology*. Alberta: Banff, 1999:13.
10. Smith R. Toward a cognitive-affective model of athletic burnout. *J Sport Psychol* 1986;8:36–50.
11. Schmidt G, Stein G. Sport commitment: a model integrating enjoyment, dropout, and burnout. *J Sport Exerc Psychol* 1991;8: 254–265.
12. Silva J. An analysis of the training stress syndrome in competitive athletics. *J Sport Exerc Psychol* 1990;2:5–20.
13. Coakley J. Burnout among adolescent athletes: A personal failure or social problem. *Sociol Sport J* 1992;9:271–285.
14. Lehmann M, Foster C, Netzer N, et al. Physiological responses to short- and long-term overtraining in endurance athletes. In: Kreider R, Fry A, O'Toole M. *Overtraining in Sport*. Champaign, IL: Human Kinetics, 1998.
15. Lehmann M, Schnee W, Scheu R, et al. Decreased nocturnal catecholamine excretion: parameter for an overtraining syndrome in athletes? *Int J Sports Med* 1992;13:236–242.
16. Morgan W, Brown D, Raglin J, et al. Psychological monitoring of overtraining and staleness. *Br J Sports Med* 1987;21:107–114.
17. Morgan W, O'Conner P, Ellickson K, et al. Personality structure, mood states, and performance in elite distance runners. *Int J Sport Psychol* 1998;19:247–263.
18. Raglin J, Morgan W. Development of a scale to measure training induced distress. *Med Sci Sports Exerc* 1989;21:60.
19. Kentta G, Hassmen P, Raglin J. Training practices and overtraining syndrome in Swedish age-group athletes. *Int J Sports Med* 2001;22:460–465.
20. Fry R, Morton A, Keast D. Overtraining in athletes. *Sports Med* 1991;12:32–65.
21. Lehmann M, Foster C, Keul J. Overtraining in endurance athletes: a brief review. *Med Sci Sports Exerc* 1993;25:854–861.
22. Kreider R, Fry A, O'Toole M, eds. *Overtraining in Sport*. Champaign, IL: Human Kinetics, 1998.
23. Lehmann M, Foster C, Gastmann U, et al. *Overload, Fatigue, Performance Incompetence, and Regeneration in Sport*. New York: Plenum, 1999.
24. Kellmann M. *Enhancing Recovery*. Champaign, IL: Human Kinetics, 2002.
25. Kuipers H, Keizer H. Overtraining in elite athletes: review and directions for the future. *Sports Med* 1988;6:79–92.
26. Urhausen A, Kindermann W. Diagnosis of overtraining. *Sports Med* 2002;32(2):95–102.
27. Halson S, Bridge M, Meeusen R, et al. Time course of performance changes and fatigue markers during intensified training in trained cyclists. *J Appl Physiol* 2002;93(3):947–956.
28. Meeusen R, Duclos M, Gleeson M, et al. Prevention, diagnosis and treatment of the overtraining syndrome: ECSS position statement task force. *Eur J Sports Sci* 2006;6(1):1–14.
29. Kentta G, Hassmen P. Overtraining and recovery: a conceptual model. *Sports Med* 1998;26(1):1–16.
30. McCann S. In: Kellmann M. *Enhancing Recovery*. Champaign, IL: Human Kinetics, 2002.

31. Knuttgen H, Saltin B. Muscle metabolites and oxygen uptake in short-term submaximal exercise in man. *J Appl Physiol* 1972; 32(5):690–694.

32. Karlsson J, Saltin B. Oxygen deficit and muscle metabolites in intermittent exercise. *Acta Physiol Scand* 1971;82:115–122.

33. Hultman E, Bergstrom J. Mucle glycogen synthesis in relation to diet studied in normal subjects. *Acta Physiol Scand* 1967; 182(1):109–117.

34. Bompa T. *Periodization: Theory and Methodology of Training*, 4th ed. Champaign, IL: Human Kinetics, 1999.

35. Brooks G, Fahey T, White T, et al. *Exercise Physiology: Human Bioenergetics and Its Applications*, 3rd ed. Mountain View, CA: Mayfield Publishing Company, 2000.

36. Ames C. Chemistry of marathon running. *J Clin Pathol* 1989;42:1121–1125.

37. Sher K, Wood P, Gotham H. The course of psychological distress in college: a prospective high-risk study. *J Col Student Devel* 1996;37:42–51.

38. Johnson J, Flamino Y. Can coaches predict the exertion of swimmers? *Am Swim* 2002;2:21-24.

39. Hogg J. Debriefing: a means to increasing recovery and subsequent performance. In: Kellman M. *Enhancing Recovery*. Champaign, IL: Human Kinetics, 2002.

40. Kellmann M, Patrick T, Botterill C. The Recovery-Cue and its use in applied settings: practical suggestions regarding assessment and monitoring of recovery. In: Kellmann M. *Enhancing Recovery*. Champaign, IL: Human Kinetics, 2002.

41. Halson S, Jeukendrup A. Does overtraining exist? An analysis of overreaching and overtraining research. *Sports Med* 2004; 34(14):967–981.

42. Rowbottom D, Keast D, Morton A. Monitoring and preventing of overreaching and overtraining in endurance athletes. In: Kreider R, Fry A, O'Toole M. *Overtraining in Sport*. Champaign, IL: Human Kinetics, 1998.

43. Matveyev L. In: Nadori L, Granek I. Theoretical and methodological basis of training planning with special considerations within a microcycle. Lincoln, NE: National Strength and Conditioning Association, 1989:11.

44. Norris S, Smith D. Planning, periodization, and sequencing of training and competition: The rationale for a competently planned, optimally executed training and competition program, supported by a multidisciplinary team. In: Kellman M. *Enhancing Recovery*. Champaign, IL: Human Kinetics, 2002.

45. Balyi O. Planning, periodization, integration and implementation of annual training programs. *Presentation to and in proceedings of the Australian Strength and Conditioning Association National Conference*. Gold Coast, Australia, 1995.

46. Fleck S, Kraemer W. *The Ultimate Training System: Periodization Breakthrough!* New York: Advanced Research Press, 1996.

47. Gandelsman A, Smirnov K. *Physiologicheskie osnovi metodiki sportunoi trenirovki*. Moscow: Fizkultura I Sport, 1970.

48. Knox S, Theorell T, Malmberg B, et al. Stress management in the treatment of essential hypertension in primary health care. *Scand J Prim Health Care* 1986;4:175–181.

49. Rowland T. Developmental aspects of physiological function relating to aerobic exercise in children. *Sports Med* 1990;10(4): 253–266.

50. Schoner-Kolb I. *Das verhalten ausgewahlter physilogischer, biochemischer und physchologischer parameter wahrend und nach einem ubertrainingsversuch an normalpersonen in alter von 23-30 jahren*. Doctoral thesis. German Sport University, Cologne, 1990.

51. Noakes T. *Lore of Running*. Champaign, IL: Human Kinetics, 1991.

52. Nudel D, ed. *Pediatric Sports Medicine*. New York: PMA, 1989.

HEALTHY ATHLETES

Conditioning Athletes

Upon reading this chapter, the coach should be able to:

1. Understand the typical response and adaptation to single and repeated exercise sessions.

2. Be aware of the basic principles of conditioning including overload, individuality, and specificity.

3. Know the difference between sport and metabolic specificity.

4. Identify the basic energy systems utilized in sport.

5. Design an exercise program to train the three energy systems.

6. Provide rationale for the importance of sport specific training.

7. Understand that humans are composed of different fiber types and that specific fiber recruitment is dependent on exercise intensity.

Brian's junior year on the ski team was one of his best. He was a slalom specialist and had won the conference and qualified for the national championships. He was elected team captain. Following the ski season Brian saw an advertisement for the Marine Corps Marathon scheduled the next fall in Washington, DC. He thought this would be a good way to stay in shape during the off-season and decided to start training for the marathon. His roommate was a distance runner at the college and he started running with him. He ran all spring and summer, occasionally long runs of 20 miles. His aerobic fitness was superb; his running program was working. He even lost 12 pounds and completed the marathon in a little over 3 hours. He continued his running program and believed he was in the best shape of his life as preseason for skiing started.

But Brian was not in shape for skiing. On the first day of ski practice he scored miserably on the vertical jump and just as badly on the agility tests. He had lost the power and agility necessary for top level slalom skiers. His first day on the slopes was an embarrassment. Unfortunately, he had become hooked on distance running and could not give up his running program. In fact, the more he ran, the worse he got at skiing. Luckily, Brian didn't get hurt his senior ski season, but he had his worst performance ever.

Slalom ski racing is a relatively brief event, lasting only about a minute. Excellent leg power, agility, technique, and balance are required for top level performance. Slalom racing is primarily an anaerobic activity. Brian's off-season training program was almost entirely aerobic, designed to train the slow twitch endurance fibers. Long–slow distance training is just the opposite preparation that an anaerobic athlete needs. What happened to Brian can happen to many athletes; they train the wrong energy system and the wrong muscle fibers. For many athletes, such training often leads to injury as well as inferior performance.

Training and conditioning athletes for competition is one of the primary responsibilities of the coach. Physical conditioning not only prepares athletes for competition, it helps prevent injury (1). As suggested in Chapter 2, the strategies and practices adopted to prevent injury are not dissimilar from the prepara-

Fast Moves

One of our colleagues recently had to transport one of his athletes to the emergency room. Fortunately, the athlete was not badly injured but did require medical care. As he was conversing with the physician in the treatment room, he noticed that several patients were wearing softball cleats. Upon inquiring, the physician said, "Didn't you know? Adult softball leagues started today." What made this event more interesting is that the coach recognized several of the injured players as regular joggers on our outdoor running trail. They thought they were in good shape for softball since they ran regularly. But joggers do not *sprint* to first base or *race* around the bases, trying to turn a single into a double. Jogging uses slow twitch muscles and sprinting uses fast twitch muscles. They may have been jogging around a running track but they were not prepared for fast moves.

tion of athletes for performance. The best preparation for competition is also the best method of preventing injury. Coaches should acquire up-to-date information regarding the fundamentals of conditioning. A top quality physical conditioning program requires planning, is based on scientific foundation, and is flexible to meet the various needs of the athlete. The well rested, well-fed, and physiologically prepared athlete is ready for competition, will perform better, and will be less susceptible to injury.

TRAINING BASICS—RESPONSE AND ADAPTATION

Before we get into the specifics of training, it is important to understand some of the basic foundations of training. Humans can adapt to stressors that they systematically encounter. With regard to athletic training, the stress is in the form of exercise. Top level performance is the result of adapting to the stress of exercise training. A classic way to look at training involves response and adaptation. Physically, we exist in a fairly constant state, called biological homeostasis (2). We remain reasonably stable from day to day. Now presume that an athlete is presented with a specific exercise stress. The activity can be anything the athlete is not normally used to doing, such as a long run, lifting a heavy weight multiple times, or performing a series of calisthenics. Fatigue is the *response* to this exercise stimulus, a temporary decrement in the ability to perform (Fig. 7.1). Fatigue is specific to the exercise. For example, fatigue due to a long run results in a decreased ability to run. Following exercise, the athlete starts to recover. Part of recovery is that the athlete compensates slightly. The athlete gets better. The compensation is specific to the stress. The stress of running makes one a better runner, not a better weight lifter. Bompa has called this brief increase in ability supercompensation (2).

One exercise stimulus is not enough to bring about adaptation. The goal is to present another stimulus following recovery (and slightly compensated). Repeated exercise sessions result in *adaptation*—a higher biological state—and a more fit individual. Figure 7.2 represents a theoretical model in which the athlete slowly adapts to the repeated stress of exercise. While Figure 7.2 appears relatively simple in this diagram, what actually happens is not always easy to discern. Classic training theory suggests that exercise should be repeated when recovery is complete. But the exact moment of compensation is almost impossible to identify. And even if we could identify it, athletes are not normally available on an unlimited basis. High school and collegiate athletes operate on a school schedule and normally

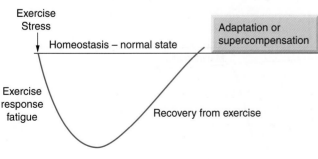

■ **FIGURE 7.1** Classic response to exercise stimulus.

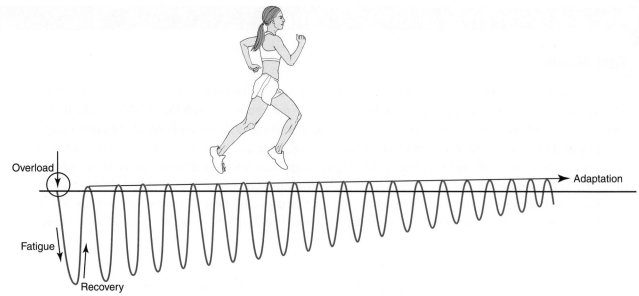

■ **FIGURE 7.2** Ideal model of exercise overload resulting in adaptation.

will train at the same time every day (fully recovered or not). Additionally, as suggested in Chapter 6, athletes must contend with stresses other than training that affect recovery. Recovery from stress is not just physiological but involves all aspects of athletes' lives (3).

Careful examination of this classic theory suggests that coaches can make two general errors. For example, if coaches adopt a "get-tough" approach and present considerable exercise stress day after day, athletes do not have time to recover (Fig. 7.3). The result of underrecovery is fatigue and a decrement in performance, just the opposite effect of the training goal. Further, when athletes are too fatigued to perform, training is compromised. Another possible problem is that the exercise stimulus is too easy. Coaches can plan too little training. This can be the result of disorganized practice, too much standing around, an overly strategic practice. Bad weather, academic conflicts, and injury can all interfere with training. Athletes who are not trained will return to their pretraining state. Ideally, athletes need the appropriate amount of exercise stress followed by recovery to continue to adapt; to improve.

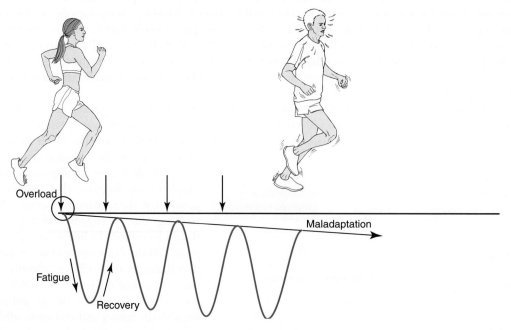

■ **FIGURE 7.3** Exercise stress prior to recovery results in maladaptation.

The Wrong Kind of Fatigue

When athletes exercise to a point where they lose coordination they become very prone to injury. The coordinated contraction of muscles stabilizes and protects joints and provides for the rhythmic contraction and relaxation of muscles. A local ski coach required his team to run to the top of a nearby mountain and back as part of training. (Note: this is only good training if there are no ski lifts!) One member of the team was so fatigued coming down that he tripped, fell, and lost several teeth. The athlete was simply too tired to maintain his balance.

ENERGY SYSTEMS—AN OVERVIEW

Understanding human energy production is one of the most important concepts in the training of athletes. Athletic events are dynamic events; they require energy. Coaches train athletes to be able to use this energy effectively; to improve the ability of the athlete to work. Athletes who cannot expend energy or work at a high rate may not perform as well as someone better trained. When athletes run out of energy they become fatigued and susceptible to injury. An understanding of energy production also provides us with information about fatigue and recovery, nutrition, and weight control.

Athletes engage in a wide range of activities ranging from just a few seconds to an event that may take hours to complete. Fortunately, the human body has three energy systems capable of providing energy for events that require rapid bursts of energy (e.g., the shot put) to events that require a moderate energy output for an extended time. In order for a training program to have the most beneficial effect, athletes must train the energy system required for their sport. In our case study, Brian trained the wrong energy system, actually compromising his ability.

To identify and train the different energy systems, one needs an awareness of the basics of energy transfer.

- Energy is the capacity to perform work. All dynamic activities require energy.
- Energy for movement (kinetic energy) in the human is the transformation of stored energy into kinetic energy.
- The primary form of stored energy in the human is in the form of carbohydrate, fat, and protein (see Fig. 9.1).

While we have thousands of calories waiting in storage, converting these calories into kinetic energy takes time. Oftentimes, we need immediate energy for activity. Activities such as a high jump or a rebound in basketball require immediate energy. Fortunately, we have an additional, but limited, source of high energy fuels located in the muscle and ready to deliver immediate energy. These are in the form of high-energy phosphagens and represent our first energy system.

The Immediate Energy System—ATP-PC

The immediate source of energy in the human body for muscular contraction is adenosine triphosphate (ATP) (4). ATP is composed of three phosphate molecules attached to adenosine. When the phosphate bond is broken, energy is released for muscle contraction (as well as many other energetic events). ATP breaks down to release adenosine diphosphate (ADP), an inorganic phosphate (P), plus the most important ingredient—energy for movement (Fig. 7.4). In fact, the energy for all muscular contractions comes from the breakdown of ATP.

This important source of fuel is located in the muscles and is readily available to be turned into energy for movement. Unfortunately, the amount of ATP is very limited and is also localized in each muscle. But it is possible to produce more. As shown in Figure 7.4, the arrows in the equation indicate that the reaction can go in either direction. Adding energy to the right side of the equation actually produces ATP. In fact, the production (phosphorylation) of ATP is constantly occurring. As ATP is broken down for energy, other fuel sources provide the energy to synthesize it.

A second reaction allows ATP to be produced almost instantaneously by a second high energy phosphate compound, phosphocreatine. Phosphocreatine (PC) is also located in the muscle and is more plentiful that ATP. The reaction shown below indicates that PC donates a phosphate group and its energy to produce ATP as soon as it breaks down (5).

$$PC + ADP \rightarrow ATP + C$$

The combination of these two high energy phosphagens is usually called the ATP-PC energy system. This is a great energy system since ATP and PC are already in the muscle and break down immediately to release energy for movement. We can appreciate the importance of this energy system when we realize the many sport activities that require immediate energy. Unfortunately, we only possess enough ATP and PC for about 8 seconds of maximal work. The ATP-PC system is immediate, powerful, but short-lived. Athletes who participate in quick, high-explosive activities need to develop their ATP-PC energy system. As the stored phosphagens become depleted, energy to make more ATP must come from other sources.

The Intermediate Energy System—Lactic Acid

The energy to produce ATP comes from two additional sources. The faster of these is the anaerobic metabolism of carbohydrate. This is technically known as anaerobic glycolysis, since carbohydrate is metabolized anaerobically—without oxygen. Typically, stored carbohydrate, in the form of muscle glycogen, un-

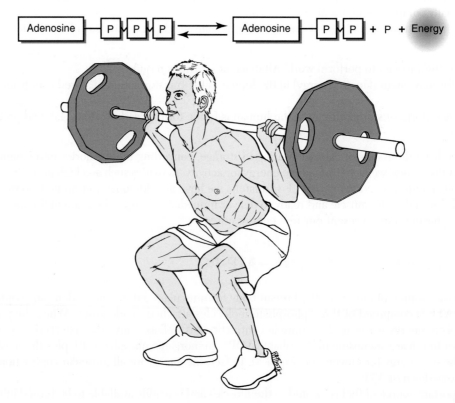

■ **FIGURE 7.4** ATP Breakdown to release energy for muscle contraction.

dergoes a relatively rapid transformation within the muscle, releasing energy. As shown in Figure 7.5, the released energy then joins with ADP and P to produce ATP. A byproduct of this process is lactic acid. Since lactic acid is produced during this process, this energy system is commonly called the lactic acid system.

The lactic acid system is relatively quick because oxygen is not involved. However, it is not as fast as the ATP-PC system since the breakdown of carbohydrate in muscle involves multiple chemical reactions. A major drawback of this energy system is the production of lactic acid. Skeletal muscles can produce fairly large quantities of lactic acid during the anaerobic metabolism of carbohydrate. The lactic acid moves into surrounding fluids and the blood stream and tends to lower the pH (makes surrounding fluids more acidic). The increased acidic environment tends to negatively affect metabolism, resulting in muscle fatigue (6). The lactic acid system is quite essential, since it tends to bridge the gap between the highly powerful (and fast) ATP-PC energy system and the relatively slow aerobic system. The lactic acid system is primarily used for activities that last longer than 8 to 10 seconds and tends to be less productive after about 3 minutes.

The Long-Term Energy System—Aerobic

Carbohydrates can also be completely metabolized aerobically. When carbohydrates are metabolized in the presence of oxygen lactic acid is not produced and considerable energy is available to produce ATP. Fats are always metabolized in the presence of oxygen as there is no metabolic pathway to yield anaerobic energy from fat. Carbohydrates are stored in the body as blood glucose, liver glycogen, and muscle glycogen, but the majority of stored carbohydrate is muscle glycogen. Since muscle glycogen is actually stored in the muscles that are used, it is a fuel that is readily available. Fats are stored throughout the body and tend to enter the muscle after exercise begins via the blood stream.

As shown in Figure 7.6, oxygen arrives at the muscle via the bloodstream, enters the mitochondrion, and combines with either fat or CHO to produce energy, carbon dioxide, and water. The energy produced

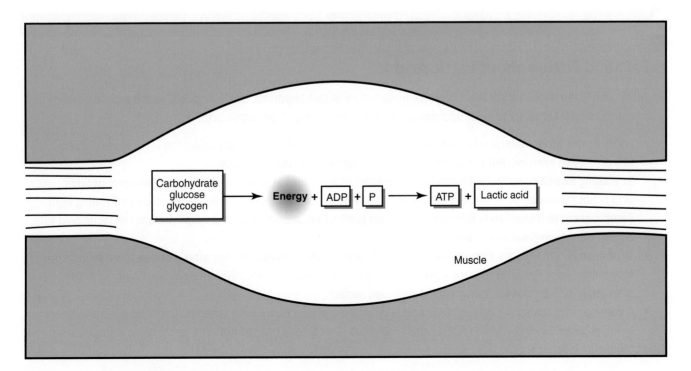

■ **FIGURE 7.5** Anaerobic metabolism of carbohydrate to make ATP and lactic acid.

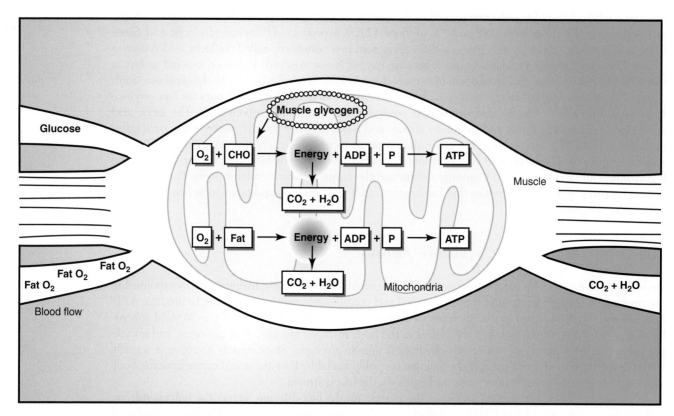

■ **FIGURE 7.6** Aerobic metabolism of carbohydrate and fat (note the entrance of oxygen and fat from the bloodstream).

Fact and Fiction about Lactic Acid

Lactic acid is the byproduct of the anaerobic metabolism of carbohydrate. Lactic acid is also the source of many misconceptions. Let us try to clear up some of the misconceptions about lactic acid.

- Lactic acid is often mentioned as a cause of muscle soreness. Lactic acid may affect the immediate discomfort of intense exercise, but is not responsible for long-term muscle soreness.
- Stretching exercises are occasionally recommended as a method of removing lactic acid. Removal of lactic acid is not facilitated by stretching exercises. However, removal of lactic acid is improved by performing light aerobic exercise immediately following lactic acid production. Aerobic exercise helps metabolize lactic acid to carbon dioxide and water and energy.
- Occasionally, athletes are encouraged to participate in a light workout the day after a competition to help remove lactic acid. Removal of lactic acid takes about 60 minutes—at most 90 minutes. Exercising 24 hours after lactic acid production has no effect on blood lactate.
- A common misconception is that lactic acid is only being produced by unfit athletes. Lactic acid is always being produced even by well trained aerobic athletes. Aerobically trained athletes just remove it faster, metabolizing it for energy.

FOCAL POINT

Fats Versus Carbohydrates

Both fats and carbohydrates are great aerobic fuels but fat is much more plentiful. A person weighing around 150 pounds is composed of approximately 80,000 calories of fat and only 2,000 calories of CHO. Most of the CHO is stored in the muscle as glycogen. Although glycogen is an excellent fuel, it is not mobile and must be utilized for fuel in the muscle in which it is stored. Aerobically trained athletes typically have more muscle glycogen than anaerobic athletes. Fat is a great fuel since it is very dense, and mobile. When exercise begins hormones signal stored fat to break down and enter the bloodstream to be delivered to the muscle for energy. Fat in the blood will go where it is needed. The muscle's selection of fat and CHO is not random but based upon the exercise condition. Typical conditions are:

- Humans tend to burn a combination of CHO and fat at all times.
- Higher intensity exercises tend to burn CHO.
- Low intensity exercise tends to burn fat.
- Long duration exercise tends to select fat.
- Endurance trained athletes tend to burn more fat.
- Individuals on high CHO diets burn more CHO.
- Individual on low CHO diets burn more fat.

is then used to synthesize ATP. The great thing about the O_2 (aerobic) system is that there are no byproducts (such as lactic acid) that hinder performance. The aerobic system depends on the delivery of oxygen to the muscle cell. Since it takes time for oxygen to travel from the air, through the lungs, and then to the heart to be pumped into the bloodstream to the muscle, the aerobic system is slower. Therefore, we need the ATP-PC and Lactic Acid systems for the initial energy production. After about 3 to 4 minutes of exercise, oxygen is being regularly delivered to the muscle and the majority of energy is delivered via the aerobic system. As exercise time increases, almost all of the energy is delivered via the aerobic system. Table 7.1 summarizes the three energy systems.

TABLE 7.1	**Characteristics of the Energy Systems**		
Characteristic	**ATP-PC**	**Lactic Acid**	**Aerobic**
Aerobic/Anaerobic	Anaerobic	Anaerobic	Aerobic
Fuel	ATP-PC	Muscle Glycogen	Fat/CHO
Speed of ATP production	Very Fast	Fast	Slow
Endurance	Very Low	Low	High
Exercise Example	Shot Put	400 meter dash	10,000 meter run
Positive Factors	Provides immediate energy for sport.	Provides intermediate energy and is faster than aerobic system.	Provides almost limitless energy without fatiguing byproducts.
Negative Factors	Short-lived	Lactic acid is produced which causes muscle fatigue.	The slowest of the energy systems.

FROM THE ATHLETIC TRAINING ROOM

The Power of the Aerobic System

During aerobic metabolism oxygen combines with fats and carbohydrates to synthesize ATP. Since we rarely run out of fat and carbohydrate (see Fig. 9.1), the rate limiting factor of this system is oxygen delivery. The power of an athlete's aerobic energy system is dependent on how fast oxygen can be delivered to the muscle. The faster oxygen can be delivered to the muscle, the faster ATP can be synthesized aerobically.

Maximum oxygen consumption, $VO_{2\,max}$, is the common measure of aerobic power. Endurance athletes need a good $VO_{2\,max}$ to compete well, since they primarily use the aerobic energy system during competition. Genetics plays a large part in determining $VO_{2\,max}$. However, $VO_{2\,max}$ can be improved with aerobic training.

Maximum oxygen consumption is often related to cardio-pulmonary health. First, oxygen must be inhaled into the lung to join with hemoglobin in the blood stream. Secondly, the heart must then pump oxygenated blood throughout the body. A healthy, powerful heart can pump vast quantities of blood (filled with oxygen) very quickly throughout the body. For this reason, we often relate cardiovascular health and VO_{2max}.

TRAINING PRINCIPLES

Exercise scientists have seriously studied training for many years. Even the early Greek Olympians, over 2,000 years ago, had athletic trainers. One result of this study is a compilation of principles that have withstood the test of time. Since conditioning programs should be based on these principles, an examination of each of these principles is central to understanding proper training.

Overload

As described in Figure 7.1, the stress of exercise results in fatigue followed by recovery. For adaptation to occur the exercise must involve sufficient stress, overload, that is beyond the athlete's normal activity. If the overload is presented in a systematic and progressive schedule, adaptation occurs (6). Overload can typically be increased by manipulating volume, intensity, and frequency. Volume may be increased by having an athlete perform a typical workout longer, running five miles instead of four. Intensity can be increased by changing the pace; frequency can be increased by running more times per week. While these procedures all overload the athlete, the overload should depend on the goal of the exercise.

Overload Must be Progressive

The athlete adapts and then must be presented with a new overload if higher fitness is the goal. To reach a new level there must be additional stress. For example, suppose an athlete has been performing three sets of 10 repetitions of the bench press with 200 pounds. Now presume that we overloaded our athlete by having him lift 210 pounds. At first, the athlete can only lift the weight seven times. But after 2 weeks of training he is up to performing three sets of 10 repetitions each. He is ready to progress to a new overload. But keep in mind that the human body is not capable of unlimited improvement. Sometimes additional stress results in maladaptation. As discussed in Chapter 6, coaches should design programs so that athletes reach their potential at the appropriate time and then actively rest before training is resumed.

Individuality

All athletes are different and will not respond to the training stimulus in an identical way. The appropriate stress for one athlete may not be an overload for another. In fact, one athlete's overload may injure another athlete. You cannot expect all athletes to improve at the same rate. For instance, an athlete who is out of condition will show much more improvement than an athlete who is already fit. Athletes must also believe they are being treated as individuals and that the coach is aware of their specific level of fitness.

Hard/Easy

Repeated hard exercise does not allow the athlete to recover. A workout that presents considerable stress to the athlete should be followed by an easy workout. Naturally, the harder the workout the longer it takes to recover. An intense workout that creates considerable fatigue should be followed by an easy workout, possibly focusing on tactics or strategy. In this manner, the athlete maintains their fitness and is ready to handle another hard workout. As described in Chapter 6, recovery must be planned into the conditioning system.

Specificity

One of the most important principles for successful athletic performance is specificity. The adaptation athletes experience is highly specific to the imposed stress. Playing soccer makes us better soccer players but it probably does little for our ability to play volleyball. Likewise, high resistance exercises make us stronger while endurance training improves stamina. Two types of specificity are generally considered to satisfy proper training:

SPORT SPECIFICITY

The vast numbers of movements many sports require are specific to each sport. Athletes must practice the exact tasks they will encounter while playing. Basketball players must have good anticipation when catching a basketball. But it is highly unlikely that this anticipation will help them catch a fly ball in baseball. Basketball players need to practice basketball. We are also suspicious of many accessories used to teach sport. For example, we encountered a basketball player who insisted on practicing every day wearing garden gloves. His theory was that this practice would improve his feel for the ball. We suggested that this practice would only help if everyone was required to wear garden gloves. Neuromuscular control is highly sport specific. The exact manner in which muscle fibers are recruited to perform specific sport activities is specific to each sport. Practicing these activities improves performance.

METABOLIC SPECIFICITY

Not only do athletes need to practice the specific activity in which they compete, they must train the energy system to be utilized as well. Metabolic specificity is training the specific energy system(s) to be utilized in competition. Athletes who participate in anaerobic sports must train anaerobically. Each sport and activity has specific metabolic requirements. Coaches need to know the predominant energy system(s) utilized in their sport and how to improve each system.

ENERGY SYSTEMS—HOW TO PREDICT

Training methods for each energy system is different. Extensive training of the aerobic system does not improve the ATP-PC or the Lactic Acid system. In fact, it has been frequently argued that such training can compromise the faster energy systems. For example, Brian (the skier mentioned at the beginning of this chapter) trained aerobically for an anaerobic sport. Brian not only trained the wrong energy system, he got slower. Athletes need to specifically train the energy system(s) that are used for competition.

Identifying the Energy System

Time is the primary variable used to determine which energy system is being utilized. Intensity is also important. For instance, brief high-speed activities are going to utilize the ATP-PC system. However, a brief activity that is performed at a slow speed is more aerobic than anaerobic. How long does the athlete actually compete? The question is not related to how long the game lasts but what the athlete actually does in the game. A football game might last over 2 hours but the game mainly consists of brief spurts of high energy activities. For this reason, football players need extensive training of their ATP-PC energy systems.

Figure 7.7 divides the energy systems into zones based upon time. The potential for power output is also part of this figure. As performance time increases, the power output (speed) of the athlete naturally decreases. This phenomenon is highly related to the energy systems that are utilized. Further, energy systems are not exclusive as athletes often rely on a combination of the three energy systems. Energy systems do not turn on and off but are constantly in action. Table 7.2 indicates the energy system most involved as a function of time. Activities in zones 1 and 5 are fairly straightforward since they are on the opposite end of the spectrum, but most sports use combinations of the energy systems. For example, a considerable amount of time in basketball is spent in low-intensity activity. One study found that every 21 seconds, basketball players perform a high-intensity run of about 1.7 seconds (7). But there are times when basketball players must run at high speed for much longer than 1.7 seconds. For this reason, basketball players use all three energy systems.

Table 7.3 presents a suggested prediction of energy system contribution by sport. Keep in mind that these are predictions and that the actual energy system contribution for players may vary considerably. Soccer mid-fielders will have a higher energy expenditure than defensive players and probably need more aerobic training (8). The requirements of playing wide receiver in football obviously differ from the offensive guard. Which energy system is used? There are no fixed answers but Table 7.3 does attempt to provide coaches with a hierarchy of emphasis.

As we examine Figure 7.7, we can observe that the aerobic system is not a major contributor for most sports. Most athletes continue to need some aerobic training. Just because the athletic event does not require a highly developed aerobic system for competition, all athletes need a reasonable aerobic system

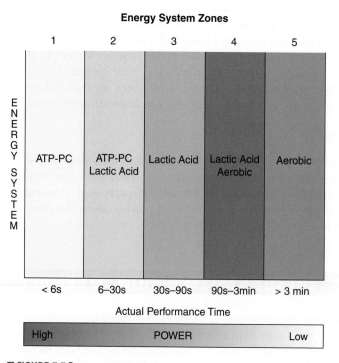

■ **FIGURE 7.7** Energy system zones.

TABLE 7.2 Energy System Zones

Zone	Performance Time	Major Energy System	Examples
1-Short bursts of high energy	0–6s	ATP-PC	Shot put 40 m dash base stealing volleyball spike
2-High energy activities at slightly slower pace typical of basketball and soccer.	6–30s	ATP and Lactic Acid	200 m dash 25 m freestyle long point in tennis soccer play defensive series in basketball
3-Performance at high speed but not at maximal speed.	30s to 2 min	Lactic Acid	400 m dash 200 meter swim
4-Slightly reduced speed—often related to last half of a longer race	2–3 min	Lactic Acid O_2	800 m run Last half of 1,500 m run
5-Usually a steady pace activity with sprint at the end.	>3 min	O_2	1,500 m run 400 m swim row 2,000 m

just to withstand the rigors of a long practice and a long season. A 2-hour practice takes a considerable toll on an athlete and reasonable aerobic training helps the athletes postpone fatigue so that they can engage and recover from intense training activities. Knowledgeable coaches learn this and condition their athletes accordingly.

ENERGY SYSTEMS—HOW TO TRAIN

Time and intensity are key aspects of energy system training. Brief, high intensity exercises stress the ATP-PC system, while long, lower intensity exercises are primarily aerobic. Once the energy system(s) for competition are identified, then the specific muscles to be utilized in competition should be trained accordingly.

Interval Training

Since the 1950s exercise scientists have known that more high quality exercise can be performed with interval training than with continuous training (9–11). Interval training is a series of repeated bouts of exercise interspersed with relief periods. Table 7.4 briefly describes the components of interval training. The duration and intensity of each work period is manipulated (along with the rest period) to stress each energy system (or combinations of systems). Table 7.5 indicates some general guidelines for energy system training. Careful attention must be given to the speed of the activity as well as the activity being performed. Activities must be performed at a speed that will utilize the energy system being trained. Simply performing an exercise for 10 seconds does not mean it is an ATP-PC activity. The intensity of the task must be high or another energy system is being utilized.

The examples presented below are quite brief and limited in number. Keep in mind that there are many methods of scheduling interval training as well as some excellent resources on interval training (12,13). As stated earlier, the energy systems are not exclusive. For example, training the lactic acid system often involves having athletes perform intervals lasting 30 to 90 seconds. Such intervals utilize the other systems as well. If the interval is 30 seconds long, the contribution of the ATP-PC system is fairly large. Likewise, if the interval is 90 seconds long, the contribution of the aerobic system is fairly large. An

TABLE 7.3   Suggested Contribution of Energy System By Sport*

Activity	ATP-PC	Lactic Acid	Aerobic O$_2$
Crew Race 2,000 m	L	M	H
Basketball	H	H	M
Field Hockey forward	H	H	M
Football lineman	H	M	L
Football receiver	H	M	M
Lacrosse mid-fielder	H	H	M
Soccer mid-fielder	H	H	M
Soccer goalie	H	L	L
Squash	H	H	M
Swim 100 meters	H	H	L
Swim 400 meters	L	M	M
Tennis Singles	H	M	M
Tennis Doubles	H	L	L
Track 100 meters	H	L	0
Track 400 meters	H	H	L
Track 800 meters	L	H	H
Track 1500 meters	L	H	H
Track 10,000 meters	L	L	H
Track long jump	H	L	0
Track shot put	H	L	0
Marathon	0	0	H
Volleyball	H	L	M

*H, high; M, medium; L, low; 0, requires no capacity.

important attribute of interval training is that many combinations can be planned to replicate competitive situations.

TRAINING THE ATP-PC SYSTEM

The focus of ATP-PC training should be on high-quality, explosive exercise. A high-quality activity means that the athlete is performing at or near maximal speed. The athlete must be motivated and rested. The

TABLE 7.4   Components of an Interval Training Session

Sets	Reps/set	Training Activity	Training Distance	Training Time	Relief	Relief Activity
How many times (sets) will this sequence be repeated before extended rest?	How many total repetitions will the athlete perform in this set?	What will the athlete do? Run, jump, swim, agility drills, and calisthenics are examples.	Distance is one method of determining the length of the repetition. For instance, run 60 yards.	Time is a second method of determining the repetition. For example, perform repetitive vertical jumps for 8 seconds.	How much rest is provided—usually measured in time.	What does the athlete do during the recovery? Example—walk or jog slowly.

TABLE 7.5 General Guidelines for Energy System Training

Energy System	Intensity	Duration	Rest Activity
ATP-PC	Very High	3–10 seconds	Rest
ATP-PC—Lactic Acid	Very High to High	10–30 seconds	Light Exercise
Lactic Acid	High	15-60 seconds	Light Exercise
Lactic Acid—Aerobic	Medium to High	30s–3 minutes	Light Exercise
Aerobic	Medium	>3 minutes	Rest or Light Exercise

jumping and plyometric drills presented in Chapter 3 are typical activities that can be utilized. Additionally, Chapter 8 presents activities designed to improve strength and power. Interval training is well suited for high intensity training. Table 7.6 presents two examples of an interval training program for the ATP-PC system.

The first example indicates that the athlete will perform 10 running sprints of 20 yards, each followed by 45 seconds of rest. This activity would be repeated three more times during practice for a total of 40 sprints. The second example has the athlete performing repeated tuck jumps for 10 seconds followed by 45 seconds of rest to be repeated five times. In this instance the athlete will perform 60 seconds of tuck jumps and then possibly switch to another jumping drill.

TRAINING THE LACTIC ACID ENERGY SYSTEM

Interval training is well suited for training the lactic acid energy system. Table 7.7 presents two examples. In the first example, the athlete runs four 200 meter dashes, each followed by 90 seconds of walking and jogging. This set of four sprints should be repeated three more times for a total of 16 200-meter sprints. The second example utilizes a basketball dribbling drill in which the athlete dribbles at high speed around cones for 45 seconds followed by 90 seconds of walking and drilling before repeating.

Training the lactic acid energy system is tough on the athlete. Due to the incomplete recovery, as well as the speed of the task, there is considerable accumulation of lactic acid. Lactic acid production is one goal

FROM THE ATHLETIC TRAINING ROOM

The Lactate Threshold

Athletes performing in endurance events need a good $VO_{2\,max}$ for successful performance. Just having a good $VO_{2\,max}$ is not enough since athletes must be trained as well. Lactate threshold is also important and positively affected by training. Blood lactate remains fairly constant as athletes slowly increase the pace of their running. However, there reaches a point where the amount of lactic acid in the blood rises exponentially, the lactate threshold. Performing at a pace above this intensity is difficult to maintain for long periods. This appears in un-trained athletes at about 50% to 60% of $VO_{2\,max}$ but in trained athletes around 65% to 80% of $VO_{2\,max}$ (1). Aerobic training not only improves $VO_{2\,max}$, such training improves lactate threshold as well. Further, training intensity, rather than volume, may be more important when improving $VO_{2\,max}$ and lactate threshold (2). Since interval training allows athletes to perform more intense work, aerobic interval training is often the method of choice for improving both of these important variables.

1. Gollnick P, Bayly W, Hodgson D. Exercise intensity, training, diet, and lactate. *Med Sci Sports Exerc* 1986;18:334–340.
2. Costill D, Thomas R, Robergs R, et al. Adaptations to swimming training: Influence of training volume. *Med Sci Sports Exerc* 1991;23(3):371–377.

TABLE 7.6 Interval Training Example for ATP-PC System

Sets	Reps/set	Activity	Training Distance	Training Time	Relief	Relief Activity
4	10	Sprint	20 yards		45s	Rest
1	6	Tuck Jumps		10s	45s	Rest

of this training method. Intense training of this energy system should probably not be conducted more than once or twice a week. Further, since considerable lactic acid accumulates, intervals should be scheduled toward the end of practice, allowing some time for light aerobic activities to facilitate lactic acid removal.

AEROBIC TRAINING

A vast number of texts have been written solely about endurance training. We highly recommend the works of Daniels (14) and Sleamaker (15) for those coaches primarily involved in training endurance athletes. Interval training for aerobic development has been successfully utilized for many years. For example, presume you want athletes to run three miles during a practice. One method is to mark off a 3-mile course and have them run continuously. The interval technique has them run six half-mile runs, but at a faster pace, with about 2 minutes rest between each run.

Interval training should not be the exclusive method of training the aerobic system. Continuous training is an effective method of improving the aerobic system and can be conducted at different speeds dependent on the duration of the exercise. Rowers often end a tough day of interval work with a continuous cool-down, returning to the dock in a recovered state. Similar techniques are used for swimmers and runners. Continuous running is also helpful as a warm-up.

Muscle Fiber Recruitment

An important aspect of the specificity of training is fiber type recruitment. Running requires the sequential contraction and relaxation of quadriceps and hamstring muscles but the actual fibers utilized within those muscles are dependent on exercise intensity. Throughout the body, individual muscles are composed of a combination of fast twitch (FT) and slow twitch (ST) fibers. Additionally, there are at least two types of fast twitch fibers. FTa fibers have some of the characteristics of FT and ST fibers while FTb are truly fast twitch. Table 7.8 indicates the basic characteristics of fast and slow twitch fibers.

ST fibers are generally small fibers that are recruited for aerobic events. ST fibers have an excellent blood supply and are full of enzymes for aerobic activity. ST fibers resist fatigue. FT fibers are larger and tend to be utilized more for anaerobic activities. FT fibers do not have a good blood supply and do not have plentiful aerobic enzymes. But they do have plentiful anaerobic enzymes and are very powerful. FT fibers tend to fatigue quickly.

The training of those fibers to be utilized in competition is an important consideration for conditioning and injury prevention. For example, the softball players mentioned in Focal Point: Fast Moves had trained their slow twitch fibers (jogging) for a fast twitch sport (softball). When the softball players started to sprint, they recruited their untrained fast twitch fibers rather than their trained slow twitch fibers. The result was a muscle strain. Not only must we be aware of the various muscles to be used in competition, we must con-

TABLE 7.7 Interval Training Example for Lactic Acid Energy System

Sets	Reps/set	Activity	Training Distance	Training Time	Relief	Relief Activity
4	4	Run	200 meters		90s	Walk or light jog
4	4	Basketball dribble around cones		45s	90s	Walk and dribble

TABLE 7.8   General Characteristics of Slow Twitch and Fast Twitch Muscle Fibers

Characteristic	Type I	Type II
Speed of Contraction	Slow	Fast
Force Production	Low	High
Fatigability	Slow to fatigue	Quick to fatigue
Typical energy system	Aerobic	Anaerobic
Fiber Recruitment	Low-power, repetitive activities	High-power explosive activities
Size	Small	Large

sider the fibers that are to be recruited within those muscles. Intensity is the basic predictor of fiber type recruitment. High intensity activities (Fig. 7.8) recruit fast twitch fibers while low intensity activities recruit slow twitch fibers. Athletes must train at the same intensity they utilize for competition.

SPORT-SPECIFIC TRAINING

The teaching of sport skills, as well as the development of tactics and strategy, is beyond the scope of this text. Coaches need to be well aware of how to teach motor skills and should not simply imitate how they were taught. Martens' guide to coaching is an excellent starting source of information (16). Similar to the presentation in this text, Martens is a strong proponent of sport specific practice. For example, Martens questions whether drills actually prepare an athlete for competition. The goal is to prepare athletes for competition. For example, football players are often seen running through tires or ropes, even though they never run through tires or ropes during the game. Does such a drill really make them better football players?

Coaches should be able to answer the following question. "What are the physical demands of the sport you coach?" Once you can answer this question you determine how to train your athletes. Many sports have been analyzed, but keep in mind the subjects studied. A study of the physical demands of playing World Cup soccer is only marginally useful for the junior high soccer program. This analysis should also be the basis of the preseason training program. For example, in the study referred to earlier on the demands of basketball, the average sprint lasted 1.7 seconds (7). As also mentioned, some sprints last longer, but we rarely see an athlete sprint the length of the gym (or even half the length) even though this is a common training technique. Training should replicate competition.

The well planned practice should result in physiological conditioning as well as skill development. The development of skill and tactics are an important part of any training, but such training should not result in a reduced physiological capacity. For instance, if too much practice time is utilized for slower repetitions of skills, extended periods of instruction, and a lot of down time, athletes lose opportunities to improve or maintain fitness. Practices must be organized so that the benefits of high-energy activities are not left out.

Drills

All athletes need to practice skills but repeatedly performing drills at speeds that are not used in competition is less effective. Putting drills into context is very important for retention and transfer (13). This means that drills should be less continuous and more game-like. Remember that the actual muscle fibers recruited for an activity are dependent on the intensity (speed) of

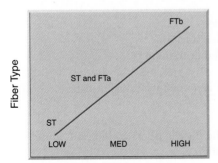

■ FIGURE 7.8 The relationship between exercise intensity and fiber type recruitment.

the task. Repeatedly performing a drill at a slow speed does not prepare the competitive muscle fibers. Athletes need to be motivated to perform drills at competitive speed. In this manner, sport specific drills will imitate competition and properly prepare the athlete. Some of the basic factors involved in a good drill are:

- Make directions clear and simple and reduce talking. Athletes learn sport skills by doing rather than listening.
- Keep the athletes busy and not waiting in long lines to perform a brief task.
- Make drills similar to competition.
- Provide enough recovery time so that athletes can perform at high speed.
- Make drills fun.

Scrimmage

One of the most common methods of practice is the scrimmage. This can be a great form of training since the activities being performed are normally the exact activities to be performed in competition. The problem with such training is that scrimmages are often done at a reduced speed. Coaches frequently interrupt play, reducing the training effect. When it is necessary to interrupt play, make your comments succinct, and get on with the scrimmage. Often the first team competes against the second team and the play is less competitive. The creative coach can adapt scrimmages so that they are done at high speed. Create games in which unequal teams can be competitive. Reduce/increase the size of the field. Change the number of players. Many techniques can be utilized to create game-like conditions that improve the physiological conditioning.

A study by Hoff et al is of interest (8). They created two soccer specific drills designed to improve the maximal oxygen uptake of teenage soccer players. One drill used a "dribbling track" where athletes dribbled a soccer ball for set durations. A second drill involved a modified soccer game played by a small group of players. They found that both soccer tasks were intense enough to improve $VO_{2\,max}$. Hoff concluded by saying, "By using small group play and a specifically designed dribbling track, soccer players, who are more readily motivated by playing with a ball, no longer need to carry out plain running to improve their maximal oxygen uptake" (18). Interestingly, Helgerud et al have found that improved $VO_{2\,max}$ resulted in a 20% increase in distance covered during a soccer match, a 24% increase in the number of involvements, and a 100% increase in the number of sprints (19). Effective physiological training can be conducted utilizing sport specific drills.

SUMMARY

- Preparing athletes for competition also helps prevent injury.
- Systematic training results in adaptation. Adaptation is the result of a systematic overload followed by appropriate recovery.
- Training involves systematic planning. It is not haphazard.
- Three energy systems provide energy during athletic competition.
- Performance time is the primary predictor of energy system identification.
- Training is specific to the sport and to the energy system utilized in training.
- Training must be individualized.
- The nature of many sports is interval and the training for sport is normally interval in nature.
- Muscles are composed of slow twitch and fast twitch fibers.
- Recruitment of muscle fibers is speed/intensity specific.
- Training for competition must be conducted to train the specific muscle fibers within each muscle.
- Athletic drills should replicate the activities utilized in competition.
- Sport specific practice can improve fitness and improve skill.

References

1. Prentice W, Arnheim D. *Arnheim's Principles of Athletic Training*, 13th ed. Dubuque, IA: McGraw-Hill Companies, 2008.
2. Bompa T. *Periodization, Theory and Methodology of Training*, 4th ed. Champaign, IL: Human Kinetics, 1999.
3. Kallus K, Kellmann M. Burnout in athletes and coaches. In: Hanin Y. *Emotions in Sport*. Champaign, IL: Human Kinetics, 2002.
4. Tullson P, Terjung R. Adenine nucleotide metabolism in contracting skeletal muscle. *Exerc Sport Sci Rev* 1991;19:507–537.
5. Holloszy J. Muscle metabolism during exercise. *Arch Phys Med Rehabil* 1982;63:231–234.
6. Powers S, Howley E. *Exercise Physiology: Theory and Application to Fitness and Performance*, 6th ed. Dubuque, IA: McGraw Hill, 2007.
7. McInnes S, Carlson J, Jones C, et al. The physiological load imposed on basketball players during competition. *J Sports Sci* 1995; 13(5):387–397.
8. Reilly T. Energetics of high-intensity exercise (soccer) with particular reference to fatigue. *J Sports Sci* 1997;15(3):257–263.
9. Fox E, Robinson S, Wiegman D. Metabolic energy sources during continuous and interval running. *J Appl Physiol* 1969;27:174–178.
10. Margaria R, Oliva R, diPrampero P, et al. Energy utilization in intermittent exercise of supramaximal intensity. *J Appl Physiol* 1969;26:752–756.
11. Saltin B, Essen B. Muscle glycogen, lactate, ATP, and CP in intermittent exercise. In: Pernow B, Saltin B. *Muscle Metabolism During Exercise*. New York: Plenum Press, 1971.
12. Fox E, Mathews D. *Interval Training*. Philadelphia: W.B. Saunders, 1974.
13. Foss M, Keteyian S. *Fox's Physiological Basis for Exercise and Sport*, 6th ed. Dubuque, IA: McGraw-Hill, 2001.
14. Daniels J. *Daniels' Running Formula*, 2nd ed. Champaign, IL: Human Kinetics, 2005.
15. Sleamaker R. *Serious Training for Endurance Athletes*, 2nd ed. Champaign, IL: Human Kinetics, 1996.
16. Martens R. *Successful Coaching*, 3rd ed. Champaign, IL: Human Kinetics, 2004.
17. Bortoli L, Robazza C, Durigon V, et al. Effects of contextual interference on learning technical sports skills. *Percept Mot Skills* 1992;75(2):555–562.
18. Hoff J, Wisloff U, Engen L, et al. Soccer specific aerobic endurance training. *Br J Sports Med* 2002;36:218–221.
19. Helgerud J, Engen L, Wisloff U, et al. Aerobic endurance training improves soccer performance. *Med Sci Sports Exerc* 33(11): 1925–1931.

Strength and Power Training

Upon reading this chapter, the coach should be able to:

1. Explain the difference between muscle strength, muscle endurance, and power.
2. Know the specific adaptations to resistance training.
3. Design a basic resistance program to develop muscular strength, power, and endurance.
4. Design functional training activities applied to sport.
5. Create a periodized resistance training program.
6. Develop a plyometric exercise program.

Luke was almost 13 when he saw the movie Pumping Iron. *Luke had suffered from asthma since birth and was never without his inhaler. He liked sports, was well-coordinated, but was also afraid that his asthma would kick in and he would have to head for the sideline. He had the normal apprehensions about moving to junior high school; bigger boys to compete against, athletic teams, and a completely new environment were unknowns. School was a continuous struggle. He asked his dad, a local physical education teacher, about weightlifting. His dad supported his efforts, bought him a beginning barbell set, and taught him proper lifting technique.*

Luke thrived on weightlifting, even taking his set along to the family's summer cottage. His asthma did not interfere with his weightlifting. Luke started getting stronger and more confident. Puberty, combined with the weightlifting, resulted in significant growth that first summer. He went out for junior varsity football and made the squad. Luke's asthma did not go away but his coach was very supportive, keeping Luke's inhaler in the medical kit. He knew Luke had the tools to excel in sport. Luke continued with the weightlifting, bought an Olympic set, and a good weight bench. He was ready for high school and varsity football. In the spring of his freshman year he won the bench press competition by pressing 140 pounds over 40 times. Weightlifting gave him confidence to compete against older boys and the strength to succeed.

But Luke's weightlifting program was not supported by everyone. Comments such as:

- *"You'll stunt your growth if you start lifting too early."*
- *"You shouldn't start lifting weights until you're in high school."*
- *"You're going to get hurt lifting weights."*
- *"You're going to get muscle bound."*

None of these fears were based on fact. Luke continued to grow, did not get hurt, and was perfectly flexible and coordinated. We now know that weightlifting is fine for 12 and 13 year old boys and girls. Approval of resistance training for youth is widely accepted in the scientific community. The following organizations have all issued statements indicating the effectiveness and safety of properly supervised resistance programs: The American Academy of Pediatrics (1), The American Orthopedic Society for Sports Medicine (2), and The National Strength and Conditioning Association (3). A well-supervised program emphasizing proper form and technique is safe and effective for young people.

The improvement of muscle strength, especially for young athletes, may be more important now than in past generations. Our increased mechanized society has reduced the need for physical labor. Unfortunately, the reduced need for physical labor has not resulted in increased physical activity for children. Reduced physical labor is accompanied by more passive forms of entertainment such as video and computer games. Further, for a variety of reasons the independent mobility of children has diminished (4). Decreased physical activity leads to reduced strength and an increased risk of injury for those children who take up competitive athletics. Indeed, strength training is a great aid for most young athletes.

STRENGTH TRAINING SHOULD BE FUNCTIONAL

As described in Chapter 2, muscles protect joints and help prevent injury. But strength developed in the weight room must be transferable to the playing field. Functional strength training is one key to injury prevention and enhanced performance. Resistance programs should be multifaceted, incorporating multi-joint weight training exercises with whole body exercises such as calisthenics and plyometrics. Athletes need symmetrical development of their bodies to provide equal training on opposite sides of joints. Exercises should be matched. For instance, every pushing exercise should have a complementary pulling exercise. Strength alone is not sufficient to stabilize joints. Agility drills, jumping drills, balance drills, sprinting, medicine ball throws, and hill running should all be part of training.

In Boyle's text on functional training he suggests that functional training is purposeful training that makes sense (5). For example, few sports are played in a sitting position but many machine-based resistance machines require one to sit. Since most athletic activities require balance and coordination, the resistance program should train these same variables. Functional training usually involves multi-joint training. Since sport activities are multi-joint, an intense focus on single-joint activities like triceps extensions or bicep curls seems wasteful. The resistance program should match the sport as well as the athlete. Power sports require power training. Weak athletes need specific development for success and injury prevention.

STRENGTH, POWER, OR ENDURANCE?

Muscle strength and power are frequently labeled as the same variable. Although strength and power are related, the definition is different. Strength is often measured as the maximum amount of force one can exert. For example, people are typically labeled as strong if they can bench press or lift a huge weight off the floor. Strength does not have the element of time. Simply lifting the weight is all that is necessary to demonstrate strength. Power is work divided by time. A powerful athlete is not only able to lift a large weight, but can do it quickly. Athletes who are powerful are able to do a lot of work in a short period of time. Time is one of the most important variables in athletics. The person who crosses the finish line in the least amount of time wins. The person who gets to the ball first gains control. Since power is time dependent, power is often a more important variable than strength.

Muscular endurance is the ability to perform a moderately vigorous task multiple times without undue loss of strength. An athlete who can perform many repetitions without loss of power has good muscular endurance. A freestyle swimmer will perform about 40 to 50 contractions of each shoulder to swim 100 meters. Swimming 400 meters will require about 200 movements of each arm. Rowers will perform about 240 strokes to row 2,000 meters. While swimmers and rowers need power, muscular endurance is very important.

FOCAL POINT

Strength Versus Endurance

Do strong people have more muscular endurance? This depends on your method of measuring endurance. Jane and Kelly are taking a weightlifting class together and were both tested for muscular endurance. Jane is stronger

(continues)

Strength Versus Endurance *(continued)*

than Kelly and is able to bench press 120 pounds while Kelly can only manage 90 pounds. They were each asked to bench press 75 pounds as many times as possible. Kelly could only manage 5 repetitions while Jane did 22 repetitions. Jane had more *absolute* muscular endurance than Kelly. She could do more total work than Kelly. On a second day the instructor had each student lift 75% of their max as many times as possible. Both Jane and Kelly were able to perform 10 repetitions before stopping. Each student had the same relative muscular endurance. Stronger individuals have more absolute muscular endurance but not more relative muscular endurance.

Athletes frequently need a balance of power and endurance. Swimmers need explosive leg power on starts and turns and a balance of power and endurance to maintain cadence. Throwers, such as javelin and baseball athletes, primarily need power development in the upper and lower body as well as excellent scapula stability. Coaches need to assess the requirements of the athlete when designing resistance programs. Training for power is different than training for endurance. A basic strength training program is the place to start to train for both power and endurance. Develop strength first and then fine tune the training to bring about the desired goal.

ADAPTATIONS TO RESISTANCE TRAINING

The goal of resistance programs should be to improve performance and reduce injury. While the most obvious adaptation to resistance training is an increase in strength, performance improvement is the real goal. Increased strength results from a program of systematically applied stress in the form of high resistance. Many forms of resistance training (e.g., surgical tubing, calisthenics, and manual resistance) increase strength. Strength gains range as much as seven to 45% and often even greater (6). Many factors influence the actual strength changes reported in the various studies. Some of the obvious reasons are the subject's familiarity with resistance training, a possible genetic predisposition for strength gains, age, gender, length of training, and the motivation of the subject. Humans adapt to resistance training by physiological and neurological changes.

Muscle Fiber Size

Hypertrophy (increased size) has long been described as a typical adaptation to resistance exercise (7,8). Individual muscle fibers get larger resulting in greater muscle mass. Larger muscles are normally stronger muscles. Muscle hypertrophy is not uniform since fast twitch fibers tend to gain more than slow twitch fibers (9). In fact, this may be one reason why certain people tend to hypertrophy more than others. It has been suggested that individuals with a high percentage of fast twitch fibers may have more potential for muscle growth (10). An important aspect in the design of resistance training programs is muscle recruitment. For example, muscles are recruited for exercise according to the size principle (11). That is, smaller muscles are recruited before larger muscles. Since fast-twitch fibers are often needed for high powered athletic activities, heavy resistance training is necessary to train the larger fast-twitch fibers.

Connective Tissue

The effects of resistance training go beyond just muscle tissue. Since tendons attach muscles to bones, they withstand the repeated strain of muscles during contraction. While the majority of research related to tendon adaptation has been conducted with laboratory animals, there is little doubt that human tendon adapts to vigorous physical exercise as well (12). Kubo et al found that tendon stiffness increased significantly as a result of strength training (13). Reeves et al found similar effects in older individuals and suggested that increased stiffness may reduce the risk of tendon injury and has implications for improved contractile force during motor tasks (14). Since tendons make positive adaptations to resistance exercise, such training should also help with injury prevention.

Neural Adaptation

Individuals who start resistance training programs always seem to make great progress in the beginning. This seems particularly true for novice lifters. This progress is not the result of muscle hypertrophy but is related to the individual's increased ability to recruit muscles. As the athlete learns to recruit muscles in a more synchronous manner, they gain strength. Further, individuals become less inhibited as they become familiar with the movements. This combination of decreased inhibition and improved muscle recruitment leads to rapid improvement (15). Figure 8.1 illustrates a typical adaptation pattern for individuals beginning resistance training programs. Neural adaptations occur first followed by actual changes to the muscle. If hypertrophy is one goal of training, resistance programs should not be short term but should last for several months (6).

RESISTANCE TRAINING VARIABLES AND CONCEPTS

The terminology of resistance training has been developing for many years. Many terms have become standardized but some are still being developed. A brief review is required before any specific recommendations can be made.

The Repetition Max (RM)

If an athlete can bench press 150 pounds 10 times (but not 11) then he is performing a 10RM. The athlete is exercising to failure. A 1RM is the maximum amount of weight an athlete can lift one time. Individuals are often assigned to exercise with a specific percentage of their 1RM. For example, an intensity of 60% of the 1RM is frequently recommended as a minimal resistance for strength training (16). We will describe some methods of determining the 1RM later in this chapter.

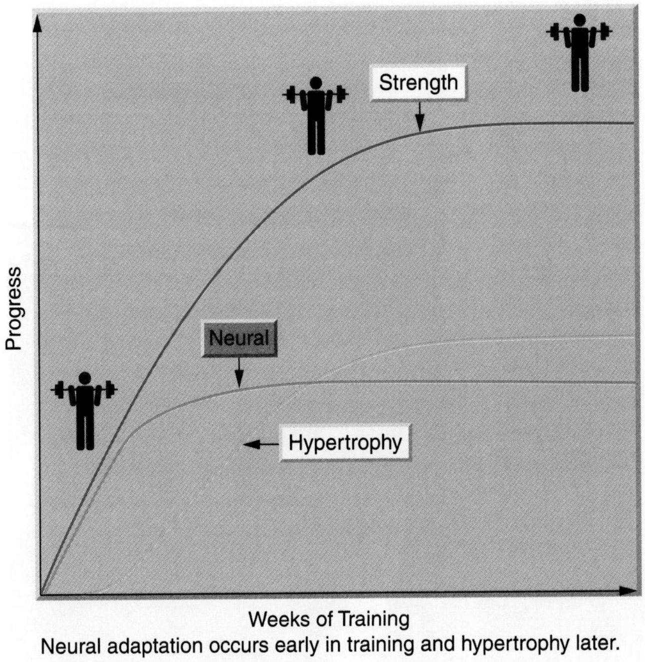

Sets

A set is a group of repetitions continuously performed and separated by a rest period of indeterminate length. The number of sets recommended for strength training has received considerable debate in the past few years. For instance, studies have shown that one set is sufficient to stimulate strength gain (16,17). However, untrained individuals experience maximal strength gains utiliz-

Neural adaptation occurs early in training and hypertrophy later.

■ **FIGURE 8.1** Neural adaptation to resistance training.

ing four sets per training session (18). This is not to say that one must perform four sets to increase strength, but that four sets result in greater gains. Multiple sets are normally recommended for athletes (19,20).

Rest Period

The amount of rest between sets varies with the goal of the exercise and the experience of the athlete. Novice lifters require more rest so they can maintain form and control. If muscular endurance is the goal then the rest period is often reduced. When performing high power/strength exercises utilizing very heavy weights (1 to 3RM for example) use a longer rest period approaching 3 minutes. Typical sets of strength exercises in the range of 6 to 10 RM require a rest period of about 2 minutes. Remember that there are no fixed rules here; these are just general guidelines. Athletes need enough rest to lift and control the weight.

Repetitions

Reps refer to the number of repetitions an individual performs in each set. The repetition max (RM) only refers to a set of repetitions that end in failure. Simply performing 10 reps and stopping is not considered a 10RM. Although RM's are generally considered the goal, most sets are completed before failure.

Multi-joint Versus Single-Joint Exercises

Multi-joint exercises refer to those exercises that utilize more than one joint. The squat exercise utilizes muscles that cross the ankle, knee, hip, and lower back. Compare this with an exercise such as a knee extension machine that only utilizes the knee extension muscles. Exercises, such as the bench press, push up, pull up, overhead press, and power clean are all multi-joint exercises. Tricep extensions, arm curls, and leg curls are all single-joint exercises. In general, multi-joint exercises are more functional and recommended in this text. Further, since time is frequently an issue for athletes, multi-joint exercises simply exercise more muscle groups with each repetition. Single-joint exercises are more useful when overcoming specific weaknesses or for rehabilitation.

Variable Resistance Machine (VRM)

Humans are not equally strong throughout a range of motion (ROM). The angle of insertion of the tendon to the bone changes as the joint moves. As well, muscle length also changes, both affecting the ability of the muscle to rotate a joint. As the name implies, a VRM machine varies the resistance (torque) throughout the range of motion. The typical procedure is to use a cam (Fig. 8.2) to change the resistance. Companies (e.g., Nautilus and Cybex) produced VRM's, manipulating resistance through a cam or pulley system. The goal is to increase or decrease resistance to accommodate the pattern of strength of the individual, offering more resistance where the individual is stronger and less at weaker positions. The wide variety of individual differences (especially height) makes this design very difficult. VRM's have been

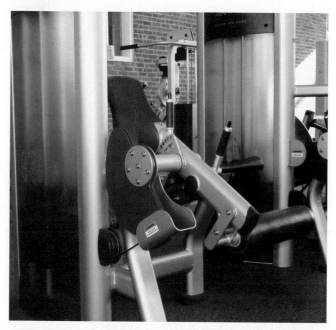

■ **FIGURE 8.2** A variable resistance machine with cam.

an excellent addition to resistance training because of their ease of use and support. However, studies have shown that they do not always work as advertised (21).

Free Weights

Free weights generally consist of barbells and dumbbells. Manufacturers of free weights have made free weights easier to handle. Many pieces of apparatus are also manufactured to accompany free weight use. We recommend small (1.5 pound) increments for weight rooms commonly utilized by women and children. Many weight rooms only have 2.5 pound plates. This sets the minimum change on a barbell at 5.0 pounds. This may not seem like much to a stronger person, but if an individual goes from 45 to 50 pounds, they are increasing their intensity by 11%. Now presume that someone is lifting 250 pounds. An 11% increase requires the addition of 27.5 pounds—a significant amount of increase.

Concentric and Eccentric

Muscles contract concentrically and eccentrically (Fig. 8.3). Concentric muscle contractions occur when the muscle exerts tension and shortens. This type of contraction is typically against gravity and is the movement normally described in an exercise. Arm curls require the biceps muscle to contract and shorten in order to lift a weight. Returning the weight to its starting position requires a lessening of tension in the biceps resulting in biceps lengthening (eccentric). Gravity actually pulls the weight down. Eccentric contractions are often used to decelerate and control a movement. Humans are stronger eccentrically than concentrically. Eccentric contractions also result in much more soreness than concentric contractions. Since athletic activities require athletes to perform both forms of contraction, athletes should train both concentrically and eccentrically. For instance, jumping requires strong concentric contractions of the quadriceps muscles, but landing requires strong eccentric contractions of the quadriceps. For this reason, we recommend both forms of training.

Ballistic Exercise

A high velocity joint movement is normally the result of a ballistic muscle contraction. Throwing, jumping, and kicking are typical examples of ballistic activities. A ballistic muscle contraction is initiated by an initial powerful concentric contraction of the required muscle groups causing acceleration. After sufficient velocity has been attained the muscle then relaxes, allowing momentum to maintain the movement. Deceleration of the movement (to protect the joint) is accomplished by eccentric contraction of the contralateral muscle. For example, many muscles are involved in overhand throwing but the triceps are involved in rapid extension of the elbow. The biceps muscle contracts eccentrically to slow down the rapid extension, one reason why baseball players have sore biceps in the early season.

Isometric Contractions

A static contraction of a muscle in which there is tension in the muscle but no movement is also an isometric contraction. We often perform static contractions for postural support. Deep abdominal and back muscles are frequently undergoing mild static contractions to maintain our upright posture. The trunk stability exercises demonstrated in Chapter 15 are isometric exercises.

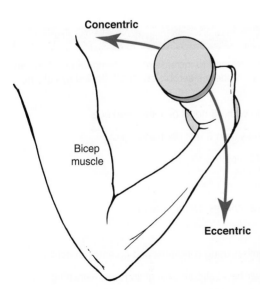

■ FIGURE 8.3 Concentric and eccentric exercise.

TABLE 8.1	Recommended Volume and Intensity of Resistance Training		
	Frequency per Week	**Volume—Sets per muscle group**	**Percentage of 1 RM**
Untrained Individuals	3	4	60
Recreational Athletes	2	4	80
Competitive Athletes	2	8	85

Exercise Order

In what order should athletes perform exercise routines? A general recommendation is to perform multijoint exercises before single-joint exercises. Exercise the large muscle groups first. If athletes are going to lift a very heavy weight for a particular exercise, perform this early in the routine (after a proper warm-up).

STRENGTH TRAINING BASICS

Hundreds of strength training studies have been conducted since the 1950s. Various recommendations have come forth regarding the number of sets, reps, and the intensity of resistance training needed for strength gain. However, these recommendations have been quite broad and fairly nonspecific. In many respects, most have indicated that if one routinely and progressively performs relatively high resistance training they will get stronger. But the research has become more sophisticated as the emergence of sports conditioning has increased in importance. Research has also become more systematic and repeatable. Clearly, the "dose" of resistance affects the "response" to that training. Two investigations have recently summarized and reviewed 177 strength training studies (using meta-analyses) (18,22). One interesting finding is that the dose-response relationship is different for diverse populations. Table 8.1 indicates three populations: untrained individuals, recreational athletes, and competitive athletes. The intensity and volume of training recommended for untrained individuals is different from recreational athletes and competitive athletes.

A Basic Program

The program identified in Table 8.2 is based upon the two summaries above as well as recommendations by Bachle and Groves (23). Unless athletes are highly familiar with resistance training, we suggest start-

TABLE 8.2	Basic Resistance Training Recommendations
Warmup	Start out with a general warm-up designed to increase muscle temperature. This can be in the form of 10–15 minutes of moderate aerobic exercise followed by light repetitions of various exercises.
Frequency	2 days per week per muscle group with 48 hours between workouts
Volume	4 Sets per muscle group for 4 weeks then 8 sets per muscle group.
Intensity	First 2 weeks: 70% 1 RM = 10–12 reps Second 4 weeks: 80% 1 RM = 8 reps Thereafter: 85% of 1 RM = 6 reps
Rest	2 minutes between each set unless athletes start to lose form.
Exercise Order	Start with large muscle groups.
Types of Exercises	Focus primarily on multi-joint exercises using concentric and eccentric exercises.
Primary Muscle Groups	Shoulders, chest, upper back, lower back, abdominals, quadriceps, hamstrings.
Cool Down	Dynamic and static stretching.

FROM THE ATHLETIC TRAINING ROOM

Weight Belts or Not?

Go into most Home Depot stores and you will find many employees wearing supportive belts around their waist. Likewise, Olympic weightlifters on television frequently wear abdominal belts. Should athletes wear weight belts when lifting free weights? Stuart McGill, a recognized authority on lower back injury, summarized research on weight belts.

1. Individuals who have not had a previous back injury appear not to need the additional protection of a belt.
2. Belts tend to give people the perception that they can lift more. The belt may allow one to lift more. Individuals who have been injured when wearing a belt tend to risk a more severe injury. Further, belts increase intraabdominal pressure and blood pressure.
3. Individuals who wear a belt tend to change their lifting styles, possibly not preparing them for when they do not have belt.

McGill concluded that belt wearing is not recommended for routine exercise participation.

McGill S. Abdominal belts in industry: a position paper on their assets, liabilities and use. *Am Ind Hyg Assoc J* 1993;54:752–754.

ing with a program more geared toward recreational athletes and then to increase the volume and intensity. Complete novices should probably start as untrained individuals. A closer examination of the variables in Table 8.2 is in order:

Warm-Up. The warm-up should last approximately 10 to 15 minutes. Start with about 5 minutes of easy aerobic exercise and progress to light skipping, hopping, arm and leg swings, lunges, jogging backward and sideways. End the warm-up with a few light repetitions of exercises similar to those planned for the session. The warm-up should not exhaust the athletes but they should be perspiring. We do not recommend static stretching during the warm-up.

Frequency. Two sessions per week per muscle group is the recommendation. Studies indicate that more than two is time wasted. However, this does not mean that athletes should not perform resistance training more than twice a week. When time is sufficient, we recommend splitting workouts between muscle groups. Two common techniques often utilized for splitting are listed in Table 8.3. One routine involves splitting workouts between upper and lower body activities. A second routine involves pushing exercises (such as dumbbell presses and push-ups) on one day, and pulling exercises (such as bent-over rowing and pull-ups) on the following day.

Volume. Start out with four sets per muscle group and progress to eight sets. Although initial observation may appear excessive, the key to this recommendation refers to muscle groups and not one specific exercise. For example, an athlete can perform four sets of the bench press and four sets of weighted push-

TABLE 8.3	**Common Split Workouts**						
	Sun	**Mon**	**Tue**	**Wed**	**Thu**	**Fri**	**Sat**
Lower Body/ Upper Body	Rest	Lower	Upper	Lower	Upper	Plyometrics Medicine Ball Agility	Rest
Push/Pull	Rest	Push	Pull	Push	Pull	Plyometrics Medicine Ball Agility	Rest

Each of these programs involves two training sessions per week per muscle group followed by plyometrics, ballistic medicine ball activities, and agility drills.

TABLE 8.4   Some Common Exercises by Muscle Group

Exercises	Muscles Involved	Example
Bench Press with barbell Bench Press with dumbbell Varied push-ups Chest flys	Pectoralis Major Coracobrachialis Anterior Deltoid Triceps	
Overhead Press with barbell Overhead press with dumbbell Inclined Press with barbell Overhead press with dumbbell	Trapezius Serratus Anterior Deltoid Triceps Supraspinatus	
Dumbbell Row Inverted Pull-up One-leg Pulley Row Bent-Over Row	Rhomboid Posterior Deltoid Infraspinatus Teres Minor Biceps	
Wide variety of Squats Various lunges One-leg box squat	Quadriceps Hamstrings Gluteus Maximus	

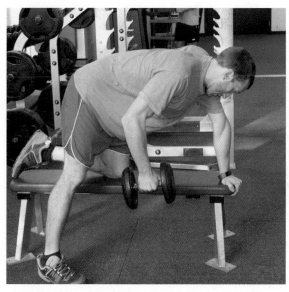

■ **FIGURE 8.4** Dumbbell pull.

ups and satisfy the eight set recommendation. While no two exercises provide identical stress, Table 8.4 provides a few examples of similar muscle group exercises. Figures 8.4 to 8.6 illustrate three exercises that all involve the same muscle group. To strengthen the upper back and shoulder plus the biceps, the athlete can use a variety of these.

Intensity. Unless the athlete is highly involved and familiar with strength training, we recommend a fairly conservative start. Start at around 70% of the 1RM for 2 weeks and then increase to 80% of the 1RM if the athlete is comfortable and performs with good form. Otherwise, take additional time. If you do not want to take the time to measure the 1RM, use the guideline that athletes should be able to perform the following number of repetitions before failure at each percentage of the 1RM (24):

- 10 to 12 repetitions at 70% of the 1RM
- 8 repetitions at 80% of 1RM
- 6 repetitions at 85% of 1RM

Increase or decrease weight accordingly to reach the desired number of repetitions. As the athlete strengthens add weight, but do this rather slowly at the beginning. Baechle and Groves recommend that once an athlete can lift more than two repetitions beyond the goal in 2 successive days then weight can be added (23). Add 2.5 to 5.0 lbs for weaker movements and 5.0 to 10.0 lbs for stronger movements such as the dead lift or squat.

PERIODIZED STRENGTH TRAINING

The basic program recommended in Table 8.2 works very well. During a program lasting 6 to 8 weeks very positive results should occur. When athletes can participate in a program lasting at least 2 to 3 months we recommend a sequence that is slightly more periodized. Periodized strength training has become more popular in the United States and studies have shown superior results (25,26). The manipulation of volume and intensity to achieve specific training goals is the root of periodized

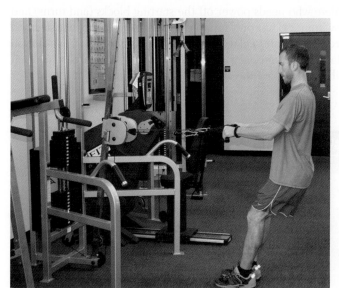

■ **FIGURE 8.5** Two-arm pull on cable pulleys.

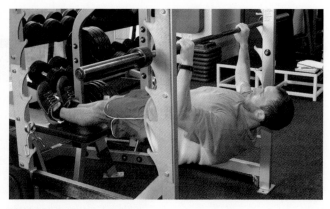

■ **FIGURE 8.6** Inclined pull-up.

training. As discussed in Chapter 4, rest and recovery periods are planned into the program. Secondly, periodized programs offer more variety, relieving some of the boredom from ones with unchanging volume.

Periodized Programs for Strength and Muscular Endurance

Long term year round strength training is probably the best form of strength training. The original periodized plans were designed to be year round, requiring the athletes to cycle through a periodized schedule several times a year. They were also designed for world class athletes participating in only a few championship events a year. In our experience, such programs are normally impractical for typical high school and college athletes. But effective periodized plans can be created for shorter periods. The basics remain the same; volume and intensity are manipulated to bring about the goal of each period.

Table 8.5 is our recommendation for a 12 week periodized program designed for an athlete to gain strength and power. Our program is based upon several classical models but also designed to fit into an academic schedule (16,25). Multiple periodized models can be created by a coach and this is only one recommendation. For example, you may want to increase or decrease the time spent on each phase. You can easily plan a program in which the athlete cycles through this program several times, usually starting each cycle a little stronger.

Keep in mind the basics presented earlier. Aim for approximately eight sets per muscle group twice a week. If there is time for strength training several days a week, use some form of splitting the workouts between muscle groups. Allow at least 48 hours rest between workouts. Training more than this is unnecessary and can lead to overuse injuries and burnout.

PERIODIZING MUSCULAR ENDURANCE

Tudor Bompa, one of the early advocates of periodization in North America, has discussed the conversion of strength to muscular endurance (27). One suggestion is to develop strength first and then shift more toward muscular endurance. As mentioned earlier, some athletic events require an athlete to repeatedly contract the same muscles in a rhythmic fashion, attempting to maintain form without undue loss of power. Resistance training programs should prepare athletes to perform the activity required in competition. If muscular endurance is required then muscular endurance should be developed. The suggested program outlined in Table 8.6 allows for hypertrophy and strength training first followed by muscular endurance. Rhea et al found a similar periodized program to elicit a 73% improvement in muscular endurance (28).

COMBINED PROGRAMS

Observe a swimmer and you will see an athlete who needs power off the starting blocks (and turns) and muscular endurance while swimming. The swimmer is just one example of an athlete who needs strength and power in one part of their body and strength and muscular endurance in another part. The solution is power training for muscles involved in starting and muscular endurance training for muscles involved in swimming. Such a combined program will help prepare the athlete for competition.

TABLE 8.5	Twelve Week Periodized Program for Strength/Power				
Goal of Period	**Hypertrophy**	**Strength**	**Power**	**Peaking**	**Active Rest**
Weeks	4	3	2	2	1
Sets/Exercise	3–5	3–5	3–5	1–3	
Reps	8–12	4–8	2–4	1–3	
Intensity	Low	Moderate	High	High	
Volume	Very High	High	Moderate	Low	

TABLE 8.6 Twelve Week Periodized Program for Muscular Endurance

Goal of Period	Hypertrophy	Strength	Muscular Endurance 1	Muscular Endurance 2	Active Rest
Weeks	3	3	3	3	1
Sets/Exercise	3–5	3–5	3–5	3–5	
Reps	8–12	4–8	15–20	20–25	

RESISTANCE TRAINING BY SEASON

Many variables must be prioritized as part of seasonal competition (Table 8.7). During the competitive season sport specific practice must take precedence over resistance training. The competitive season is not the time to develop strength and power. The goal should be to maintain gains from earlier resistance training. Fortunately, strength adaptations tend to persevere. One recommendation is to schedule 1 to 2 resistance training sessions a week during the competitive season (24). Strength training sessions during the season should be low in volume and high in intensity. Following a warm-up the athlete should simply rotate from one exercise to the next, performing one intense set of each. Such a procedure will only take about 15 minutes and help maintain strength. Unless an athlete needs to overcome some particular weakness, the exercises should all be multi-joint exercises.

Problem Sports

Sports that start in the fall are problematic with regard to resistance training and overall conditioning. Not only are student athletes not supervised in the summer, they often work and live where training facilities are sparse. Of all the fall sports, football is particularly troublesome because of the high level of physical contact and relatively high injury rate. Coaches recommend summer workouts and usually provide extensive workout information for their incoming athletes. Unfortunately, such information does not insure that athletes adhere to a workout regimen.

FOCAL POINT

Power Endurance or Muscular Endurance

Muscular endurance may fall into more than one category. For example, running at high speed for 50 seconds (e.g., 400 meter dash) requires over 100 muscular contractions of each leg. However, each of the contractions is composed of a brief stretch-shortening cycle followed by a ballistic muscular contraction. A swimmer may perform the same number of muscular contractions but the contractions are less ballistic (requiring continued contraction throughout the range of motion). The ballistic form of muscular endurance is more power oriented while the more uniform muscular contraction (like in swimming or rowing) is traditionally labeled muscular endurance. Bompa suggests that the training methods for each of these activities should be different. He recommends that the load for power-endurance should be 15 to 30 repetitions with about 50% to 70% of maximum weight. The speed should be very dynamic with rest intervals of 5 to 7 minutes. For traditional muscular endurance, Bompa suggests using a lighter weight of 50% to 60% and performing medium to fast repetitions for 30 to 60 seconds. He recommends repeating this 3 to 6 times with rest periods of only 60 to 90 seconds.

Bompa T. *Periodization Training for Sports*. Champaign, IL: Human Kinetics; 1999.

TABLE 8.7   Prioritizing Training Variables by Season

Season	Resistance Training	Sport Specific Training	
Off-season	High priority	Low Priority	Basic hypertrophy is the goal—first 4–5 weeks of a periodized plan
Early preseason	Medium priority	Medium Priority	Strength and Power development
Preseason	Low Priority	High Priority	Complete periodized training
Competitive Season	Low Priority	High Priority	Resistance train only 1–2 times per week with 1 intense set each of core exercise program

One solution (although not ideal) is to have the athletes complete a solid periodized resistance program in the spring. Athletes should be encouraged to repeat this program during the summer. During preseason football athletes should participate in some moderately intense resistance training sessions focusing on strength and power. This is not the time for a periodized program. Fall sport athletes such as field hockey and soccer players can best use their time by sport specific practice. We also recommend the activities in Chapter 14 designed to reduce the incidence of lower limb injuries.

IMPLEMENTING A RESISTANCE TRAINING PROGRAM

Implementation and maintenance is the key to success for any resistance program. Resistance training only works if athletes regularly engage in a progressive program designed to generate specific changes. You can have the finest facilities, the perfect combination of sets and reps, and wonderful periodized plans. But if the athletes do not participate, the best laid plans fail. We have seen a number of schools build elaborate fitness facilities that showcase the school but are unwilling to staff such facilities with professional personnel. We often find fitness facilities almost completely run by students.

Trained supervisors are the most important part of a resistance program. The typical high school and college athlete does not possess the knowledge (and often the motivation) to create and maintain a successful program. Coaches are often willing and able to incorporate sound resistance programs but are limited by NCAA and high school athletic federations. Collegiate coaches are usually limited to 18 to 19 weeks/year of coach-athlete contact. Many state high school athletic associations have similar rules. The appointment of a strength and conditioning coach is one answer. Otherwise, coaches may give suggestions for resistance training but cannot directly supervise or direct athletes out of their allotted time.

Assessment

Before selecting specific activities for athletes, some form of assessment should be conducted. Remember that the purpose of resistance training is to improve performance and prevent injury; improvement in some strength activity unrelated to the athlete's sport is a waste of time.

REQUIREMENTS OF THE SPORT

Consider the individual needs of each athlete when planning a program. This includes the specific weaknesses of the athlete as well as the needs of the sport. If a sport requires significant sprinting, then lower body power activities should be part of the program. Is upper body strength a requirement? Do big players have an advantage? Is there considerable lateral movement, backward movement?

Most athletes will benefit from a resistance program that strengthens the basic joints of the body: shoulder, upper back, chest, trunk, hip, knee, and ankle. As mentioned earlier, we strongly recommend symmetrical development of muscles around joints. Many sports place specific stress on certain joints.

Creating Successful Athlete Directed Resistance Programs

We surveyed coaches and asked how they were able to encourage athletes to participate in self directed resistance programs. Two ideas were generally used that seemed quite successful. Many coaches establish either training partners or small training groups during out of season. Students are grouped according to schedule and interest and meet on a regular schedule to work out. Coaches try to put at least one athlete in each group who tends toward leadership, motivating the athletes to work together. One coach used three person groups, allowing one student to train while the other two spot for exercises like squats and bench presses. Bonnie May (retired volleyball and softball coach at Smith College with over 800 wins) said she liked to put her players in teams of two. "When you are responsible to one person for your workout, you know you have to be there. Each athlete spots the other." Some coaches used web-based workouts, providing athletes choices of exercises that they might wish to use. Assigning specific exercises is normally against policy but coaches can provide suggestions.

Wrestlers and football players need strong necks. Baseball players need excellent trunk rotation and high jumpers need power and flexibility. Coaches are generally aware of the specific needs of their athletes. Some general guidelines by sport are listed in Table 8.8.

INDIVIDUAL ASSESSMENT

One program will not meet the needs of every athlete. Students often come to a sport with great differences in experience. As mentioned in Chapter 2, we now find athletes who have been competing and training since a very early age. Some athletes have been under the supervision of personal trainers, and many have attended sport camps where they were coached by professional athletes. And there are great potential athletes who have never trained or played on an organized team. Such individual differences present an interesting challenge to the coach. Start slowly and allow yourself to get to know the needs of each athlete. Some questions you might ask are:

- Does the athlete have any particular weaknesses? If so, then the resistance program should be designed to overcome these.
- Does the athlete need to get bigger? You'll occasionally see athletes who have excellent skills but are pushed around a lot. Usually they just need to get a bit bigger and a program of exercise and proper nutrition can be designed to result in additional hypertrophy.
- Is this athlete new to resistance training? Create a simple program for this athlete designed for success. Use more VRM training than free weight training and limit the program to only a few exercises. Do not overload them with a wide variety of exercises.
- Has this athlete had a lot of experience with resistance training? Use this athlete as an example for demonstrations. Athletes with experience should be rewarded. Let them teach the other athletes but also present them with challenges. Periodize their training.
- Is this an athlete with significant strength and little skill? Some athletes get really hooked on weight training and want to spend all their time in the weight room. Coaches know that strength training only goes so far and these athletes need to spend much more time on the playing field. Encourage these athletes to get involved in pick-up games. Encourage them to play intramurals or to get involved with community leagues. Find them a practice partner.

Measuring Strength

The 1RM is the standard measure of muscle strength. Many training protocols use a percentage of the 1RM to assign resistance. However, we seriously question the need to know 1RM strength at the begin-

TABLE 8.8 Specific Needs of Athletes by Sport	
Baseball Softball	Good trunk rotation, shoulder strength and flexibility. Need power and not endurance.
Basketball	Rebounding players need size and the ability to get off the ground quickly. Power training of the legs and trunk is essential.
Divers	Need good leg power off the board plus core strength. Specific strength exercises for the neck should be included.
Field Hockey, Soccer, Lacrosse	Less attention to upper body and more to lower body for these athletes. Extensive focus on knee stability is required.
Football	Because of the extensive contact and body size of football players, resistance training is very important. Most football players need hypertrophy. Besides a solid resistance program for the major muscle groups, neck stability is important.
Rowing	Trunk stability is very important for these athletes with more attention to lower than upper body.
Skiing (Alpine)	Skiers need power and endurance of lower body with special attention to quadriceps and hamstrings.
Swim (freestyle, butterfly, backstroke)	Focus is on strengthening and maintaining shoulder joint muscles. Swimmers tend to overdevelop swimming muscles and to neglect contralateral muscles. Resistance programs should include both. Special attention must be given to those muscles that stabilize the scapula: trapezius, rhomboid, serratus anterior, and pectoralis minor.
Swim (breaststroke)	Less shoulder flexibility is required but breaststroke swimmers need more work for knee and hip stabilization
Tennis	Need to maintain shoulder flexibility during resistance training—careful attention to full ROM exercises. Tennis players also need good forearm and wrist strength. Similar to swimmers, they need strong scapula support.
Track (sprinting)	Sprinters need symmetrical upper and lower bodies. Strong legs must match strong arms. Focus should be on multi-joint power exercises.
Track (hurdling)	Hurdlers need a program similar to sprinters but with improved flexibility of lower body.
Track (middle and long distance)	Middle and distance runners need symmetrical upper and lower body. Hypertrophied upper bodies are normally a detriment.
Track (jumpers)	Resistance training for these athletes must focus on power development through multi-joint activities.
Track (throwers)	Most throwers benefit by hypertrophy. Discus and javelin throwers also need good flexibility. Similar to jumpers, throwers need extensive power development with little attention to single-joint exercises. Wrist and hand strength development are important.
Wrestlers	Need excellent strength but must maintain good shoulder flexibility. Strong necks are imperative.

ning of a program. Athletes often come to a program untrained and unfamiliar with proper lifting protocol. Testing the unfamiliar athlete is inaccurate and places the athlete in a vulnerable position. Establishing the appropriate resistance for each lift is not that difficult. The first priority should be to allow the athlete to become familiar with the proper form. As technique develops simply add weight until the desired resistance is found.

Strength testing can be an excellent motivational tool for athletes. Athletes frequently want to know how they compare to other athletes on the team. Athletes can estimate their 1RM by performing maximum repetitions with a weight they can lift more than once but less than ten times. The National Strength and Conditioning Association has presented equations to predict 1RM from 2 to 15RM (24).

TABLE 8.9	Predicting 1RM from Repetitions to Failure
% 1RM	**Number of Repetitions to Failure**
100	1
95	2
93	3
90	4
87	5
85	6
83	7
80	8
77	9
75	10
70	11
67	12
65	15

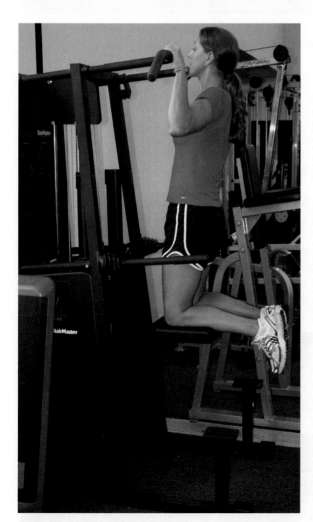

■ **FIGURE 8.7** Assisted pull-up.

Table 8.9 provides an estimate of the percent of 1RM an individual can achieve when performing 1 to 10RM. As with all predictions, there is error in this method. However, this is one place to start before testing for 1RM strength. We believe the 1RM test should be reserved for athletes who are thoroughly familiar with technique. Baechle et al present an excellent 1RM testing protocol (24).

Although the 1RM is a standard test, Boyle recommends the use of body resistance exercises to measure functional strength. How well do athletes handle their own bodies? As Boyle suggested, an athlete may be able to bench press 350 pounds, but if they weight 350 they are only lifting their body weight (5). Pull-ups, chin-ups, push-ups, inverted rows, and one-leg box squats can be used to measure functional strength and muscular endurance. Boyle recommends pull-ups (palms forward) for men and chin-ups (palms facing) for women. Since many female athletes cannot perform multiple pull-ups, many coaches use assisted pull-ups (Fig. 8.7) as an alternative. Most of these exercises are fairly familiar to athletes and can be administered rather easily. Regardless of how strength is measured, standardized procedures should be utilized. Athletes must utilize proper form and complete every repetition. Also, it is a waste of time to measure strength if the results are not utilized. Do it right or do not do it at all.

RESISTANCE TRAINING ACTIVITIES

Since most sports are played in a standing position, we recommend a preponderance of activities in which athletes must support themselves (i.e., they are standing). Most fitness centers have an array of fixed motion, variable resistance machines. In general, we do not recommend a program that relies heavily on variable resistance machines. But there are times when such machines can be quite useful.

We strongly support accompanying traditional strength training exercises with body weight exercises (Fig. 8.8). Body control is a huge factor in athletic performance and injury reduction. Athletes play sports in an unstable environment. Even a seemingly perfect grass playing field is uneven. This coupled with team members and opponents all vying for the same space creates instability. Therefore, perform some resistance training in an unstable environment (Fig. 8.9).

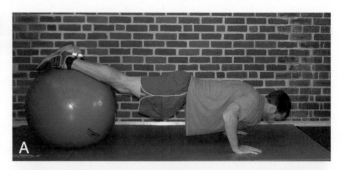

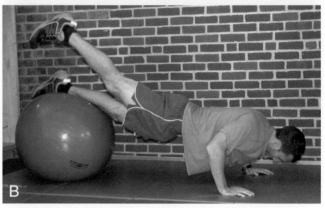

■ **FIGURE 8.8 A.** Push-ups on stability ball: two leg balance. **B.** Push-up on stability ball: one leg balance.

Free Weights versus VRMs

Exercise scientists have debated the pros and cons of free weights and variable resistance machines for many years (Table 8.10). An athlete who systematically participates in a resistance program using either free weights or VRMs will get stronger. Both methods of resistance training work and there are advantages to each.

The most common advantage often mentioned for free weights is the need to balance and support the weight. Take a look at an exercise like the squat. In the free weight version, the athlete must balance and support this weight throughout the entire range of motion, stabilizing the weight with trunk muscles. The squat exercise with a free weight is much more than an exercise for the legs and hips. This same exercise performed on a VRM (usually called the leg press) involves little balance and the athlete's trunk is often supported by the machine. One might say that the squat should only be performed with free weights. But the exercise on the VRM requires no spotting and the athlete can do this quickly and without supervision.

Novice athletes can perform the leg press without fear of tripping or falling. Go into almost any weight room and you will see far more people performing leg presses on VRM machines than squats with free weights.

We recommend a combined program of free weights and VRMs. Some muscles (such as the latissimus dorsi) are difficult to train with free weights. Do not think of free weights as just barbells since dumbbells can frequently be used. Novice athletes are less intimidated by dumbbells and can learn balance and control before moving to more complicated barbell ex-

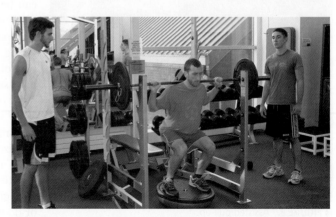

■ **FIGURE 8.9** Squat on Bosu ball—an advanced functional exercise.

TABLE 8.10 Advantages and Disadvantages of Free Weights and VRMs

	Free Weights	VRMs
Cost	Free weights cost less but large squat racks and lifting platforms are not cheap.	
Ease of Use	Takes longer to learn how to use free weights.	Very easy to use
Speed of Use	Athletes take considerable time removing and adding weights.	Resistance and body position are quickly changed and athletes can rotate through a series of VRM exercises quickly.
Balance and Support	Free weights require athletes to move in a balanced fashion and to often support a weight with their entire body.	VRM usually requires little balance or support. This may be a good thing for novice lifters.
Allowance for acceleration	Free weights allow an athlete to accelerate a weight through a range of motion.	Most VRMs must be performed at a fairly constant velocity.
Coordinated Movements	Free weights allow more coordinated movements such as a clean—requiring sequential chain-like muscle contractions similar to sport requirements.	Far less coordination is required.
Transition to Performance Activities—Functionality	From the specificity viewpoint, free weights more closely resemble athletic movements and provide better transfer.	

ercises. As athletes become more familiar with weight training, there should be increased emphasis on free weight training. Free weights require more balance, control, and stability; all of which may help prevent injury. Figure 8.10 represents a transition from supported exercise on a VRM to a more functional squat using a free weight. Figure 8.10A illustrates a leg press during which the trunk is supported. Figure 8.10B demonstrates a squat exercise in the upright position with less support, while Figure 8.10C shows a squat in an unsupported position.

Pulley Weights

One of the weaknesses of VRMs is the requirement of a fixed plane throughout the range of motion. Several manufacturers now produce excellent resistance machines using free standing weights that are moved with various pulley attachments. These machines are highly adaptable to a wide variety of movements requiring stabilization and balance. These free standing systems allow a quick change of resistance as well as the ability to imitate many athletic movements. Figure 8.11 illustrates an athlete performing a multi-joint exercise that is difficult to replicate with machines or free weights. Figure 8.12 shows an athlete performing a standard pulling exercise on one leg, requiring good balance and core strength.

POWER TRAINING

Athletes must be able to produce force quickly for athletic success. Joint stability also requires muscles to contract quickly and synchronously. Power is an important attribute for both performance and injury prevention. Studies have shown that strength training can improve power, but not all strength training is the same (6). From the standpoint of specificity, resistance exercises performed slowly would tend to have less transfer than faster resistance exercises (29). Many free weight exercises can be performed at higher speed. Resistance exercises using one's own weight can often be performed quickly. VRMs often call for steady paced exercises at slower speeds. Athletes can enhance power by moving resistance at higher speeds.

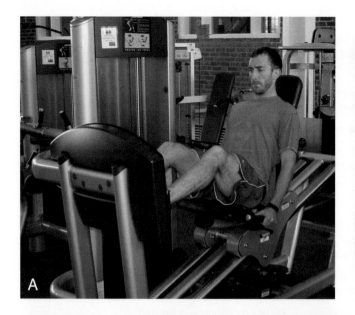

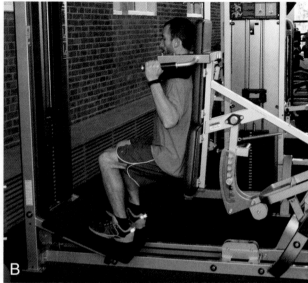

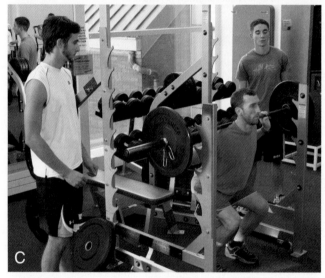

■ **FIGURE 8.10** Three Squat transition with decreasing support. **A.** Leg press on VRM. **B.** Upright squat on fixed motion machine. **C.** Upright squat with free weights.

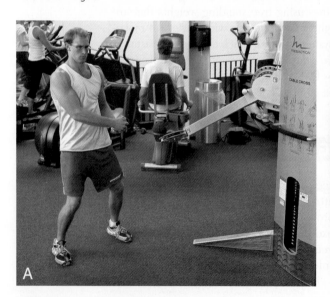

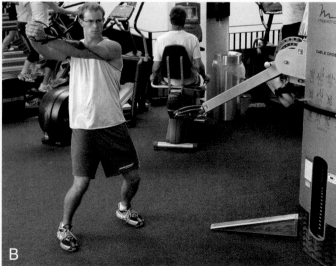

■ **FIGURE 8.11** A functional exercise using a free motion pulley machine.

Core Training

In recent years there has been increased interest in core exercises. Stability is one of the important functions of the core (torso). As discussed in Chapter 15, the stability of the trunk is vital for injury prevention. Core strength is also essential for performance. The key to optimal performance in many sports is the transfer of force from the ground through the body. Kicking, throwing, and jumping activities all use this transfer of force through the body, the kinetic chain. The torso is a critical part of the kinetic chain since force from the ground must travel through the trunk. If the trunk muscles are weak, part of the force generated from the ground is lost. We recommend good core strength for athletes in all sports, but rowers, throwers and hitters require excellent core strength. For example, rowers must transfer force through their trunk to the hands gripping the oar. If the trunk tends to collapse, force is lost. Likewise, the trunk rotation needed to throw and hit is critical for top level performance. The number of core exercises is vast but exercises in which athletes must support themselves tend to develop core strength. The lower back exercises illustrated in Chapter 15 are good examples. Also, Figures 8.5, 8.6, 8.8, 8.9, and 8.12 require core strength.

To develop power we encourage coaches to supplement typical strength training programs. The various jumping activities described in Chapter 3 are all designed to improve power. Brief spurts of high speed running on a track or up a hill train muscles to contract quickly and strongly. Plyometric exercises develop power, especially when conducted in conjunction with strength training (29). Although there are many suggestions in the training literature, we will examine three common ways to supplement basic strength training with power activities.

High Power Resistance Exercises

Perform high-power resistance exercises by decreasing the weight and increasing the speed of movement. High power resistance exercises are almost always performed with free weights (barbells and dumbbells) and are usually multi-joint movements. Exercises like the bench press, overhead press, dead lift, and the squat can all be performed at a higher speed, attempting to replicate sport movements against resistance. You will need to experiment with this a bit to determine the perfect resistance, but athletes will benefit from the training and enjoy the variety. Athletes need good lifting skills with skilled spotters before this type of training.

A good example of high-power resistance training is the power clean (that is how it got its name). A successful clean cannot be performed at slow speed. The clean is also an exercise that involves a synchronization of muscle contractions (the kinetic chain) transferring force from the ground to the bar. Observe an athlete performing a vertical jump and you see an example of the kinetic chain in action. Throwing, kicking, and striking all involve the kinetic chain. Cleans are fairly complex maneuvers and require good coordination, but several forms of cleans can be performed from the fairly complex to simpler versions. Proper form must be first taught with light weights. Performing exercises with speed and control against resistance is a great way to train for power.

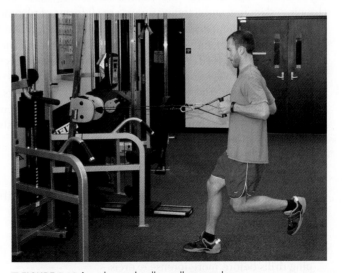

■ **FIGURE 8.12** An advanced pulley pull on one leg.

Medicine Ball Activities

Training with medicine balls has been around for many years. But the popularity of using medicine balls waned, relegated to boxing workouts and therapeutic exercise. One problem was that medicine balls were often a bit too large and difficult to adapt to sport. Manufacturers now produce medicine balls of different weights and sizes; balls that rebound, some even with handles. The popularity of medicine ball use has accompanied the increased interest in training functional strength and power.

One recognized benefit of medicine ball training is the ability to stress the kinetic chain. The kinetic chain almost always involves the transfer of momentum from the ground up through the trunk. Power activities for hip and trunk rotation are difficult to simulate with standard resistance training and medicine ball training can easily be designed to stress these movements. Medicine ball training is an excellent transition from strength to power, allowing athletes to accelerate through kinetic chain movements. Such movements replicate many athletic activities as well as providing resistance.

Extensive research on the effect of medicine ball training on strength and power has not been conducted. In one study researchers had high school baseball players simply swing a bat 100 times per day. One group supplemented their bat swinging with medicine ball rotation exercises. They found that torso rotational strength and power was significantly improved with medicine ball rotational training, and that such training was superior to bat swinging only (30). Some studies have not shown medicine ball training to be effective (31). Medicine ball training should not take the place of traditional resistance training techniques. However, we support the supplementation of traditional resistance training with medicine ball training; especially that training that focuses on trunk rotation.

Plyometric Exercise

Athletes frequently land from a jump and immediately rebound into the next movement. Watch a basketball player jumping for a rebound and you will observe a quick flexion of the knee and hip just prior to the rapid extension required for jumping. Since muscles and tendons tend to contract immediately after being stretched (the stretch reflex), humans naturally use this reflex to exert greater tension. This is classically referred to as the "stretch-shortening cycle" (SSC) and is composed of three phases (32).

- Phase 1 is the eccentric phase in which the muscle and tendon are stretched.
- Phase 2 is the period of time between the eccentric phase and the subsequent concentric contraction—also called the transition or amortization phase.
- Phase 3 is the concentric contraction of muscles that were just stretched. These contractions normally result in tension that is greater than a contraction without prestretching.

Plyometric exercise was designed to specifically train the stretch-shortening cycle. Most coaches are aware of plyometric training and often associate this form of training with box or "depth" jumping. But any exercise that involves the stretch-shortening cycle can be considered as a plyometric activity. Hopping, skipping, and standing jumps are all forms of plyometric training. Many plyometric activities require little equipment and are easy to implement. In addition to training the SSC, many plyometric activities also focus on landing skills. As discussed in Chapter 3, the improvement of landing skills is one of the strategies recommended for preventing ankle and knee (specifically ACL) injuries.

Plyometric exercises place considerable stress on joints and muscles and athletes must be strong enough to withstand these stresses. Athletes with weak legs, knees, and backs should undergo a basic strength training program prior to starting plyometrics, particularly higher intensity plyometrics. Research has shown that the combination of plyometric exercises and strength training is superior to either method individually for improving power (33).

CONDUCTING A PLYOMETRIC PROGRAM

Introduce plyometric exercises in a progressive fashion, starting with low intensity activities. Table 8.11 presents a list of plyometric exercises of increasing intensity. The following are some general considerations for developing your plyometric program:

- Athletes should warm up properly with aerobic exercise, dynamic stretching, light skipping and hopping drills before more intense exercises.

TABLE 8.11	Plyometric Jumps of Increasing Intensity
Activity	**Description**
Standing Jumps	These jumps emphasize only the vertical component of jumping by having the athlete repeatedly jump into the air. There are many forms of these jumps such as tuck jumps or squat jumps. These jumps can also be done with turns. See Chapter 3 for landing suggestions.
Standing Jumps on One Leg	Repeat jumping straight up is one example.
Horizontal Hopping	Repeatedly hopping on two legs across a field or gym mat stresses the vertical and horizontal component. Using cones or barriers provides a target and motivation.
Bounding	Bounding can be an exaggerated form of running in which the athlete attempts to cover as much distance as possible on each bound. Provide a target distance. Bounding on one leg is quite difficult and places considerable stress on the knee and ankle. Start off one-legged bounding slowly.
Depth (Box) Jumping	Increasing the vertical distance traveled prior to jumping increases the eccentric phase of the SSC. A simple box jump is to have an athlete jump off and on the same box for a short time period. Add a horizontal component by jumping off one box onto another. After the athletes are comfortable with this place boxes of different heights in a row and have then travel through it as fast as possible.

- Start with activities such as standing jumps before moving to more intense activities such as bounding or box jumps.
- Use cones and flexible hurdles for jumping.
- The landing area for plyometric activities should be soft. Grass, gym mats, or cushioned runways work best. Never use concrete as a landing surface.
- Plyometric activities should be brief and intense. Remember that these are not endurance activities. Provide ample rest and focus on high quality activity.
- Considerable muscle soreness is expected at the beginning since there is substantial eccentric stress on muscles.
- Modify the program for athletes who tend to continuously have sore knees, ankles, or hips.
- Boxes for depth jumping must be stable and provide a high friction landing surface.
- Normally, plyometric exercises should be performed twice a week at least 48 hours between sessions. During the competitive season, we recommend plyometrics no more than once a week.

Upper Body Plyometrics Plyometric exercises are typically designed for the lower body. Skipping, hopping, and jumping are all natural lower body exercises that involve the stretch-shortening cycle. Plyometric exercises for the upper body have been designed and most (but not all) include the use of a medicine ball (34). As suggested earlier, medicine ball activities have not been studied in detail. Currently, reports from studies utilizing upper body plyometrics are mixed. Some have not supported upper body plyometrics (30,35), while some studies have shown positive results from upper body plyometrics (36,37). Although the efficacy of upper body plyometrics is somewhat unclear, we suspect that specific athletes, such as throwers, may benefit from upper body plyometrics. While we do not recommend upper body plyometrics as a replacement for upper body strength training, medicine ball training appears to be very functional and a reasonable supplement to resistance training.

COMPATIBILITY OF AEROBIC TRAINING AND RESISTANCE TRAINING

Resistance training specifically improves the ability of muscles to contract with greater force. Locally, aerobic training improves aerobic enzymes and blood flow to muscles. Aerobic training does not make you stronger. The adaptation to training is specific to the stimulus. But what if an athlete wants to pursue extensive aerobic and resistance training? Will the training adaptations be compromised?

Maximum Box Height

"How high should the boxes be?" This is often the most frequent question coaches ask when planning depth jump training. The height of the box is directly related to the strength and power of the athlete. If an athlete jumps off a box and tends to collapse, the box is too high. You will need a reasonable number of shorter boxes to give athletes time to adapt to box jumping. Short boxes can be interspersed into a long line of boxes. We determine the maximum box height by first measuring vertical jump. Now have your athletes jump off boxes of increasing heights. Athletes should be able to repeat their maximum vertical jump off the box; if not, the box is too high. This method determines maximum box height as well as the jumping ability of the athlete!

In an early study conducted in 1980, Hickson had subjects perform endurance exercises, strength exercises, or a combination of both (38). Strength training did not affect aerobic improvements but aerobic training compromised gains in strength. Subjects in this study only trained for 8 weeks and the training program was quite arduous. Researchers have argued that the subjects in this study were simply overtrained (6). Since this first study on incompatibility in 1980, several have studied this same question. Not all have agreed with Hickson's original finding. Additionally, studies have also addressed the effect of aerobic training on power (39–41). Although additional research is still needed, some general findings of these studies are:

- Strength training does not seem to compromise aerobic training.
- Extensive aerobic training may negatively affect gains in strength.
- Extensive aerobic training probably has more negative effects on higher velocity resistance movements required for power events.

Since power is one of the desired attributes of sport, we do not recommend significant aerobic training for power athletes. Strength and power athletes need a preponderance of strength and power training, not aerobic training.

SUMMARY

- Resistance training is a safe and effective method of improving strength.
- Muscles play an important role in joint stability and stronger muscles result in stronger joints.
- Some athletes such as swimmers and rowers require considerable muscle endurance for success.
- Many athletes require high velocity muscle contractions (power) for success.
- A basic strength training program should precede specific muscular endurance or power training.
- Individuals initially adapt to resistance training by neural adaptation. As training continues the muscle fibers increase in size (hypertrophy).
- Although single set training improves strength, athletes who need excellent strength should perform multiple sets.
- Strength training for competitive athletes should involve eight sets per muscle group twice a week.
- Vary the exercises to stress the same muscle group.
- Multi-joint exercises are preferred over single-joint activities.
- Periodized resistance training is superior to straight set training.
- Successful resistance training programs require supervision.
- Power training such as plyometrics and high velocity resistance training should supplement basic strength training.
- Concurrent strength and aerobic training may compromise the development of power.

References

1. The American Academy of Pediatrics. Strength training by children and adolescents. *Pediatrics* 2001;107(6):1470–1472.

2. American Orthopaedic Society for Sports Medicine. *Proceedings of the Conference on Strength Training and the Prepubescent.* Chicago: American Orthopaedic Society for Sports Medicine, 1988.

3. National Strength and Conditioning Association. Youth resistance training: position statement paper and literature review. *J Strength Cond Res* 1996;18:62–75.

4. Armstrong N. *Young People and Physical Activity.* New York: Oxford University Press, 1997.

5. Boyle M. *Functional Training For Sports.* Champaign, IL: Human Kinetics, 2004.

6. Fleck S, Kraemer W. *Designing Resistance Training Programs,* 3rd ed. Champaign, IL: Human Kinetics, 2004.

7. Goldberg A, Etlinger J, Goldspink L, et al. Mechanism of work-induced hypertrophy of skeletal muscle. *Med Sci Sports Exerc* 1975;7:248–261.

8. Sale D, McDougall J, Alway S, et al. Voluntary strength and muscle characteristics in untrained men and women and body-builders. *J Appl Physiol* 1987;62:1786–1793.

9. Hather B, Tesch P, Buchanan P, et al. Influence of eccentric actions on skeletal muscle adaptations to resistance. *Acta Physiol Scand* 1991;143:177–185.

10. Hakkinen K, Alen M, Komi P. Changes in isometric force- and relaxation-time, electromyographics and muscle fiber characteristics of human skeletal muscle during strength training and detraining. *Acta Physio Scand* 1985;125:587–600.

11. Sale D. Influence of exercise and training on motor unit activation. *Exerc Sport Sci Rev* 1987;15:95–151.

12. Jablecki C, Heuser J, Kaufman S. Autoradiographic localization of new RNA synthesis in hypertrophying skeletal muscle. *J Cell Biol* 1973;57:743–759.

13. Kubo K, Kanehisa H, Fukunaga T. Effects of different duration isometric contractions on tendon elasticity in human quadriceps muscles. *J Physiol* 2001;536(2):649–655.

14. Reeves N, Maganaris C, Narici M. Effect of strength training on human patella tendon mechanical properties of older individuals. *J Physiol* 2003;548(3):971–981.

15. Sale D. Neural adaptation to resistance training. *Med Sci Sports Exerc* 1988;20:135–145.

16. Fleck S, Kraemer W. *The Ultimate Training System: Periodization Breakthrough.* New York: Advanced Research Press, 1996.

17. American College of Sports Medicine. The recommended quantity and quality of exercise for developing and maintaining cardiovascular and muscular fitness in healthy adults. *Med Sci Sports Exerc* 1990;22:265–274.

18. Rhea M, Alvar B, Burkett L, et al. A meta-analysis to determine the dose response for strength development. *Med Sci Sports Exerc* 2003;35(3):456–464.

19. Marx J, Ratamess N, Nindl B, et al. Low-volume circuit versus high-volume periodized resistance training in women. *Med Sci Sports Exerc* 2001;33:635–643.

20. McGee D, Jessee T, Stone M, et al. Leg and hip endurance adaptations to three weight-training programs. *J Appl Sports Sci Res* 1992;6:92–95.

21. Johnson J, Colodny S, Jackson D. Human torque capability versus machine resistive torque for four Eagle resistance machines. *J Appl Sports Sci Res* 1990;4:83–87.

22. Peterson M, Rhea M, Alvar B. Maximizing strength development in athletes: a meta-analysis to determine the dose-response relationship. *J Strength Cond Res* 2004;18(2):377–382.

23. Baechle T, Groves B. *Weight Training: Steps to Success,* 2nd ed. Champaign, IL: Human Kinetics, 1998.

24. Baechle T, Earle R, Wathen D. Resistance training. In: Baechle T, Earle R. *Essentials of Strength Training and Conditioning,* 2nd ed. Champaign, IL: Human Kinetics, 2000:395–425.

25. Stone M, O'Bryant H, Garhammer J. A hypothetical model for strength training. *J Sports Med Phys Fitness* 1981;21:342–351.

26. Willoughby D. The effects of mesocycle length weight training programs involving periodization and partially equated volumes on upper and lower body strength. *J Strength Cond Res* 1993;7(1):2–8.

27. Bompa T. *Periodization Training for Sports.* Champaign, IL: Human Kinetics, 1999.

28. Rhea M, Phillips W, Burkett L, et al. A comparison of linear and daily undulating periodized programs with equated volume and intensity for local muscular endurance. *J Strength Cond Res* 2003;17(1):82–87.

29. Harris G, Stone M, O'Bryant H, et al. Short-term performance effects of high power, high force, or combined weight-training methods. *J Strength Cond Res* 2000;14(1):14–20.

30. Szymanski D, Szymanski J, Bradford T, et al. Effect of 12 weeks of medicine ball training on high school baseball players. *Med Sci Sports Exerc* 2004;36(5):S207.

31. Newton R, Murphy A, Humphries B, et al. Influence of load and stretch shortening cycle on the kinematics, kinetics and muscle activation that occurs during explosive upper-body movements. *Eur J Appl Physiol* 1997;75(4):333–342.

32. Cavagna G, Dusman B, Margaria R. Positive work done by a previously stretched muscle. *J Appl Physiol* 1968;24:21–32.

33. Fatouros I, Jamurtas A, Leontsini D, et al. Evaluation of plyometric exercise training, weight training, and their combination on vertical jumping performance and leg strength. *J Strength Cond Res* 2000;14(4):470–476.

34. Chu D. *Plyometric Exercises with the Medicine Ball,* 2nd ed. Livermore, CA: Bittersweet Publishing Company, 2004.

35. Wilson G, Murphy A, Biorgi A. Weight and plyometric training: effects on eccentric and concentric force production. *Can J Appl Physiol* 1996;21:301–315.

36. Fortun C, Davies G, Giangarra C, et al. Computerized isokinetic testing of patients with rotator cuff impingement syndromes demonstrates specific RTC external rotators power deficits. *Phys Ther* 1997;77:S106.
37. Schulte-Edelmann J, Davies G, Kernozek T, et al. The effects of plyometric training of the posterior shoulder and elbow. *J Strength Cond Res* 2005;19(1):129–134.
38. Hickson R. Interference of strength development by simultaneous training for strength and endurance. *Eur J Appl Physiol* 1980;45:255–263.
39. Dudley G, Djamil R. Incompatibility of endurance and strength training modes of exercise. *J Appl Physiol* 1985;59:1446–1451.
40. Hennessy L, Watson A. The interference effects of training for strength and endurance simultaneously. *J Strength Cond Res* 1994;8:12–19.
41. Sale D, MacDougall J, Jacobs I, et al. Interaction between concurrent strength and endurance training. *J Appl Physiol* 1990;68: 260–270.

Nutrition and Performance

Upon reading this chapter, the coach should be able to:

1. Describe why good nutrition supports optimal athletic performance.
2. Explain why an adequate intake of carbohydrate supports energy production during physical activity, and describe ways to optimize muscle glycogen stores.
3. Explain why athletes have higher protein needs than sedentary people, and estimate protein needs for their teams.
4. Discuss how vitamin needs change only a little with an increase in physical activity, and give advice on whether or not an athlete should consider a multivitamin and mineral supplement.
5. Describe which athletes are most likely to be at risk for iron-deficiency anemia.
6. Provide athletes with guidelines for optimal fluid intake during practices and competition.
7. Offer athletes general guidelines for consuming a nutritious diet.
8. Give athletes advice on pregame meals and snacks, how to eat and drink well for optimal recovery from exercise, and eating during daylong competitions and endurance events.
9. Find nutritious meal options while traveling with their teams.

Ryan joined his high school's lacrosse team during his sophomore year. His team was very competitive, and Ryan's soccer training and athletic ability helped him excel at this new sport. Although he had not done much exercise over the winter, he responded quickly to the strenuous training sessions and felt himself getting stronger each day. Ryan was looking forward to the competitive season.

Several of the team's competitions consisted of tournaments that lasted all day, or sometimes all weekend. The team attended their first weekend tournament just a few weeks after they began training.

Ryan's team did well the first day, winning all three games. At home that night Ryan's parents were out. Ryan was so tired he had no appetite, but knew he should eat something, so he grabbed a little leftover beef stew and went to bed early. The next morning he awoke late, almost missing the bus to the tournament. No time for breakfast, he wolfed down a sports bar on the ride.

A steady cool drizzle greeted the team as they disembarked from the bus. As predicted, the games were more challenging today as Ryan's team advanced to the semifinals. Ryan played hard and well during the first game. Hungry, he grabbed a banana during the half hour break before the second game, and drank plenty of water.

Ryan started to feel really hungry and tired during the second game. He called for a sub when he could, but the coach kept sending him right back in on the next point. During the second half of the game, Ryan felt like he was in a dream. Time slowed down; he felt dizzy and disoriented. His head began to ache, and he couldn't concentrate on the game. Although he willed his legs to move, they felt like lead, and he missed the ball twice in a row. The coach pulled him out of the game after the opposing team scored another point. After the lunch break Ryan started to feel a little better, but still shaky and his head continued to pound. He was disappointed in himself, and was forced to watch the last game of the day from the sidelines.

Good nutrition plays a supporting role in sports training and performance. Food provides us with fuel and the substances our bodies need to make energy, to grow, to repair damage, and to maintain good health. While good nutrition cannot make a great athlete, inadequate nutrition can interfere with training and prevent athletes from performing up to their abilities. Ryan's story illustrates the devastating effects that can result from poor nutrition.

Coaches must encourage their players to eat well so they can play well. Good nutrition, along with a generally healthful lifestyle, helps keep athletes in the game. Well-fed athletes have the energy and strength, both physically and mentally, to achieve their personal best. Well-nourished athletes are less likely to get "run down." They have stronger immune systems, which means fewer colds and flus, and thus fewer missed practices and contests. Good nutrition helps prevent fatigue, a leading cause of sports injury. In addition, good nutrition contributes to lifelong good health, and coaches can provide a positive influence on young people as they establish eating habits that may last a lifetime.

But let's admit it: coaches have limited power when it comes to influencing athletes' daily food choices. You are limited in the amount of nutrition advice you can give (See Focal Point: Nutrition Advice: How Much Can Coaches Give). In addition, athletes do most of their eating when they are away from you, except when you are traveling together. This means that you, the coach, have two nutrition jobs. First, give your athletes good sports nutrition guidelines and use your persuasive influence to encourage them to eat well on a daily basis. And second, feed your athletes well when they are in your care.

This chapter begins with basic sports nutrition information that will help you apply nutrition science to sports performance. Along the way we will address the questions about food and nutrition that coaches

FOCAL POINT

Nutrition Advice: How Much Can Coaches Give?

Coaches often field questions about nutrition, weight control, and lifestyle recommendations for peak performance. As a coach, you must remember that the type of nutrition and weight control advice that you may give is limited. Your scope of practice, what you are allowed to do in your profession, is proscribed by several different institutions, including your employer, your state, your certification organization, and your sport governing body.

Your employer may set limits on how much nutrition advice coaches may give. If you have any questions about your employer's policies in this area, be sure to discuss these with your athletic director. Your organization may be limited by state regulations, and be concerned about liability issues.

Your state governs the licensure of nutrition professionals. Some states, such as Ohio and Florida, mandate that only licensed professionals, such as registered dieticians, may provide nutrition advice for monetary gain. State regulations trump guidelines from other organizations. Lifestyle Management Associates summarizes state laws regarding who can give nutrition advice on their helpful website, http://lifestylemanagement.com/state_law_pages.

Your certifying organizations and sport governing bodies may also provide guidance for you regarding scope of practice. Many certification programs, such as the National Strength and Conditioning Association, include some basic sports nutrition information in their programs, and allow professionals with certain certifications to provide basic nutrition information to athletes. If you are certified, check with your organization to review their limitations regarding how much nutrition advice you may give your athletes.

(continues)

Nutrition Advice: How Much Can Coaches Give? *(continued)*

Most institutions and organizations allow coaches to give mainstream, scientifically sound, basic nutrition advice that promotes the health and well-being of their athletes. For example, you may encourage athletes to eat by the Food Guide Pyramid (explore www.mypyramid.gov), and reinforce basic messages such as consume more vegetables, fruits, and whole grains, and fewer foods high in saturated fats. You can teach your athletes how to read food labels. You can share handouts with general nutrition information from reputable writers and organizations. You may encourage athletes to drink plenty of fluids and to replenish fuel stores with carbohydrates and proteins following workouts.

Coaches should never diagnose health problems or prescribe treatments, including dietary supplements. You should also avoid acting as a psychotherapist. Be ready to refer your athlete to a licensed nutritionist or dietician, or other health care provider, if:

- You suspect your athlete has disordered eating or exercise behavior.
- Your athlete has a lot of questions about his or her diet that go beyond "general information."
- Your athlete has a medical condition, such as diabetes.
- Your athlete wants to follow a restrictive diet.
- Your athlete wants specific daily meal plans.

Helpful websites:

American Dietetics Association. www.eatright.org

Lifestyle Management Associates. http://lifestylemanagement.com/state_law_pages

United States Department of Agriculture. Mypyramid.gov: Steps to a Healthier You. www.mypyramid.gov

commonly field from their athletes. The second part of this chapter will discuss more specific coaching issues such as pregame meals, eating on the road, and nutritional support for day-long events.

UNDERSTANDING NUTRIENTS

A nutrient is a substance that the body must obtain from food in order to maintain good health. Your body needs over forty different nutrients. Scientists classify nutrients into six categories. Carbohydrates, proteins, and fats provide the chemical bond energy that your body captures and converts into usable energy. (You can also obtain energy from alcohol, but since alcohol is not required by the body, it is not considered a nutrient.) These energy nutrients also provide chemical units from which the body builds the molecules and tissues it needs. Carbohydrates, proteins, and fats are called macronutrients because your body needs them in relatively large amounts. When we talk about the amounts of these nutrients in food, you will see we measure them in grams.

Vitamins and minerals are called micronutrients because we need them in smaller amounts, and they are usually measured in smaller units such as milligrams (mg). Vitamins provide chemical units that participate in thousands of important biochemical reactions in the body. For example, vitamin D is essential for packing calcium into bone tissue. Many B vitamins play important roles in energy production. Minerals have many different functions. Calcium and phosphorus, for example, give strength to bones and iron gives hemoglobin the power to carry oxygen in the bloodstream. Like vitamins, minerals also participate in hundreds of biochemical reactions.

The sixth nutrient, water, always seems to come last on the nutrient list, even though it is the most essential nutrient for both sports performance and for staying alive. Most athletes already know that bodies function at their best when optimally hydrated.

Carbohydrates

One of the most important training goals for athletes in many sports is to maximize their ability to produce energy quickly and efficiently. You need energy for muscular contraction, oxygen delivery, and for thinking. Athletes in sports that require a great deal of energy for training and/or competition have the most to gain from optimal fueling, and the most to lose when they, like our lacrosse player Ryan in the story above, are running on empty.

GLYCOGEN

Your body's primary sources of energy for physical activity are glycogen, a carbohydrate stored in the muscles and the liver, and fat, stored in the muscles and throughout the body. Muscle glycogen provides fuel for muscle contraction, while liver glycogen provides a steady supply of glucose to maintain optimal blood glucose (blood sugar) levels. Your brain relies primarily on glucose delivered by the blood for fuel, so when blood glucose levels fall you may feel disoriented, spacey, or confused. That's your brain in trouble.

Your body relies heavily on glycogen for moderate to high intensity exercise. Low intensity activities such as walking rely primarily on stored fat for energy, while low to moderately intense activities such as jogging use both fat and glycogen for fuel.

On average, people can store only about 800 to 2,000 calories of energy in glycogen (1,2). Figure 9.1 summarizes the energy contained in the body's energy stores. You can see why liver and muscle glycogen stores can run low after a couple hours of endurance activity. And keep in mind that glycogen stored in nonexercising muscles is not readily available to the exercising muscles. This means that your body can't really access all of the stored muscle glycogen.

Endurance athletes are particularly concerned about maximizing glycogen stores for training and performance. Your body can make fat from just about anything you eat, but optimal glycogen stores depend on an adequate intake of dietary carbohydrate.

DIETARY CARBOHYDRATE

The dietary carbohydrate family includes sugars, starches, and dietary fiber. Sugars, also called simple carbohydrates, are relatively small molecules that are quickly absorbed following digestion. Sugars occur naturally in the plant foods we eat: fruits, vegetables, and grains. Milk contains a sugar called lactose (many people have difficulty digesting this sugar—see Focal Point: Milk "Allergies"). Sugar is also added to many food products, such as desserts and beverages. During digestion and absorption, your body breaks down all of these various sugar molecules into glucose.

Starches are made up of hundreds of glucose units strung together in various formations (Fig. 9.2). Starches, also called complex carbohydrates, are found in plant foods and their products. Especially high in starch are grains and grain products, such as breads and pasta; root vegetables such as potatoes, beets, and carrots; and vegetables that are plant seeds, such as corn, peas, and beans (think energy storage). Your body digests starches into glucose.

Dietary fiber cannot be broken down by your digestive system. It remains in the digestive tract, and forms the bulk of the stools. Fiber slows digestion and the absorption of nutrients. A good fiber intake (25 g per day) keeps your digestive tract healthy and prevents constipation. Too much fiber consumed at the wrong time, however, can cause discomfort and diarrhea during physical activity, especially activities that require continuous running.

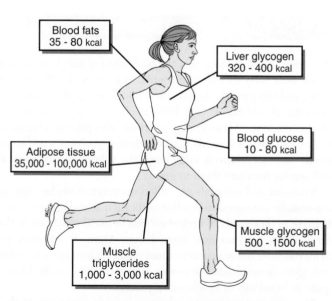

■ **FIGURE 9.1** Energy stores. Approximate caloric value of various energy storage sites. Adipose tissue energy stores vary widely depending upon person's size, muscle fiber type composition, and body composition.

FOCAL POINT

Milk "Allergies"

Do you have athletes who say they are allergic to milk? In most cases, their "allergies" are not true allergies, which are an immune system response, but actually lactose intolerance, a problem with milk digestion. Some people lack the digestive enzyme lactase that breaks down milk sugar, also known as lactose. When lactose is not well digested, people experience excess gas, bloating, and abdominal cramps. Not good for optimal performance! Most lactose intolerant people become very good at avoiding the foods that cause discomfort.

Caucasians are one of the few groups that continue to digest milk in adulthood. A majority (greater than 80%) of Hispanics, African Americans, Asians, and Native Americans are lactose intolerant.

Some athletes avoid milk because they believe it causes extra mucus production or triggers asthma. Scientific evidence does not support this claim. While milk does leave a coating in the mouth and throat, this is from the milk itself, and is not extra mucus and is not related to allergies (1). Swallowed food is rarely a cause of asthma. Food allergies are almost always marked by systemic symptoms such as anaphylaxis, swelling of the throat or tongue, severe hives, or symptoms of shock, such as a drop in blood pressure.

1. Pinnock CB, Arney WK. The milk-mucus belief: sensory analysis comparing cow's milk and a soy placebo. *Appetite* 1993;20(1):61–70.

FOCAL POINT

Fast and Slow Carbohydrates: Glycemic Index

Your digestive system breaks down the carbohydrate stored in foods at different rates. This rate depends upon many factors, including the molecular configuration of the carbohydrates and the other foods with which the carbohydrate is consumed. Dietary fats and fiber slow down the digestion and absorption of carbohydrates.

The glycemic index of a food is a measure of how quickly the carbohydrate in that food is digested and absorbed as blood glucose; in other words, how quickly glucose appears in the bloodstream following consumption of that food. Another measure, glycemic load, represents a more accurate picture of a food's influence on blood sugar, because it takes into account both glycemic index and the amount of carbohydrate present in that food. Carrots, for example, have a high glycemic index, but because a serving of carrots has a relatively low carbohydrate content, their glycemic load is not so high. Tables listing food's glycemic indices and loads can be found at www.mendosa.com/gilists.htm and www.glycemicindex.com (1,2). These are great sites for people who want to learn more about glycemic index and glycemic load.

Most athletes do not need to be concerned with glycemic index or load. A few exceptions include the following:

- Athletes experiencing hypoglycemia (low blood sugar)—these athletes need a food or beverage that will get sugar back in the bloodstream quickly. Most sports drinks deliver sugar quickly.
- Athletes with diabetes, or other problems with blood sugar regulation—these athletes may regulate carbohydrate intake to minimize spikes in blood sugar following food intake, and thus look for food and food combinations lower in glycemic load. Diabetic athletes should include protein and high-fiber foods with snacks and meals to slow carbohydrate absorption.

(continues)

Fast and Slow Carbohydrates: Glycemic Index *(continued)*

- Athletes looking for ways to refuel during physical activity or who must refuel quickly before the next work-out—high glycemic foods will have a faster impact on blood sugar. Fruit juices, sports beverages, and other high-sugar foods low in fat and fiber allow carbohydrate to enter the bloodstream quickly.
- Athletes looking for pregame foods that will release glucose into the bloodstream more slowly—lower glycemic foods may be more helpful here. Pasta dishes, smoothies (yogurt-fruit drinks), and bananas are common pregame foods.

1. Mendosa D. Revised international table of glycemic index (GI) and glycemic load (GL) values, 2002. Available online at www.mendosa.com/gilists.htm. Accessed June 28, 2007.
2. University of Sydney. GI database, 2005. Available online at www.glycemicindex.com. Accessed June 28, 2007.

AVOIDING AN ENERGY SHORTAGE

Maintaining good muscle and liver glycogen stores is not too hard for most well-fed athletes. Most of us automatically include carbohydrate foods in every meal; that is just how people in almost every culture tend to eat. Nutritionists recommend that active people, including athletes, consume between 55% and 65% of their calories as carbohydrates. Endurance athletes who use a great deal of glycogen during practices or contests should shoot for the higher figure. For someone who eats about 2,000 calories a day, this comes to 1,100 to 1,300 calories of carbohydrate, or 275 to 325 grams of carbohydrate (each gram of carbohydrate is worth about 4 calories of energy). Someone who needs 4,000 calories a day would need twice as much, or 550 to 650 g of carbohydrate. Fortunately, you do not have to search too hard to find carbohydrate food choices! Common breakfast carbohydrate foods include cereal, toast, bagels, pancakes, waffles, milk, and fruit. Lunch often features bread in sandwiches and fruit, and dinner usually includes at least one serving of starchy foods such as pasta, rice, bread, or potatoes. Table 9.1 lists the carbohydrate content of some common foods.

Research suggests that many athletes could improve their performance by consuming larger amounts of carbohydrate (see Focal Point: Does Carbohydrate Intake Really Make a Difference?). Glycogen stores need not be depleted to be sub-optimal. Some athletes may consistently consume somewhat lower than optimal carbohydrate intakes for the energy demands of their sport.

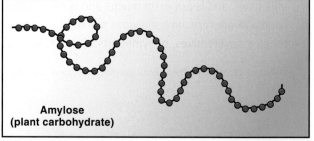

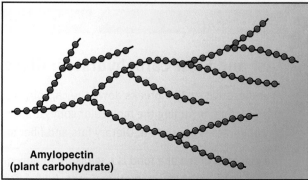

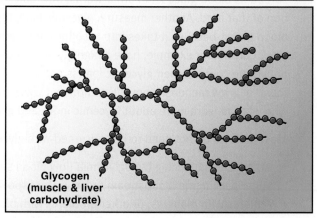

■ **FIGURE 9.2** Common forms of starch. Starches are composed of hundreds of glucose units. Pictured are two common forms of plant starch found in foods, amylose and amylopectin, and glycogen, the storage starch found in your muscles and liver.

TABLE 9.1 Carbohydrate Content of Selected Foods

Food	Serving size	Carbohydrates (g)
Soft drinks	12 oz	25–40
Apple juice	8 oz	30
Lemonade	8 oz	28
Orange juice	8 oz	26
Gatorade	8 oz	14
Milk, 1%	8 oz	13
Beer	12 oz	13
Bagel	1	57
Bread, whole wheat	1 slice	21
Waffle, Eggo	1	14
Saltines	5 crackers	10
Spaghetti noodles, cooked	1 cup	40
Pizza	4 oz slice	29
Raisin bran	1 cup	45
Rice Krispies	1¼ cup	29
Cheerios	1 cup	22
Raisins	¼ cup	31
Banana	1 medium	28
Grapes	1 cup	28
Blueberries	1 cup, raw	21
Apple	1 medium	20
Jam/preserves	1 tablespoon	14
Peanut butter	2 tablespoons	6
Hummus	1 tablespoon	3
Sugar	1 teaspoon	4
Baked potato	1 large	60
Mashed potatoes	1 cup	35
Green peas	1 cup, cooked	25
French fries	10 pieces	17
Carrots	½ cup sliced, boiled	8
Spinach	1 cup, boiled	7
Tomatoes	1 cup, chopped, raw	6
Baked beans	1 cup	55
Lentils	1 cup, cooked	40
Kidney beans	1 cup, cooked	40

Sources: Food labels and Pennington JAT, Douglass JS. *Bowes and Church's Food Values of Portions Commonly Used*. Philadelphia: Lippincott, Williams & Wilkins, 2005.

Athletes who eat inadequate calories and carbohydrates can run into serious problems. Ryan's story in the opening paragraph of this chapter is typical of less experienced athletes who have not yet cultivated good sports nutrition habits. Ryan's failure to replenish his glycogen stores led to low blood sugar and poor performance.

Athletes with hectic schedules who live on their own and may not have enough food around, or who are fatigued, sometimes fail to consume adequate calories or carbohydrates. Some athletes may not understand the importance of an adequate intake of carbohydrates, or may even be avoiding carbohydrates, possibly in an attempt to lose weight. You might find these athletes running on empty even for vigorous exercise of shorter durations, since they may begin activity with lower than optimal glycogen stores. Help educate these athletes about the importance of a balanced diet and good sports nutrition.

Are there times during the year when your athletes compete in tournaments that last 1 or more days? Or times when you hold double practices? During these periods you may need to be a little more careful that your athletes consume some extra carbohydrate calories. And if your practices and contests frequently require 90 minutes or more of vigorous exercise, then your athletes will benefit from understanding the importance of stocking and replenishing glycogen stores as efficiently as possible. Here are some suggestions for maintaining optimal glycogen stores.

- Train regularly for your sport. Training increases the ability of muscles to store and use glycogen, so the muscles required for your sport get really good at storing and using energy.
- Consume a food or drink with plenty of carbohydrate within an hour of each practice or competition. Your muscles' glycogen storage chemistry is in high gear following exercise, so give them the carbohy-

FOCAL POINT

Does Carbohydrate Intake Really Make a Difference?

Many coaches tend to believe that carbohydrate intake is only important for athletes who rely primarily on aerobic energy production. Most studies have looked at long distance runners and swimmers performing long training sessions. But adequate glycogen stores are also important in many team sports that require power and strength over an extended period of time. An interesting study of elite ice hockey players found that players who consumed diets high in carbohydrate demonstrated better performance during a game.

Like many team sports, ice hockey requires intermittent high intensity exercise. Players typically play one minute shifts interspersed with 1 to 3 minutes of recovery (1). Out of a 60 minute game, players are on the ice about 20 minutes. Does carbohydrate intake matter for these athletes?

To answer this question, Christian Akermark and colleagues recruited volunteers from two elite Swedish ice hockey teams. Half of the volunteers consumed 40% of their calories as carbohydrates (their normal diet), while the other half received a 60% carbohydrate diet for 3 days in between two games. Athletes, who were in season, trained as usual on 2 of these days. The researchers observed the following:

- Athletes on the higher carbohydrate diet had 45% higher glycogen levels at the beginning of the second game than athletes on the lower carbohydrate diet. Researchers concluded that the athletes' normal diet (40% carbohydrate) does allow for adequate glycogen resynthesis in between games.
- A motion analysis of the athletes demonstrated that those on the higher carbohydrate diets skated on average a 30% greater distance during the game, and skated faster than athletes in the other group. High carbohydrate players went in for more shifts, and spent more time on the ice than low carbohydrate players. Differences were greatest during the last period of the game, when fatigue levels typically lead to a decline in performance.

1. Akermark C, Jacobs I, Rasmusson M, et al. Diet and muscle glycogen concentration in relation to physical performance in Swedish elite ice hockey players. *Int J Sport Nutr* 1996;6:272–284.

drate they need to pack in energy for the next workout or competition. It can take 24 hours or more to replenish glycogen stores, so start right away.

- Be sure to include carbohydrate foods in meals or snacks that follow vigorous exercise. Include carbohydrate foods in other meals as well.
- Alternate hard and easy training days, and give your body at least 1 day of rest each week. Taper before important contests. Rest allows glycogen stores to build to optimal levels, in addition to allowing your body adequate time for recovery.

SHOULD YOUR ATHLETES PRACTICE CARBOHYDRATE LOADING?

Endurance and ultra-endurance athletes sometimes engage in carbohydrate loading in hopes of boosting their glycogen stores even higher than normal. In fact, another word for carbohydrate loading is "glycogen supercompensation." The idea is to make the body so eager to manufacture some glycogen that it overdoes it, and stores some extra.

How do you make the body eager to manufacture glycogen? You give it the message that energy demands are high and that current glycogen stores are inadequate. And then give it time to recharge. You can give your body this message in several ways. Early experiments in glycogen loading had athletes "strip" glycogen supplies by exercising to exhaustion a week before a major competition, and then follow this day with 3 days of a low-carbohydrate diet with moderate training. Theoretically, at this point muscles should be screaming for carbohydrate (3 days of high carbohydrate followed, with little exercise). This resulted in increased glycogen stores (3).

Most people find this procedure difficult and fatiguing. Many athletes report feeling lethargic and depressed if they train when carbohydrate intake is low (4). Researchers have also expressed concern that such extreme dietary manipulation could lead to the loss of muscle tissue and other negative health effects (3).

Fortunately, the low-carbohydrate diet phase does not appear to be essential for stimulating extra glycogen storage. A gradual combination of tapering exercise volume and increasing carbohydrate intake seems to be just as effective for improving athletic performance. Most endurance athletes who use carbohydrate loading simply taper exercise, and maintain a high intake of carbohydrates for 3 or 4 days before competition.

Some athletes have experimented with other loading methods. One interesting study had seven male cyclists perform 3 minutes of very hard cycling, and then consume a very high carbohydrate diet (10 g carbohydrate per kg) during the following 24 hours (5). The researchers found that glycogen stores doubled from the previous day's pre-exercise levels.

Individual responses to carbohydrate loading, and indeed, to any type of dietary manipulation, vary tremendously. Several studies have questioned whether any kind of carbohydrate loading, aside from providing adequate carbohydrate in the diet, improves performance (6,7). Results of carbohydrate loading in female athletes have been particularly mixed, although one recent study suggested that females generally do improve performance when extra calories along with extra carbohydrates are added to the diet several days before competition (8).

Coaches should also remember the potentially negative aspects of carbohydrate loading. Athletes must practice any type of dietary change during training, not competition. Athletes who add new foods, or change the volume or timing of food intake may experience abdominal cramps or diarrhea. Successful carbohydrate loading adds 2 to 4 pounds of body weight. This is mostly water weight, because each gram of carbohydrate is stored with three grams of water. The extra weight bothers some athletes, while others figure the water will come in handy during an endurance event.

Most coaches tell us that asking athletes to carbohydrate load is not worth the effort, unless coaches are working with elite endurance athletes who are willing to go to great lengths to practice carbohydrate loading. Simply following the guidelines presented in the previous section for optimizing glycogen stores appears to be enough dietary support for most athletes.

Protein

Protein in the diet provides building blocks called amino acids that the body then uses to make its own proteins. Much of this protein is found in muscle and other structural components, such as the collagen in tendons, ligaments, bone, and other organs. Proteins also make up the immune cells that fight infection; red blood cells that carry oxygen; neurochemicals such as serotonin that carry messages between nerve cells; and the enzymes that regulate biochemical processes, such as those responsible for energy production. In addition, the body metabolizes some amino acids for energy, especially during heavy or long bouts of physical activity or when glycogen supplies are low.

Amino acids are often likened to letters of an alphabet, and proteins to words that are spelled with those letters. In order to spell a word, you must have enough of the right letters available when you need them. Our bodies use 20 different amino acids to manufacture the wide variety of proteins we require. Given an adequate protein intake, we can make ten of the amino acids we need. The other 10 are called essential amino acids which means we must obtain them from our diet.

Our bodies do not store a large supply of amino acids, so to have the letters available when we need them, we must consume adequate protein, including all 10 essential amino acids, daily. Foods that contain all 10 essential amino acids are called complete proteins. Meat, dairy products, and eggs all contain complete protein. Plant proteins are often short one or two amino acids, but since most cultures combine plant proteins in meals (for example, consuming rice with beans, or peanut butter with bread) plant foods can provide a plentiful protein supply.

The U.S. Recommended Dietary Allowance (RDA) for protein is 46 g for average sized adult women and 56 g for adult men (9). Since protein needs vary with size, we often take body weight into account in our recommendations. Thus, the recommended protein intake for sedentary adults is around 0.8 grams per kilogram of body weight (or 0.36 g/lb). People who are significantly overweight (overfat) should base their calculations on a weight that would be healthy for them.

DO ATHLETES NEED EXTRA PROTEIN?

Much research suggests that both strength and endurance athletes need more protein than sedentary people. Protein needs increase for several reasons, including:

- To build more muscle, in response to strength training
- To repair muscle fibers damaged by training
- To increase red blood cell supply (exercise training increases blood volume)
- To replace amino acids metabolized for energy

Adolescents also need extra protein to support their growing bodies. Figure 9.3 illustrates recommended protein intakes for a variety of groups. The harder athletes train, the more likely they are to need extra protein. Athletes who train a few times a week at a fairly low intensity have only slightly higher protein requirements, about 1 g/kg body weight.

Research shows that most people in North America easily meet or exceed protein requirements. Most athletes also get plenty of protein in their diets. As energy expenditure increases, so does hunger! Athletes usually consume more protein as they eat more food. One survey of athletes found that most athletes, including a wide range of both strength and endurance athletes, males and females, consumed enough protein (10). Excess protein intake (above protein requirements) does not increase muscle mass or improve performance and may be associated with health problems (see Focal Point: Do High Protein Diets and Protein Supplements Enhance Athletic Performance?).

But there are some important exceptions. As you think about the protein needs of the athletes you coach, be aware that some individuals and certain groups of athletes may fail to consume adequate protein. Most vulnerable are adolescents who are restricting calories, especially those who are vegetarians or who consume little meat. Dancers, figure skaters, cheerleaders, distance runners, female gymnasts, lightweight rowers, and wrestlers may consume too few calories.

Restrictive diets pose a double risk for protein intake. First, fewer calories and the elimination of certain food groups tend to lead to an inadequate protein intake. And second, when carbohydrate intake is too low, the body will burn more protein to meet energy needs. Less protein supplied but more protein metabolized may create a protein deficit, and can mean loss of lean tissue and reduced muscle strength, a weaker immune system, and in females, loss of the menstrual cycle.

Athletes who severely restrict calories are at risk for numerous health problems, not to mention reduced athletic performance, and are discussed in more detail in the next chapter. Let's just say here that they probably need nutrition counseling at least, not just more protein in their diets. Athletes who do not

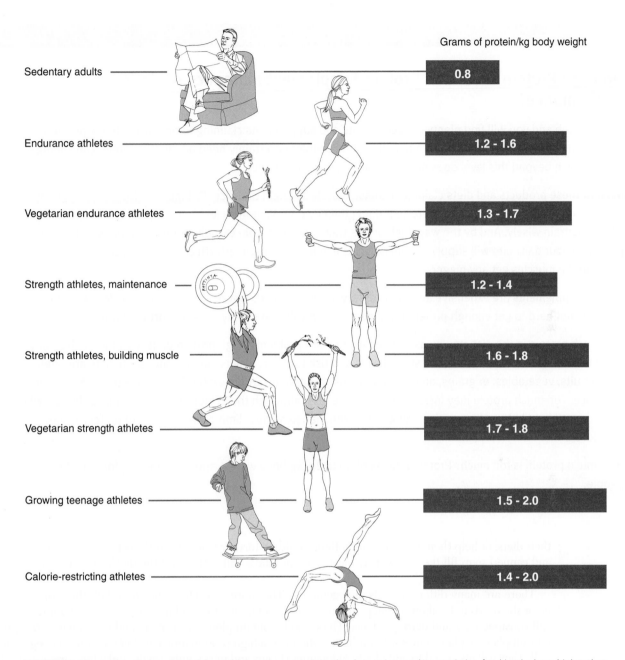

Grams of protein/kg body weight

Sedentary adults	0.8
Endurance athletes	1.2 - 1.6
Vegetarian endurance athletes	1.3 - 1.7
Strength athletes, maintenance	1.2 - 1.4
Strength athletes, building muscle	1.6 - 1.8
Vegetarian strength athletes	1.7 - 1.8
Growing teenage athletes	1.5 - 2.0
Calorie-restricting athletes	1.4 - 2.0

■ **FIGURE 9.3** Recommended protein intake. Athletes who are training hard, growing, and/or restricting food intake have higher than normal protein needs. Numbers are grams protein per kilogram body weight.

pay much attention to food choices might benefit from some good information to help them choose foods at each meal that will help them meet their higher protein needs. Table 9.2 lists some common foods and their protein content.

VEGETARIAN ATHLETES

When coaches hear that their athletes are vegetarian, they may wonder whether those athletes are getting the protein they need. But protein is not the only nutrient that may be lacking in vegetarian diets. Important vitamins and minerals may be low as well.

Vegetarian diets can be very nutritious. Many vegetarian athletes have chosen a vegetarian diet to improve their health, and in the interest of health, they educate themselves about nutrition and meal planning. Some people, however, think that simply giving up meat will automatically improve the quality of

Do High Protein Diets and Protein Supplements Enhance Athletic Performance?

Surf the web and you will find plenty of special diets and supplements claiming to enhance athletic performance. Many of these feature high protein intakes. While athletes certainly need adequate protein, consuming extra protein beyond this level does not enhance athletic performance.

Most of these products and diets claim to increase muscle strength and size. But muscle size and strength are determined more by genetics and exercise training than by diet. Your muscles may increase in strength and size when you train wisely. And by the way, fuel for this training comes from carbohydrate, not protein. Adequate protein in your daily diet will supply the amino acids needed for muscle growth and repair; excess protein will not help the muscles get any bigger.

Protein supplements are expensive and unnecessary, except in cases where athletes are truly deficient in protein. It is not hard to get enough protein from foods, which will also supply other important nutrients.

Too much protein in the diet may be associated with health problems. High protein diets are often high in saturated fats, which increase blood cholesterol levels and risk for heart disease later in life. Such diets are often low in fruits, vegetables, or grains, and may fail to supply enough carbohydrates for exercise training and performance. Too much protein may increase risk of bone loss, although the evidence for this is mixed. People who are susceptible to kidney disease, including those with diabetes, must limit protein intake to protect kidney function.

How much protein is too much? Protein intakes of up to 2g/kg body weight appear to be safe for most healthy people.

their diets, or help them lose weight. Nothing could be further from the truth! If French fries, ice cream, and canned soup fill the void left by meat, protein intake will suffer, and the diet will be too high in fat and salt.

There are many different kinds of vegetarians. The more restricted a person's diet, the more careful he or she needs to be about menu planning. Some vegetarians simply eliminate meat from their diets, but still consume eggs and dairy products. These foods contain plenty of protein, and will enhance the protein supplied by plant sources. But athletes who need a high protein intake will need more than eggs and milk; they will also need to add plenty of legumes (beans and peas), nuts, seeds, and whole grains to their diet. These foods will also help to add iron and zinc, minerals plentiful in meat.

With each food group eliminated from the diet, certain nutrients are a little more likely to be inadequate without good menu planning. A vegan diet is one of the most restrictive, since it contains no animal products. Vegan athletes must consume a variety of protein sources throughout the day to ensure adequate amino acid intake (Fig. 9.4). Vegan athletes who are trying to meet fairly high protein requirements will have to eat a lot of food. For example, a 70 kg athlete trying to consume 1.8 g/kg of protein (recommended protein intake for vegetarian strength athletes) will need 126 grams of protein. A quick glance at Table 9.2 will show you that's a lot of peanut butter, lentil soup, and soy milk!

A high intake of plant foods means a diet high in fiber. While fiber is good for your health, it may also cause digestive problems during physical activity. Protein supplements (available in vegan formulae), and fortified rice and soy beverages provide low-fiber protein options.

Protein is not the only nutrient that may be low in a vegan diet. Other nutrients of concern include:

- Vitamin B_{12}: Found only in animal products and in nutritional supplements. Vegans can obtain B_{12} from nutritional yeast, or from vitamin B_{12} fortified products such as breakfast cereal and soy milk.

TABLE 9.2 Protein Content of Selected Foods		
Food	**Serving size**	**Protein (g)**
Milk, 1% fat	1 cup	8
Yogurt	1 cup	8
Ice cream	½ cup	3
Cottage cheese, 1% fat	1 cup	6
Cheese, American	1 slice	5
Tuna, canned	2 oz	13
Cod, baked	3 oz	19
Hamburger	3 oz	22
Chicken	3 oz	25
Egg	1 large	6
Walnuts	1 oz	7
Sunflower seeds	1 oz	6
Peanut butter	2 tablespoons	7
Kidney beans, cooked	1 cup	15
Lentils, cooked	1 cup	18
Soy milk	1 cup	6
Rice, white, cooked	1 cup	4
Spaghetti noodles, cooked	1 cup	7
Bread	1 slice	3
Oatmeal, cooked	1 cup	6
Cereal, Cheerios	1 cup	3
Chocolate chip cookie, 2¼' diameter	1 cookie	1
Potato, baked	1 large	6
Broccoli, chopped	1 cup	6
Butternut squash, mashed	1 cup	3
Apple	1 medium	0
Banana	1 medium	1
Blueberries, raw	1 cup	1

Food labels and Pennington JAT, Douglass JS. *Bowes and Church's Food Values of Portions Commonly Used*. Philadelphia: Lippincott, Williams & Wilkins, 2005.

- Iron: Vitamin C triples iron absorption from plant sources, such as legumes, grains, and vegetables. Females may also need iron fortified food products, such as breakfast cereals.
- Zinc: Found in grains, nuts, seeds, and legumes.
- Vitamin D: Plant sources do not provide vitamin D, which is added to milk products to enhance calcium absorption and utilization. Vitamin D is often added to food products such as orange juice and soy milk. Regular exposure to sunlight will help prevent low vitamin D levels.
- Riboflavin: A B vitamin plentiful in milk, it is also found in dark green vegetables, and added to fortified foods.

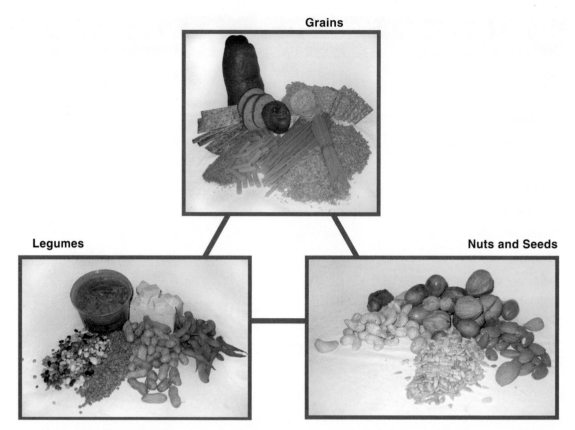

Grains

Legumes

Nuts and Seeds

■ **FIGURE 9.4** Vegan protein combinations. Vegan athletes consume no animal products and must consume a variety of protein sources throughout the day to ensure an adequate intake of the amino acids they need. Combining food from any two of the three plant protein groups supplies high quality protein. For example, a combination of peanut butter (legume group) plus bread (grain group) or rice (grain group) and beans (legume group) provides all the different amino acids your body needs.

- Calcium: Found in dark green vegetables, sesame seeds, legumes, and grains. Since daily requirement for this mineral is fairly high, it is often difficult to meet calcium needs through plant sources alone. For this reason, many vegans add calcium-fortified products such as orange juice and soy milk to their diets.

Fats

We have said that athletes need more carbohydrates and more protein than their sedentary friends. What about fat? Athletes do not appear to have an increased need for fat, except perhaps in terms of an increased need for energy (calories). Fat is a concentrated source of energy, providing 9 calories per gram versus the 4 calories per gram provided by carbohydrates and protein. Endurance and ultra-endurance athletes striving to maintain a high caloric intake to fuel their very high energy needs must have plenty of fat in their diets in order to get enough calories in a reasonable amount of food.

Both athletes and nonathletes need fat in their diets to provide essential fatty acids and add flavor to food. Fat slows the rate at which food empties from the stomach, so meals with some fat feel more satisfying. Adding fat to a meal slows the absorption of carbohydrate into the blood stream. Dietary fat helps your body absorb fat-soluble vitamins.

Fat is an important fuel for physical activity of low to moderate intensity. At low intensities we use fats from the bloodstream. These can be provided by meals or by the breakdown of fat (triglyceride) from fat cells. As exercise intensity increases, we rely more on the triglycerides stored in the muscle tissue, along with some carbohydrate. And at high intensities, little fat is burned for fuel.

Using fat for fuel is a great idea, because fat stores are much more abundant than carbohydrate stores (see Fig. 9.1). Many athletes have manipulated training methods and diets in attempts to increase their bodies' reliance on fat for fuel, hoping to spare glycogen and avoid hitting the wall. The good news is that exercise training does indeed teach the body to use more fat for fuel at a given workload. Training regularly gears up the fat-burning enzymes.

But in general, dietary manipulations have not produced much reliable change in performance. Some researchers have given athletes very high fat diets to encourage increased fat utilization during physical activity (11,12). While fat metabolism has increased somewhat in response to dietary change in these studies, performance did not improve much, and many athletes were uncomfortable on high-fat diets.

Sports nutritionists recommend that athletes get about 20% to 30% of their calories from fats, choosing healthful sources of fats as much as possible. Nuts, avocados, olive and canola oil products, and fish supply omega-3 fatty acids, the type of fats that help to prevent heart disease and reduce inflammation.

Coaches sometimes find that a few of their athletes strive for as little fat in the diet as possible, either from misguided attempts to reduce weight or because they think fat is bad for their health. Such athletes tend to follow vegetarian diets, and their diets may be low in protein and certain vitamins and minerals. These athletes need some basic nutrition education to help correct their misconceptions (such eating behaviors may also be symptomatic of eating disorders; see next chapter).

Vitamins

Vitamins are complex organic compounds that help to regulate biochemical reactions throughout the body. Questions regarding athletes' vitamin intakes have come from two different research perspectives. First, athletes and coaches have wondered whether athletes have an increased need for certain vitamins. Are athletes more likely than sedentary people to become deficient in certain vitamins? You will see in this section that athletes in developed countries tend to meet their required dietary intakes for vitamins, with a few exceptions.

The second perspective on vitamins asks whether if enough vitamins are good, could more be better? In other words, do extra vitamins enhance physical performance? Researchers in this area have tried to better understand the biochemical functions of the various vitamins as they relate to sport performance, and to experiment with large doses in both animals and people.

B VITAMINS

Many of the B vitamins play important roles in energy production. No wonder coaches worry that their athletes might need extra vitamins. Fortunately, vitamins tend to be recycled rather than used up during metabolic processes, so athletes' vitamin requirements are not much higher than the requirements for nonathletes. Some research suggests that athletes should consume somewhat higher levels of several of the B vitamins, especially thiamin, riboflavin, and B_6 (10). Athletes generally consume more food as energy expenditure increases, so the vast majority of athletes have plenty of B vitamins in their diets. Notable exceptions include athletes on low calorie diets and athletes who generally have a poor diet. These athletes would benefit from a multivitamin supplement that supplies around 100% of the daily requirement for vitamins. Excessive doses (amounts over the required dietary allowance) of B vitamins do not appear to enhance performance, except in undernourished athletes.

The B vitamins are water-soluble, and thus are not stored to any great extent in the body. This means they are needed in the daily diet, but that extra B vitamins are usually excreted, so moderately high doses are less likely to be toxic. One exception to this is vitamin B_6, which can cause nerve damage at high doses (over 80 mg/day for people younger than 19 years old, or over 100 mg/day for those 19 and older).

ANTIOXIDANTS

Several vitamins participate in biochemical pathways that protect the body from oxidative damage. These include the vitamins C and E, the mineral selenium, and the carotenoid family. Carotenoids are plant pigments responsible for the red, orange, and deep yellow colors found in many fruits and vegetables. Many dark green vegetables contain carotenoids as well, but the dark green of chlorophyll masks the lighter shades of the carotenoids. The most well known carotenoid is beta-carotene, but many others have been studied as well, including lycopene and lutein. The body can make vitamin A from carotenoids.

Early laboratory studies on the chemical properties of antioxidant nutrients suggested they might help neutralize harmful chemicals called free radicals that are produced in the body as a part of normal cellular metabolism, and in response to environmental pollution. Oxidative damage caused by free radicals is thought to increase damage to muscle tissue and blood cells; to accelerate the aging process and diseases associated with aging including Alzheimer's disease and artery disease; and to contribute to the development of cancerous cells. Because athletes experience more oxidative stress than sedentary people, researchers have wondered whether they require higher intakes of antioxidant nutrients, and whether high intakes of these nutrients might prevent injury and/or improve athletic performance.

Most research has found that athletes are rarely deficient in these nutrients. In fact, studies have found that athletes tend to have normal levels of these nutrients, despite high levels of physical activity (13). Some studies have even found that athletes have higher levels of plasma antioxidants than sedentary people, despite no difference in dietary intake of these nutrients (13). This may be explained by the fact that regular exercise trains the body's natural antioxidant systems, so that dietary antioxidants are used more effectively (14). Indeed, some researchers have proposed that higher levels of plasma antioxidants and better functioning antioxidant systems may explain some of the health benefit that is observed with regular exercise (13).

Despite a lack of evidence that athletes need to consume more antioxidant nutrients, some researchers continue to ask, could more be better? So far, there is not much evidence that increased intake of antioxidant nutrients improves performance, unless athletes are already deficient in these nutrients (15). And some research suggests antioxidant supplements may even have negative health effects (see Focal Point: Are Antioxidant Supplements Harmful?).

Since antioxidant supplements do not appear to offer a competitive advantage, and may even be associated with health risks, athletes and recreational exercisers would be better off spending their money on

FOCAL POINT

Are Antioxidant Supplements Harmful?

Many studies are examining whether or not large doses of these nutrients might forestall illnesses associated free radical damage, especially heart disease and cancer. Several of these studies have not only failed to find a benefit, but have even found that supplements containing vitamin E or beta-carotene (one of the carotenoids) may actually *increase* risk of negative health effects (1,2).

Studies of people taking beta-carotene supplements have found slightly higher cancer rates, especially for current and former smokers (1). Scientists do not know why beta-carotene might increase cancer risk. Some suggest that at the high doses found in supplements, beta-carotene may enhance the action of carcinogens, or interfere with the action of other antioxidants.

How harmful are beta-carotene supplements in healthy nonsmokers? More research is needed. What seems clear at this point is that these supplements have the potential to be carcinogenic, so athletes should consume their carotenoids in food. A diet with a variety of fruits and vegetables is the best way to get a healthful supply of carotenoids.

Research on vitamin E has shown more mixed results. While one analysis suggested a higher mortality rate for people taking high doses (400 IU or more) of vitamin E, critics have pointed out that many of the subjects in these studies were already at risk for heart disease (2). Some studies have found health benefits from taking supplements with low doses of vitamin E (improved immune response, lower risk of Alzheimer's Disease) (3).

How harmful are vitamin E supplements? Vitamin E does not appear to be harmful at low doses (less than 200 IU). Supplements made from natural mixed tocopherols may be safer, and have more health benefits, than alpha tocopherol supplements.

(continues)

Are Antioxidant Supplements Harmful? *(continued)*

Vitamin C and selenium have not been found to be harmful, but maybe new studies will come out next year! To be on the safe side, people who decide to take antioxidant supplements should consume low doses.

1. Bjelakovic G, Nikolova D, Simonetti RG, et al. Antioxidant supplements for prevention of gastrointestinal cancers: a systematic review and meta-analysis. *Lancet* 2004;364:1219–1928.
2. Miller ER, Pastor-Barriuso R, Dalal D, et al. Meta-analysis: high-dosage vitamin E supplementation may increase all-cause mortality. *Ann Intern Med* 2005;142(1). Available online at www.annals.org. Accessed December 1, 2007.
3. Greenberg ER. Vitamin E supplements: good in theory, but is the theory good? *Ann Intern Med* 2005;142(1). Available online at www.annals.org. Accessed December 1, 2007.

healthful, wholesome foods rather than supplements. Vitamin E is found in wheat germ, nuts, seeds, avocados, and their oils, as well as some vegetables and breakfast cereals. Carotenoids are plentiful in richly colored fruits and vegetables. Consuming nine servings a day of a large variety of fruits and vegetables will help you get the whole range of nutrients and other helpful components that contribute to good health. Vitamin C is found in many fruits and vegetables, including sweet peppers, citrus fruit, strawberries, and broccoli. Selenium is found in Brazil nuts, mixed nuts, halibut, tuna, turkey and many other foods.

Minerals

Minerals are simple inorganic compounds. Most of our mineral needs are easily obtained from a well-balanced diet, with a few exceptions; most notably iron but also zinc (see section on vegetarian diets, above, for good sources of these minerals). Iron is the only mineral whose dietary requirement appears to increase, and then only slightly, in response to high doses of physical training (16). Many young women fail to consume adequate calcium, thus putting themselves at risk for osteoporosis later in life. Coaches working with girls and women should encourage these athletes to consume adequate calcium on a daily basis. Good sources of calcium include low-fat dairy products; broccoli and other dark green vegetables; and calcium-fortified products such as tofu, soy milk, breakfast cereals, and orange juice.

IRON

Iron forms an important component of hemoglobin, the molecule in red blood cells that helps to bind oxygen. Athletes participating in heavy training show somewhat higher iron losses than sedentary people. These losses appear to be highest in long distance runners and have been attributed to the destruction of red blood cells as they pass along the capillaries in the sole of the foot; the high, repetitive pressure of the foot-strike injures these cells. But nonrunners involved in heavy training also appear to have higher iron needs as well, so red blood cells may have shorter lives and thus a higher turnover when metabolic rate is high, as during exercise (17).

Iron is the most common nutrient deficiency worldwide. Iron deficiency occurs when iron intake fails to meet iron losses; thus either low iron intake or high iron loss, or a combination of both can lead to iron deficiency.

Several factors increase risk for iron-deficiency anemia. The regular blood loss that occurs with the menstrual cycle puts girls and women at higher risk, and their dietary iron needs are higher than those of men and postmenopausal women. Vegetarians and people who restrict calories tend to have a low iron intake, and be more prone to iron-deficiency. If you coach young women who tend to be calorie-restricting vegetarians, look out! A sizeable percentage of your team may be at risk for iron-deficiency anemia.

Because anemia develops slowly, athletes often adjust to their reduced hemoglobin levels and do not realize anything is wrong. Suspect anemia if your athletes are tired and if their performance is declining. Other symptoms include pale skin color, irritability, weakness, headache, and unusual food cravings. Many disorders cause these symptoms however, so anemia must be diagnosed with a blood test before initiating treatment (see From the Athletic Training Room in this section). Iron supplements can be harmful, so never recommend anything more than a daily multivitamin and mineral supplement to your tired athletes. Send them to their health care providers for diagnosis and treatment.

Why Does it Take Athletes So Long to Recover From Iron-deficiency Anemia?

Iron-deficiency anemia is not usually diagnosed until iron levels have been deficient for a long time. By the time most blood tests reveal low hemoglobin levels, iron stores have become very low. After your athletes begin taking their iron supplements, it takes quite a while for hemoglobin levels and iron stores to recover. It takes at least 2 months for the body to develop adequate hemoglobin and rebuild its supply of red blood cells once more iron becomes available.

Iron-deficiency develops in three stages. In the first stage, iron stores in the liver, spleen, bone marrow, and intestinal lining begin to drop. This storage form of iron is called ferritin. No physical symptoms are associated with low ferritin levels.

The second stage of iron-deficiency is characterized by a slowing of the shuttle service that carries iron stores in the blood. The molecule that shuttles iron around is called transferrin. As transferrin levels decline, we see reduced iron transport and lower production of hemoglobin. Physical working capacity may begin to decline in this stage.

In the third and final stage of iron deficiency anemia, blood tests finally reveal low hemoglobin levels. This is the stage at which most new cases of iron-deficiency anemia are diagnosed. Athletes may have gone for a blood test because of symptoms such as fatigue, reduced performance, trouble concentrating, or frequent illnesses.

Treatment of iron-deficiency anemia begins with diagnosing the reason for the deficiency, ruling out conditions such as ulcers that might cause internal bleeding. Sometimes heavy menstrual bleeding may contribute to excessive blood (and iron) loss. Girls and women with heavy periods may use oral contraceptives to reduce menstrual blood loss.

Treatment usually includes iron supplementation, and instructions to consume more dietary sources of iron. Meat eaters have an advantage during treatment, not only because meats contain iron, but because the iron from meat sources is better absorbed than that from supplements or plants. The body generally absorbs less than 20% of the iron in our daily diet (and only 10% in a vegan diet). Athletes with anemia are counseled to avoid foods that decrease absorption (coffee, tea, fibrous foods), increase vitamin C intake, and use iron cookware.

If your athletes take their supplements as prescribed, hemoglobin levels should return to normal in a few months. Iron stores will take 6 months to a year to recover, so encourage your athletes to continue treatment until their providers are satisfied that recovery is complete.

Beard J, Tobin B. Iron status and exercise. *Am J Clin Nutr* 2000;72(2):594S–597S.
Fallon KE. Utility of hematological and iron-related screening in elite athletes. *Clin J Sports Med* 2004;14(3):145–152.

SPORTS ANEMIA

Some athletes experience low hemoglobin levels in response to an increase in training. These lower levels have no symptoms, but the "anemia" shows up on a blood test. Researchers believe that this form of anemia, known as "sports anemia" is not the result of iron-deficiency, but rather develops because of the increase in blood volume that occurs with training. The body responds to training by first increasing plasma volume, the watery portion of the blood. It takes several weeks for hemoglobin levels to catch up, and sometimes they remain a bit low. These lower levels do not appear to hurt performance or cause fatigue (3).

ELECTROLYTES

Most coaches are familiar with electrolytes as components of sport recovery beverages. Electrolytes are a type of mineral that forms electrically charged particles when dissolved in water. Sodium, chloride, potassium, and phosphorus are electrolytes that dissolve in body fluids, where they perform many important functions, including the regulation of water balance. Some electrolytes are lost in perspiration, and must be replenished by the diet. Athletes exercising vigorously for long periods of time (longer than an hour) in the heat are at risk for dehydration. Electrolytes are added to recovery beverages to assist in the rehydration process.

Water: The Most Essential Nutrient

A lean, adult body is about 60% water by weight. Water is found in every cell of the body, in the fluid between cells, and in other body fluids, including blood, cerebrospinal fluid (fluid in the brain and spinal cord), synovial fluid, and digestive juices. All of our physiological processes, including energy metabolism, muscular contraction, and temperature regulation work best with adequate hydration. A water loss of even 1% or 2% can cause a decrease in physical performance. We lose water every day through urination, bowel movements, sweating, and breathing. Any factor that increases any of these losses increases fluid requirements.

Most coaches already keep a close eye on water availability for their athletes. Physical activity increases your fluid needs in several ways. Exercise in the heat dramatically increases water loss through sweating, as the body tries to rid itself of the heat generated by muscle contraction (see Chapter 4).

Physical activity increases water loss in neutral and cold environments as well. You lose water when you breathe, especially when the air is dry, since you humidify the air in your lungs. Cold air holds little moisture, and you can lose over a liter of fluid when you exercise for several hours outdoors in winter.

In cold air or water, the blood vessels near the surface of your skin close down to prevent heat loss and blood is shunted to the core. This change in core blood volume stimulates the kidneys to make urine, another form of fluid loss. As you warm up and circulation expands back into the skin, this water needs to be replaced for optimal performance (3).

Fluid needs vary widely from person to person, depending upon several factors (18). Take these into consideration when you are planning fluid replacement strategies for your team.

- Exercise intensity and duration: The longer and more strenuous your workout or competition, the greater the water loss.
- Environmental conditions: Water losses will be much higher in the heat.
- Individual sweating rates: Males tend to sweat more heavily than females. Some athletes on your team may be very heavy sweaters and need more extra fluids than average in hot weather.
- Body size: Big people will lose more water than smaller people.

How much attention you pay to adequate hydration will depend on your sport and environmental conditions. Plenty of water should always be easily available at practices and contests, and athletes should be urged to drink before, during, and after activity. If risk of dehydration is low for your athletes, simply encouraging plenty of water may be all you need to do. If you need to encourage more fluids, provide sports drinks. Athletes tend to drink more when fluids are cool and flavored.

If dehydration is a risk for your team either because of weather or prolonged exercise, part of the training of your athletes is learning how to stay optimally hydrated for peak performance. Part of an athlete's training is to figure out how much water he or she typically loses for a given period of time under standard conditions (whatever they are for your team), and then practice staying hydrated without developing gastric distress from too much water, sports drinks, or other beverages. Make copies of the guidelines listed below (Focal Point: Guidelines: Adequate Hydration for Peak Performance) for your athletes, and encourage them to practice good hydration. Be sure a scale is available for private pre- and postpractice or contest weight checks. (Remember that weight-conscious athletes will be uncomfortable with public weigh-ins.)

Guidelines: Adequate Hydration for Peak Performance

Consuming enough fluids is essential for peak performance. The following guidelines will help you meet your fluid needs before, during, and following physical activity (1–3).

1. **Drink plenty of water before practices and competitions**. You are limited in how much water you can absorb during exercise, so it is possible to lose water more quickly than you can replace it. Therefore, it is important to begin your long workout or contest well hydrated.
   - Drink plenty of fluids during the 24 hours preceding your practice or competition.
   - Drink 2 or 3 cups of water 2 or 3 hours before the event.
   - Drink another cup 10 or 20 minutes before the event begins.
2. **Drink during exercise**. Experts generally recommend about a cup of water or sports drink every 15 or 20 minutes, more if you are larger or a heavy sweater. Water is fine for shorter (less than 1 hour) events. If you will be exercising longer, a sports drink might be helpful to keep your blood sugar levels up and replace electrolytes (especially sodium and potassium).

   If you would like more specific recommendations regarding how much to drink during exercise, try the following:
   - Practice drinking adequate fluids during training, not during a contest. Learning how to stay hydrated is especially important if you are training for an event requiring prolonged, vigorous activity, such as a marathon, or if you compete in hot weather. Part of your training is to figure out how much water you typically lose for a given period of time under standard conditions (whatever they are for your area), and then practice staying hydrated.
   - Weigh yourself before and after physical activity. Each pound of lost weight means you should have drunk another two cups of fluids before and during physical activity. Add this to your normal drinking pattern.
   - Learn which sports drinks agree with you, if you will be using sports drinks during competition. Some people find certain drinks, especially those containing fructose, cause abdominal cramps or diarrhea when consumed during vigorous exercise. Way to lose a race!
3. **Drink after exercise**. If your workout or event was quite long, you may not have been able to drink enough to keep up with fluid losses. Drink two cups of fluid for every pound of weight lost. Sports drinks are especially helpful if you have become dehydrated. Consuming fluids with carbohydrate (sports drinks, juice) after exercise will help your body replenish glycogen stores.
4. **Check the color of your urine throughout the day**. Urine should be pale in color. Dark, concentrated urine indicates dehydration. Some vitamin supplements cause deep yellow urine. If this is your case, then monitor urine volume, which should be plentiful.
5. **Do not drink too much water**. Occasionally, blood sodium levels can dip too low when sodium losses through sweating are combined with excessive water intake. Most cases occur in slow, inexperienced marathoners (over 4 hours) who exercise at lower intensities and drink too much water. If you have exercise periods of over 4 hours, drink sports drinks instead of water, add a little more salt to your food, or eat some salty snacks like chips or pretzels.

1. American College of Sports Medicine, American Dietetic Association, and Dieticians of Canada. Nutrition and Athletic Performance; Joint Position Statement. *Med Sci Sports Exerc* 2000;32(12):2130–2135.
2. Clark N. *Nancy Clark's Sports Nutrition Guidebook*, 3rd ed. Champaign IL: Human Kinetics, 2003.
3. Thompson J, Manore M. *Nutrition: An Applied Approach*. San Francisco: Pearson Education, 2006.

POWER EATING FOR PEAK PERFORMANCE

Teach your athletes that good nutrition will help them achieve their training goals and give them the energy and nutrients they need for peak performance. Carve out a few minutes of practice time every few weeks to promote good nutrition practices. Some coaches choose to spend part of a practice discussing nutrition, perhaps inviting someone knowledgeable about sports nutrition to a practice to talk with players. Perhaps one of your athletic trainers would be willing to do a short workshop on nutrition topics most relevant to your team. One workshop is rarely enough to improve your athletes' eating habits, however. You must bring up the subject several times each season, even if just for a few minutes, to remind athletes that eating habits make a difference. This section contains suggestions for helping your athletes develop eating behaviors that support peak performance.

Encourage Your Athletes to Eat Well Most of the Time

Elite athletes develop training diets that work for them and their sports. Encourage your athletes to think of their eating habits as part of their sports training. Your basic message here is to promote the selection of nutritious foods that will supply the carbohydrates, protein, fats, vitamins, minerals, and fluids that fuel sports performance. Athletes need to eat regularly and eat well.

Hopefully most of your athletes will have encountered some good nutrition instruction somewhere along the line, at least in health class. Simple advice is often the most effective. While elite athletes may take the time to calculate how many grams of protein and carbohydrates they need, keep diet records, and read books on sports nutrition, many athletes do not have this level of interest. Work with what you have on your team.

If your athletes have internet access, send them to the USDA Food Pyramid website (Fig. 9.5). This simple and helpful site asks users to enter their age, sex, and activity level, and provides a pyramid to fit that person's approximate caloric needs. Your athletes can click on "Meal Tracking Worksheet" to print a diet record form. Ask them to write down what they eat on a typical day, and compare it to the food pyramid recommendations. This exercise shows athletes what foods they need to eat more or less of.

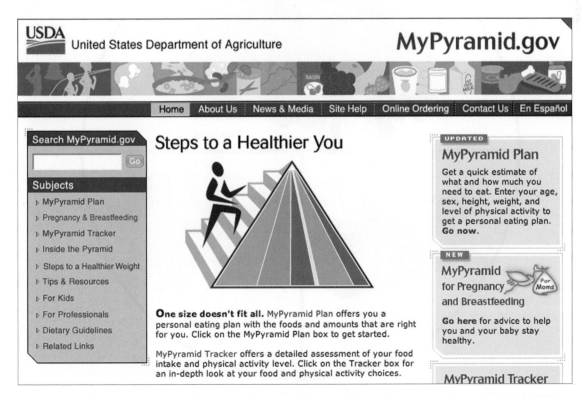

■ FIGURE 9.5 MyPyramid website. Mypyramid.gov, the United States Department of Agriculture food guide pyramid website, offers sound nutrition advice and tools for diet analysis. (Available online at www.mypyramid.gov.)

Depending upon your practices and sport, your athletes may have to add some calories to their pyramid recommendations, since activity levels only go to "over 60 minutes per day." Instruct them to spread these calories over the various food groups. If you are interested in estimating caloric expenditure, consult any of the sports nutrition books listed at the end of this chapter.

Even thinking about the pyramid may be too much for some of your athletes. An even simpler suggestion is to think of each meal as a plate (Fig. 9.6). One-fourth of the plate should contain a source of protein, one fourth a starch, and one-half fruits and vegetables. Of course the meal need not appear neatly divided in this fashion. Here are some examples:

- Meat lasagna, salad, milk, and fruit: The noodles are the starch; the meat, milk, and cheese the protein; the tomato sauce, salad and fruit are the fruits and vegetables. Make it a big salad.
- Grilled chicken sandwich with lettuce and tomato, cole slaw, fruit salad: The chicken is the protein; the bread is the starch; the lettuce, tomato, cole slaw, and fruit salad are the fruits and vegetables.
- Breakfast cereal, milk, banana, orange juice: Milk is the protein; cereal the starch; the banana and orange are the fruits and vegetables.

If one meal "plate" is a little short on a category, make a food from that category one of your snacks. For example, if lunch is a big salad with egg and tuna but little starch, grab a bagel or rice cake at snack time.

Many athletes eat a sizeable percentage of their calories as snacks. Thus, good snack choices are important, especially for athletes limiting calories. Suggest that your athletes regard snacks as small meals, and be sure food choices contain protein and carbohydrate. Instead of empty calorie foods like sodas and donuts, encourage nuts, fruits, yogurt, sandwiches, and trail mix. Treats are fine, but in moderation.

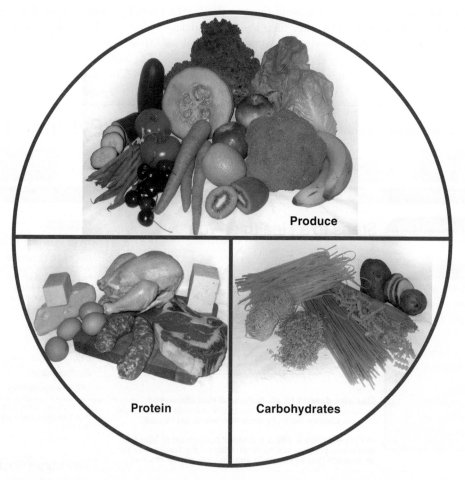

■ **FIGURE 9.6** Meal Food Choice Guide. Athletes can eat healthfully by visualizing each meal as a plate, and filling the plate as illustrated. Roughly half of the meal's volume should be fruits and nonstarchy vegetables, one-fourth other good sources of carbohydrates, and one-fourth good sources of protein.

Encourage Smart Pregame Eating

Many athletes have questions about how to eat before practice or competition. While some are looking for a magic food that will guarantee a personal best, others are simply trying to find foods that will agree with them and not cause abdominal cramps during competition or practice.

When advising your team about pregame meals and snacks, emphasize both meal content and timing. As always, athletes should practice pregame meals before practice rather than competition to be sure they know how early they can eat before activity, and what foods agree with them.

A pregame meal should be consumed at least 3 hours before activity, although smaller amounts of food closer to competition time may be fine. A meal usually takes about 2 to 4 hours to leave the stomach, a process called gastric emptying. Gastric emptying rates vary widely from person to person, and are influenced by several factors (19).

- Size of the meal—larger volumes of food take longer to leave the stomach.
- Amount of fat and calories in the meal—denser meals leave the stomach more slowly.
- Dehydration—athletes who are dehydrated experience slower gastric emptying.
- Osmolarity—fluids with small amounts of electrolytes and carbohydrates empty more quickly from the stomach than plain water, but beverages with a high carbohydrate content empty more slowly.
- Exercise intensity—the stomach continues to empty during exercise, except during high intensity exercise, when blood flow to the gastrointestinal tract declines.
- Sex—women tend to experience slower gastric emptying, and report more digestive problems during sport, than men. Women may also find that rates of gastric emptying vary with phases of the menstrual cycle.
- Stress—stress reduces blood flow to the gastrointestinal tract and delays gastric emptying.

A pregame meal should be high in carbohydrate, moderate in fat and protein, and not too big. Too much fat may "feel too heavy," and slow digestion too much, although some athletes are not bothered by this. Athletes should rely on tried and true food combinations that they know agree with them. Two or three cups of fluids should also be part of the pregame meal.

Some athletes have sensitive stomachs, or are too nervous to eat 3 or 4 hours before competition. These players should be sure to have big meals the day before. They might also try liquid meals or instant breakfast drinks for their pregame meals.

What if your athlete missed a pregame meal? Many athletes tolerate small snacks even up to an hour or less before competition. A banana, some yogurt, or a few crackers may be fine. Something is better than nothing, unless your athlete will develop abdominal cramps from eating. A sports drink with carbohydrate may help get underfed athletes through a game at least. Be sure they eat well after competition.

Urge Athletes to Eat and Drink Well for Postexercise Recovery

After prolonged exercise, glycogen storage biochemistry is all pumped up and ready to go, and your athletes may be dehydrated. Carbohydrate beverages such as fruit juice or recovery sports drinks satisfy thirst and give the body a head start on glycogen storage for the next workout or competition. Athletes who have become dehydrated should consume a beverage with electrolytes to restore fluid balance. A carbohydrate snack within an hour of exercise can also help replenish glycogen stores.

Glycogen replenishment is especially important for athletes who are burning a lot of calories each day. Most athletes have almost daily practices in season. Since it can take over 24 hours to replenish glycogen stores, consuming carbohydrate soon after a workout helps to keep an athlete's energy stores up. If you are running practices twice a day, plenty of carbohydrate in between practices is a must.

Eating During Exercise: Daylong Competitions and Endurance Events

Athletes rarely need to eat during exercise lasting less than 60 to 90 minutes. But if your athletes exercise continuously for longer than this, they will perform better if they consume some carbohydrate along with their fluids to keep blood sugar up and prevent glycogen depletion. Athletes performing prolonged endurance exercise must practice eating during training to figure out what foods and fluids agree with them.

Some athletes can tolerate fruit and candy along with sports drinks. Some will even use sports bars (and drink extra water). Help your endurance athletes figure out how they will eat during exercise.

All day competitions pose a challenge for many coaches. You need to be sure your athletes have access to good food, and to time their snacks and meals so that they do not interfere with competition. Once you have your day's schedule, plan light meals and snacks for your team around your playing times.

Many coaches must take along food for their teams. Portable meals and snacks include sandwiches; bagels, peanut butter, and jelly; muffins; fruit such as oranges, bananas, apples, and grapes; granola, cereal, and sports bars; trail mix (nuts, dried fruit, chocolate); and beverages such as smoothies, fruit juice, and sports drinks. These meals and snacks should be high in carbohydrate with some protein. Athletes should consume plenty of fluids throughout the day.

It sounds like we think athletes need to spend every free moment either exercising or eating, but of course this is not the case! Energy balance is important, and will be discussed in the next chapter. Athletes should only be replacing the calories they are burning. The calories in pregame meals and postexercise snacks should not cause weight gain (except in underweight athletes). If extra calories are consumed as part of postexercise recovery, then the next meal should be a little smaller than usual.

Growing adolescents participating in hours of daily exercise will need to consume a lot of calories to support growth, maintain health, and supply energy. But players who do not burn a lot of calories during practice (or who mostly sit on the bench during competition) need not be so concerned about glycogen depletion (see Focal Point: Fueling for Sport? Or Pigging Out?) . Try to guide your team accordingly.

Eating Well On the Road

Does your team sometimes stop for a meal while traveling to or from a contest? Eating on the road may pose a challenge to fueling your athletes, depending upon what is available in your location. Many coaches find fast food the best option for their schedules and budgets.

An occasional fatty meal will not ruin your athletes' health or prospects for your regional championship. On the other hand, if your athletes are typical of most young people, they may eat out fairly frequently. Teaching them how to eat well when dining out may benefit their sports performance and give them tools for preventing obesity in the years to come.

Most fast food establishments offer variety in their menus. Help your athletes think about choices that will increase their carbohydrate and protein intakes, while limiting their intake of fats. If limiting calories is also a concern, pay even more attention to limiting fats. Here are some general guidelines to eating well at fast-food establishments and other restaurants.

- Limit fried food. Even "healthful" meats like chicken and fish lose their health standing when fried. Remember that "crispy" is code for fried. Look for grilled and baked meats instead. While potatoes are a great food, most of their calories come from fat once they are fried. A baked potato topped with a variety of beans, vegetables, and a little sour cream, yogurt, or cheese can make a delicious meal.

FOCAL POINT

Fueling for Sport? Or Pigging Out?

Several of the coaches we have spoken with tell us their teams sometimes use sport as an excuse to overeat. A high school crew coach asks parents to help provide food for race day. "They have good intentions, but they bring tons of desserts. Come on, the race lasts for less than 10 minutes, but my athletes spend all day eating. How many calories do they really need? Now I tell them what to bring—less dessert!" A volleyball coach said she urges her team to eat well in between games during daylong tournaments. "But at the end of the day, the team practically binges on empty calorie snacks. I don't think this is healthy. There is a big difference between fueling for sport and pigging out!"

- Limit sour cream, mayonnaise, and other "creamy" additions to meals. These add fat and calories, but little protein or carbohydrates. Choose broth soups over cream-based soups.
- Sandwiches can be a great source of carbohydrates and protein. Look for lower fat fillings: turkey, roast beef, or chicken. A little cheese is fine. Add some tomato, lettuce, and other vegetables for texture and flavor.
- Avoid milkshakes unless you really need extra calories. Instead, get low-fat milk, fruit juice, a small soda, or water.
- Add fruit and salads, if your budget allows.

Eating Advice for Coaches

When we discussed our sports nutrition ideas with coaches, several suggested adding a section of advice for coaches. After all, coaching can be an endurance event! Coaches need energy to sustain them through long hours of practice and competition that often occur in the early mornings, late afternoons, or on weekends. While coaching does not usually demand the physical exertion you ask of your athletes, it demands a great deal of focus and concentration, and keeping an even temper under stressful situations.

A high energy level requires a healthful lifestyle. Food alone will not give you energy unless you are getting enough sleep and maintaining some balance in your days. If fatigue is a problem, take a look at your sleep habits and stress level along with your diet.

A well-balanced diet will help you maintain a good energy level and avoid the fatigue associated with poor eating habits. In general, small meals higher in protein foods and vegetables help you feel alert, while larger meals higher in carbohydrates can help you feel relaxed. Before a practice or contest, a small meal or large snack that is not too high in carbohydrate will give you the sustained focus and energy you need. When the contest is over and it is time to relax, join your team in a high carbohydrate meal.

But limit your calories if you tend to gain weight. Many coaches still eat like athletes, even though their physical activity levels are not what they once were. Avoid obesity by limiting portion size and avoiding empty calories. Make time in your day for exercise. Some coaches even work out with their teams when it won't detract from their coaching, for example, running warm-up laps with them.

Drink plenty of water. Remember that you lose water when you breathe; talking increases water loss even more. Keep plenty of water on hand for you as well as your athletes.

Limit caffeine. While a few cups of coffee or the equivalent do not appear to be harmful to your health, too much caffeine consumed late in the day may impair sleep quality at night. If you are frequently tired, try getting more sleep. Too much caffeine can also make you nervous and irritable.

Remember that as coach, you are a role model for your athletes. Eat the same delicious, nutritious foods you advise them to eat. Coaches need good fuel, too! And athletes respect coaches who walk their talk.

SUMMARY

- Good nutrition plays a supporting role in sports training and performance. Inadequate nutrition can interfere with training and prevent athletes from performing up to their abilities.
- Coaches may give mainstream, scientifically sound basic nutrition advice that promotes the health and well being of their athletes, but must never diagnose health problems or prescribe treatments, including meal plans or dietary supplements.
- Optimal glycogen stores help support training and performance in most sports, and require an adequate carbohydrate intake.
- Strength and endurance athletes need more protein than sedentary people, but can generally obtain sufficient protein with a balanced diet.
- Athletes should get about 20% to 30% of their calories from fats, choosing healthful sources of fats as much as possible.
- An adequate vitamin and intake is important for athletes, but extra vitamins and minerals (above the Recommended Dietary Intake) do not enhance performance.

- Coaches should give their athletes guidelines for maintaining optimal hydration to maximize performance and prevent heat injury.
- Coaches should encourage athletes to eat well most of the time, to plan smart pregame meals or snacks that will not interfere with performance, and to eat and drink well for postexercise recovery.
- Coaches traveling with their athletes should model and encourage healthful eating while away from home.

References

1. Thompson J, Manore M. *Nutrition: An Applied Approach*. San Francisco: Pearson Education, 2006.
2. Williams MH. *Nutrition for Health, Fitness, and Sport*. New York: McGraw-Hill, 2005.
3. McArdle WD, Katch FI, Katch VL. *Sports & Exercise Nutrition*, 2nd ed. Philadelphia: Lippincott, Williams & Wilkins, 2005.
4. Keith RE, O'Keeffe KA, Blessing DL, et al. Alterations in dietary carbohydrate, protein, and fat intake and mood state in trained female cyclists. *Med Sci Sports Exerc* 1991;23:212.
5. Fairchild TJ, Fletcher S, Steele P, et al. Rapid carbohydrate loading after a short bout of near maximal-intensity exercise. *Med Sci Sports Exerc* 2002;34(6):980–986.
6. Andrews JL, Sedlock DA, Flynn MG, et al. Carbohydrate loading and supplementation in endurance-trained women runners. *J Appl Physiol* 2003;95:584–590.
7. Burke LM, Hawley JA, Schabort EJ, et al. Carbohydrate loading failed to improve 100-km cycling performance in a placebo-controlled trial. *J Appl Physiol* 2000;88(4):1284–1290.
8. Tarnopolsky MA, Zawada C, Richmond LB, et al. Gender differences in carbohydrate loading are related to energy intake. *J Appl Physiol* 2001;91:225–230.
9. National Academies of Science. *Dietary Reference Intake Series*. Washington, DC: National Academies Press, 2005. Available online at www.nap.edu.
10. Manore M, Thompson J. *Sports Nutrition for Health and Performance*. Champaign, IL: Human Kinetics Publishers, 2000.
11. Burke L, Hawley J. Effects of short-term fat adaptation on metabolism and performance of prolonged exercise. *Med Sci Sports Exerc* 2002;34:1492–1498.
12. Kiens B, Helge JW. Adaptations to a high fat diet. In: Maughan R. *Nutrition In Sport*. Oxford: Blackwell Scientific, 2000.
13. Watson TA, MacDonald-Wicks LK, Garg ML. Oxidative stress and antioxidants in athletes undertaking regular exercise training. *Int J Sport Nutr Exerc Metab* 2005;15:131–146.
14. Brites FD, Evelson PA, Christiansen, MG, et al. Soccer players under regular training show oxidative stress but an improved plasma and antioxidant status. *Clin Sci (Lond)* 1999;96:381–385.
15. Powers SK, DeRuisseau KC, Quindry J, et al. Dietary antioxidants and exercise. *J Sports Sci* 2004;22(1): 81–95.
16. Akabas SR, Dolins KR. Micronutrient requirements of physically active women: what can we learn from iron? *Am J Clin Nutr* 2005;81(5):1246S–1251S.
17. Telford RD, Sly GJ, Hahn AB, et al. Footstrike is the major cause of hemolysis during running. *J Appl Physiol* 2003;94:38–42.
18. American College of Sports Medicine, American Dietetic Association, and Dieticians of Canada. Nutrition and Athletic Performance; Joint Position Statement. *Med Sci Sports Exerc* 2000;32(12):2130–2135.
19. Jeukendrup A, Gleeson M. *Sport Nutrition: An Introduction to Energy Production and Performance*. Champaign, IL: Human Kinetics, 2004.

Weight Control and Disordered Eating

Upon reading this chapter, the coach should be able to:

1. Explain the most common methods of estimating body composition, and describe how these tests are typically used in sport settings.
2. Explain to athletes how to interpret the results of body composition tests given the errors inherent in these measures.
3. Discuss the variables that influence an athlete's body fat level.
4. Refer athletes to appropriate professionals for dietary advice on weight control.
5. Discourage athletes from using very low-calorie diets to lose weight quickly, and explain why these diets are ineffective in the long run, and why they interfere with sport training and performance.
6. Caution athletes who are trying to "make weight" against the use of harmful dehydration practices.
7. Understand how dieticians construct diet plans for weight loss and weight gain.
8. Explain the variables associated with successful weight control.
9. Recognize the signs of disordered eating and develop a plan for referring athletes who are having problems to professional help, should the need arise.

Kira had always been a little heavier than many of her friends. Not surprisingly, she looked a lot like everyone else in her family: big boned, stocky, and strong. She was an excellent athlete, played a variety of sports throughout school, was pitcher for and captain of her high school softball team, and was recruited to play softball in college.

The transition to college dining hit Kira pretty hard. Kira had a healthy appetite and was tempted by the variety of food served at each meal. The "freshman fifteen" took her by surprise, however; she got out her spring clothes and found that nothing fit. And softball season was ready to begin!

Kira asked her coach about the best way to lose weight quickly. The coach herself had lost 20 pounds a few years ago on a very low-calorie diet, and gave Kira the book she had used. The diet allowed only 1,400 calories a day, and very few carbohydrates—Kira's favorite foods! Kira wondered how she would live without bread and pasta.

Nevertheless, Kira pursued the diet with the same self-discipline she used for her sports conditioning. And sure enough, she lost 5 pounds in the first week! Kira was ecstatic. But during the second week Kira's performance started to decline. Her swing lost its power, and her pitching accuracy was off. One day after a 2 hour practice, Kira felt so dizzy she had to sit down, and skip the end of practice laps.

Kira felt miserable as she sat in the shade, her head spinning. How had she gone from MVP team all star to rookie wimp in 2 weeks? She wondered why she felt so weak, and decided maybe this diet was not a good idea.

How much does a coach really need to know about weight control and eating disorders? After all, unlike the coach in the case study above, you are not going to put your athletes on weight loss diets or counsel them out of their eating disorders. But body composition is at least somewhat related to performance in most sports, so change in body composition may be a training objective for some of your athletes. Many will approach you with questions about body composition, weight, and performance. You may also need to correct misinformation that you hear regarding weight control.

This chapter opens with a discussion of body composition. We will review the most common ways to estimate body composition, and discuss how these measures are typically used in sports training situations. We will also review the many variables that work together to determine an athlete's body fat level.

Sometimes a coach may wish to nudge overweight athletes to consider reducing body fat levels. Is there a way for a coach to do this without creating problems? Can you adjust team practices to help overweight athletes burn a little more fat while training for peak performance? What diets work best for athletes? Where should you send your overweight athletes for sound weight loss advice?

Some sports, such as wrestling, boxing, and light weight rowing, have weight categories for competition. Athletes in these sports strive to "make weight" but may end up sacrificing strength, power, endurance, and coordination when their attempts lead to dehydration and glycogen depletion. If you coach one of these sports, this chapter will help you help athletes to decide what weight category is best, and guide them to make weight in ways that maximize peak performance.

What do you say to an athlete who asks for advice on gaining weight? Should you ever suggest an athlete gain weight? The next section presents advice on gaining in ways that lead to a healthy body composition, rather than extra adipose tissue that may leave your athlete saddled forever with problems related to obesity.

Body image, appearance, and weight become psychological issues for many young people, and athletes are no exception. Obesity rates continue to skyrocket in our cultures that promote overeating and sedentary lifestyles. Yet media images of perfect bodies, both male and female, have become increasingly unrealistic. Children and adolescents often struggle to figure out if they are okay, and self-esteem can suffer when they feel that they do not live up to their families', friends', and society's expectations.

Sports add another dimension to body image issues. In many cases, sports participation is protective, as athletes learn to appreciate their bodies' skill, speed, strength, and power. But in some cases, sports participation can send vulnerable athletes into patterns of harmful behaviors in attempts to change weight and size, and into the tailspin of eating disorders or drug abuse. This chapter concludes with a section on harmful weight control practices, body image, and eating disorders to help you, the coach, understand these devastating situations. As a coach, you can help prevent eating disorders among athletes on your team by emphasizing good nutrition and regular sports training, rather than "ideal weight," as the most effective means for achieving peak performance. Coaches must also be prepared to address the issue of athletes with eating disorders. It is imperative that you, the coach, are able to recognize the warning signs of disordered eating and other pathogenic weight control practices, and refer troubled athletes to professional help before it is too late.

BODY COMPOSITION AND SPORT

People come in all shapes and sizes, including athletes. As everyone knows, certain shapes and sizes confer a performance advantage in some sports. For example, being tall is an advantage if you play basketball, while a small stature is a prerequisite for racehorse jockeys. Thinness helps if you are a ballerina, whereas bigger is better for sumo wrestlers.

Much of a person's shape and size is outside our control. Athletes and coaches tend to focus on the few things they can affect, however limited: muscle size and body fat level. Many athletes are able to lose or gain several pounds with a well-balanced weight control diet and appropriate exercise. It is a mistake to believe, however, that muscle size and body fat levels are infinitely malleable. Mother nature sets limits on each person's capacities for change. Problems result when athletes believe that unrealistic change is simply a matter of having enough will power and training.

What is Body Composition?

Most people gauge whether or not they are too fat by evaluating their body weight. Weight is often evaluated in relation to a person's height. Body mass index (BMI) is one such weight for height measure (Fig. 10.1). BMI is commonly used to assess whether an individual is overweight or obese (1). A BMI greater than 25 is regarded as overweight, and a BMI of greater than 30 is classified as obese. In children and adolescents, overweight classification is based on percentiles; children whose BMI is in the upper 15th percentile for their age and sex are considered at risk for overweight, and the upper 5th percentile are classified as overweight (2).

Body weight and BMI may not provide enough information for athletes, however, especially those who are quite muscular. These athletes can be heavy for their height, and technically obese by BMI classifications, but actually very lean. Their heavy weight is composed of extra muscle, which gives them power, strength, and size advantages in many sports. When these athletes have questions about whether or not they are too fat, body composition measures are more helpful than BMI.

As you know, the body is composed of many things besides fat, but in sport, body composition is simplistically divided into two components: fat and everything else. Body composition means what percentage of a person's body mass (body weight) is fat tissue, and what percent is not fat. Researchers have a fairly rough idea of the range of body fat percentages that are healthy and normal for various population groups, including athletes (3).

A certain amount of fat, called essential body fat, is required for even the leanest individual. Fat is a component of bone marrow, nerves, the spinal cord, brain, and many other internal organs. Essential fat contributes approximately 3% to 5% of body mass (3).

Body Mass Index

The body mass index (BMI) is used to determine who is overweight.

$$BMI = \frac{703 \times \text{weight in pounds}}{(\text{height in inches})^2} \quad OR \quad \frac{\text{weight in kilograms}}{(\text{height in meters})^2}$$

BMI score is at the intersection of height and weight. A body mass index score of 25 or more is considered overweight and 30 or more is considered obese.

25 Overweight Limit   Overweight

Weight	100	105	110	115	120	125	130	135	140	145	150	155	160	165	170	175	180	185	190	195	200	205
Height																						
5·0	20	21	21	22	23	24	25	26	27	28	29	30	31	32	33	34	35	36	37	38	39	40
5·1	19	20	21	22	23	24	25	26	26	27	28	29	30	31	32	33	34	35	36	37	38	39
5·2	18	19	20	21	22	23	24	25	26	27	27	28	29	30	31	32	33	34	35	36	37	37
5·3	18	19	19	20	21	22	23	24	25	26	27	27	28	29	30	31	32	33	34	35	35	36
5·4	17	18	19	20	21	21	22	23	24	25	26	27	27	28	29	30	31	32	33	33	34	35
5·5	17	17	18	19	20	21	22	22	23	24	25	26	27	27	28	29	30	31	32	32	33	34
5·6	16	17	18	19	19	20	21	22	23	23	24	25	26	27	27	28	29	30	31	31	32	33
5·7	16	16	17	18	19	20	20	21	22	23	23	24	25	26	27	27	28	29	30	31	31	32
5·8	15	16	17	17	18	19	20	21	21	22	23	24	24	25	26	27	27	28	29	30	30	31
5·9	15	16	16	17	18	18	19	20	21	21	22	23	24	24	25	26	27	27	28	29	30	30
5·10	14	15	16	17	17	18	19	19	20	21	22	22	23	24	24	25	26	27	27	28	29	29
5·11	14	15	15	16	17	17	18	19	20	20	21	22	22	23	24	24	25	26	26	27	28	29
6·0	14	14	15	16	16	17	18	18	19	20	20	21	22	22	23	24	24	25	26	26	26	28
6·1	13	14	15	15	16	16	17	18	18	19	20	20	21	22	22	23	24	24	25	26	26	27
6·2	13	13	14	15	15	16	17	17	18	19	19	20	21	21	22	22	23	24	24	25	26	26
6·3	12	13	14	14	15	16	16	17	17	18	19	19	20	21	21	22	22	23	24	24	25	26
6·4	12	13	13	14	15	15	16	16	17	18	18	19	19	20	21	21	22	23	23	24	24	25

■ **FIGURE 10.1** Body mass index. Body mass index (BMI) score is at the intersection of weight and height. A BMI of 25 or more is overweight and 30 or more is classified as obese. (Source: *Shape Up America*. National Institutes of Health)

Females have another category of essential fat: sex-specific fat, which provides them with female body parts: breasts, hips, and thighs. The leanest of females is fatter than the leanest of males thanks to sex-specific fat. These fat stores support reproductive function. It takes a lot of calories to run the menstrual cycle and to grow and nurse a baby, so extra energy stores are part of the female body, much to the dismay of many female athletes (and nonathletes!). Sex-specific fat stores contribute somewhere between 5% and 9% of body mass in females (3).

Storage fat is found in the muscle in the form of intramuscular triglycerides, and in the larger fat storage areas, such as subcutaneous fat (the fatty layer under the skin) and visceral fat (packed around the visceral organs in the abdominal cavity). Storage fat contributes about 12% of body mass in a healthy male, and roughly 15% body mass in a healthy female (3).

In general, a body fat range of 10% to 22% is considered normal and healthy for males. For females, the healthy range is about 20% to 32% fat (4). Very lean but healthy young males have been estimated to be as low as 3% fat, while lean but healthy females can be as low as 12% fat (3). Given the error in body composition estimates, described below, keep in mind that these figures are rough averages, and may not apply to any particular athlete. They are included here to give you a general idea of how much of the body is comprised of fat.

How Closely is Body Composition Associated with Performance?

This question is a difficult one to answer. Too little or too much body fat will interfere with performance in most sports at some point, but defining exactly what is too little and what is too much is difficult. Obviously, the extremely overweight person who can barely walk will not make your team. But over the years, we have known many high quality athletes who were above "ideal" body composition who did extremely well on their college teams, even at the Division I level.

Researchers have studied the associations between both body composition and body type and sports performance, mostly among elite athletes. At elite levels, we observe that athletes in a given sport do tend toward similar body types. Body composition is most strongly related to performance in sports where extra body fat lowers economy, such as in distance running and cycling, and sports where a lean appearance contributes to a high score, such as gymnastics, diving, and figure skating. Athletes in these sports may have the most questions regarding the relationship of body composition to performance. And they may have the most to gain by losing extra body fat, if the fat is lost slowly and sensibly.

But peak performance also depends upon many other factors, including good health, strong muscles, the ability to produce energy for muscle contraction, excellent sport-specific motor skills, and good decision making under competitive pressure. Athletes need physical and psychological toughness to get the most out of their sports training and competition. Inadequate nutrition can hurt all of the above. We have often seen athletes lose a few pounds in an attempt to sharpen their competitive edge, only to see performance decline because they also lost strength, power, endurance, and focus.

So the long answer to the question of body composition and performance is that the relationship depends on several variables. In some sports, at elite levels, yes, body composition is an important variable. But many coaches place more emphasis on this variable than necessary, especially considering that there are many more important variables linked to performance that athletes can actually work on in practice. Many factors affect an individual athlete's body composition. Reducing body fat can be very difficult, and your overweight athlete may already be struggling with food, weight, and body image issues.

How is Body Composition Measured?

Body composition can only be directly measured by cadaver dissection, a measure that interferes with sport performance. However, estimates of body composition can be made using a variety of techniques to measure variables such as body density and thickness of subcutaneous fat. The most common body composition tests used by sports teams include the following:

- Underwater weighing: The more people sink when placed in water, the greater their density. By calculating density from water weight, you can calculate approximately what percentage of a person's mass is fat (Fig. 10.2). Error occurs in this test because density of nonfat tissue varies somewhat from

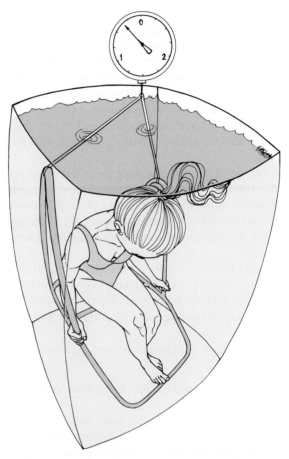

■ **FIGURE 10.2** Underwater weighing. The underwater weighing procedure provides an estimate of body composition based on a person's body density.

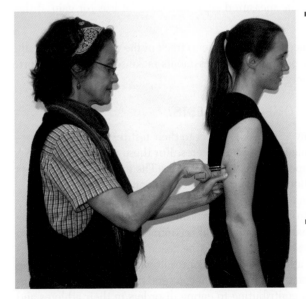

■ **FIGURE 10.3** Skinfold measurement. Body composition may be estimated from skinfold measurements.

person to person, yet the test calculations rely on an average value. The test is also difficult to administer, especially for people who have trouble exhaling completely underwater. Residual lung volume (the amount of air remaining in lungs after a complete exhalation) should be measured, since this air contributes to a person's buoyancy, but often test administrators use a predicted value instead.

- Skinfold measurements: Skinfold thickness is measured with calipers at several standard anatomic sites (Fig. 10.3). These measurements are then entered into an equation that predicts percent body fat, based on the observation that about one third of a person's body fat is stored subcutaneously (4). Skinfold measures are most accurate when performed by an experienced test administrator, since measures taken on the same person can vary widely among test administrators. If you have ever tried to take skinfold measures, you have probably observed how difficult it can be to standardize your technique. In addition to measurement error, prediction equations may over- or under-predict for any given individual, since patterns of fat deposition vary from person to person.

- Circumference measurements: A tape measure is used to measure circumferences at various body sites, such as upper arm, waist, and hips. Circumference measures are then entered into an equation that predicts percent body fat, sometimes along with skinfold measurements. Like predictions from skinfolds, predictions from circumferences are based on population averages and may not apply to a given individual.

- Bioelectrical impedance analysis (BIA): BIA is based on the fact that fat conducts electricity more slowly than nonfat tissue, which contains quite a bit of water. A weak current is sent through the body, and its speed reflects relative fatness. BIA measurement assumes a constant body water content, but people vary somewhat from this assumption. Anything that changes hydration level will affect body fat estimates, including dehydration, premenstrual water retention, food in the stomach, and elevated muscle glycogen levels (remember glycogen is stored with extra water).

- Air displacement: Instruments such as the Bod Pod estimate body composition from air displacement. The heavier you are for a given size, the denser and less fat you are. Like underwater weighing, the Bod Pod predicts body fat from body density. Individual variations in tissue density reduce the accuracy of body fat predictions.

Because body fat results are expressed as a number (e.g., 16% fat), they sound scientific. To most people, a number implies measurement precision, like height and weight. It is important to realize, however, these numbers are imprecise. Even when performed under ideal circumstances, most of these tests have a prediction error of at least 3% or 4% body fat (5). This means that an athlete found to be 16% fat may actually be anywhere from 12% to 20% fat. Many times test circumstances are far from ideal, and assumptions underlying the test may not be true for certain athletes (3,6,7). In these cases the measurement error is even greater. This huge range introduces a measure of uncertainty into any calculations your athletes may be making about how much body fat they can afford to lose. Some experts recommend reporting results as a range rather than a single number in order to give athletes a more accurate picture of what test results really indicate (8).

Wrestlers are especially vulnerable to errors in body composition estimates, since these tests are used in weight certification procedures to calculate minimum wrestling weight, and wrestlers' lowest allowable weight classes they can wrestle in without physician's consent. Most wrestling teams use skinfold measures or underwater weighing to estimate body composition, since some research (but not all) has found more error to exist with bioelectrical impedance estimates, and equipment using air displacement methods is not yet widely available at most schools (6,9–11).

Wrestling coaches must be aware of the error inherent in body composition estimates. A theoretical minimum weight may not be achievable for a given athlete. Similarly, some athletes may weigh in at a very low (even negative percent fat) body composition due to measurement error. Fortunately, NCAA and the National Federation of State High School Associations wrestling rules allow these athletes to wrestle with physician's permission (12,13).

Although body composition tests have a large margin of error, error can be reduced in several ways (11,14).

- Tests given by experienced professionals tend to be more accurate, and the results more accurately explained.
- If athletes have body composition assessed, the same test should be used each time. So, for example, if athletes were measured initially using a skinfold test, be sure the exact same test is given (by the same person, if possible) for the followup test. Then, even though the percent fat number may not be accurate, a change in value will reflect a real change in body composition.
- Be sure athletes understand that body composition tests have limited accuracy, and that it is important to follow all instructions carefully. All tests assume adequate hydration, so athletes should not be tested if they are dehydrated.
- Athletes may wish to consider using skinfolds and circumferences as stand alone measures. Changes in skinfold thickness, if the test is performed repeatedly by the same highly qualified person, will indicate changes in the thickness of subcutaneous fat at the measured sites, and thus, fat loss (or gain, if the numbers get larger) (15).

Always remind your athletes that it is performance that counts. Keep track of the numbers that really matter: performance times, goals, assists, whatever performance assessments make sense for your sport. Getting stuck on body fat numbers is a waste of energy.

WHEN SHOULD COACHES ADMINISTER BODY COMPOSITION TESTS?

Because of their limited accuracy and because many athletes overreact to their test results, body composition tests have limited usefulness and can be damaging to some athletes. For these reasons, the NCAA recommends against team weigh-ins and body composition assessments (16). (The exception is for sports such as wrestling where weight and body composition must be determined for competition.)

Coaches should not administer body composition tests to their teams or to individual athletes, but refer individual athletes seeking advice on weight control to the athletic trainer, strength and conditioning coach, exercise physiologist, or nutrition professional for advice and, if recommended, body composition analysis. This recommendation is important for several reasons. First, the coach should avoid getting entangled in disordered eating issues with individual athletes, and this can result when you start evaluating body composition. A coach who focuses too much on body composition can send the wrong signals to athletes. In some cases, coaches have been accused of contributing to eating disorders in their athletes and exceeding their scope of practice. Second, body composition tests should generally be followed up with advice on setting weight control goals and losing weight, if necessary, and the coach should not be doing these things. Third, even if the coach has received training in performing body composition analysis, the time invested in evaluating body composition will probably not pay off in terms of improving performance. Performing these tests takes too much time away from your priorities: planning and conducting practices, planning for competitions, and so forth.

You can still recommend healthy eating consistent with currently accepted guidelines without conducting body composition analyses. Eating for peak performance is important regardless of weight loss goals.

HOW ARE BODY COMPOSITION TESTS USED IN SPORTS TRAINING?

Wrestlers must undergo body composition tests at the beginning of their season to determine minimal wrestling weight. Determining minimal wrestling weight is required for both collegiate and high school wrestling. This requirement was implemented to prevent harmful weight reduction practices. If you coach wrestling, you will work closely with your athletic training staff and school medical team to evaluate each athlete and come up with the most sensible wrestling weight goal and category for him or her. Be sure to follow the guidelines provided by your institution. College coaches should consult the NCAA Wrestling Rules and Interpretations rulebook (12), and high school coaches should consult their state high school athletic association guidelines (13). Good information is also available at the National Wrestling Coaches Association website (14).

Body composition tests may also be used in sports training situations for individual athletes who are seeking advice about whether losing or gaining weight might be helpful for performance. Tests should be administered by someone qualified to work with athletes on weight control concerns (for example, athletic trainers, strength and conditioning coaches, exercise physiologists, or sports nutritionists).

Body composition tests should always be followed up with counseling regarding sensible weight control practices. Just as a medical test should never be given unless knowledge of the results will affect treatment decisions, a body composition test should never be given unless follow-up treatment, i.e., weight control programs, are part of the package if needed.

Body composition tests are especially helpful for large athletes who wonder if they are too fat. A body composition test may show that although they are "overweight," they are not overly fat. Such athletes might have a very hard time losing weight, and their attempts may not only be unsuccessful but detrimental to performance. Body composition estimates can help nutrition professionals working with overweight (over fat) athletes estimate feasible weight loss goals.

Body composition assessments may also be helpful for lean athletes who think they are too fat. When such analyses are performed by experienced nutrition professionals, body composition tests may reassure lean athletes that their body composition is right where it should be.

Athletes (with the exception of wrestlers) should never be forced to undergo body composition tests (8). Tests should be offered, if available, to athletes with questions about weight control who are motivated to discuss body weight issues with a qualified professional.

FROM THE ATHLETIC TRAINING ROOM

Helping Athletes Set Realistic Weight Loss Goals

Body composition estimates help athletic trainers and nutrition professionals set weight loss goals for athletes who could benefit from losing weight. If you know an athlete's weight and current percent fat, you can calculate what he would weigh at a healthy body composition. Recognizing the error in body composition scores, it is often preferable to calculate a healthy weight range, rather than a single number.

Weight history sometimes helps in determining a realistic weight goal. For example, if an athlete has only recently gained weight, and was at a healthy weight until then, a goal of returning to her prior weight is probably realistic. An athlete who wants to reach a low weight he has never actually weighed before may be disap-

(continues)

Helping Athletes Set Realistic Weight Loss Goals *(continued)*

pointed. Even if body composition tests suggest that the low weight would be a healthy one, that weight may not be achievable.

Setting a goal weight is tricky, because weight loss rarely proceeds as it should, even with extra exercise and dieting. Some athletes just cannot get down to their "ideal" level. Researchers suggest that obese people forget about ideal weight or weight range and only try to lose 5% to 10% of their weight (1). Unrealistic weight loss goals can be discouraging, as people diet but fail to reach their goals (2,3). Failure can lead to frustration, anger, disappointment, and depression. If the athlete is an emotional eater, which obese people often are, dieting failure may even lead to weight gain, when dieters overeat to assuage negative feelings.

Sometimes coaches and athletic trainers get questions from very lean athletes who are seeking weight loss advice. Some of these athletes want to improve performance in sports such as running and cycling, where less extra body fat can translate into faster times. Others want to achieve a lean physique to enhance their ratings in sports where appearance is part of the evaluation, such as gymnastics, diving, figure skating, or body building. Some may need to reach a specific weight to qualify for an activity, such as light weight rowing, or a lower weight class in wrestling. And some athletes may just be obsessed with food and weight. Coaches should refer these athletes to a nutrition professional. Nutrition professionals, in turn, can help these athletes determine how much weight loss is feasible and monitor performance and health to be sure weight does not go too low. Nutrition professionals can also help screen these athletes seeking minimal weight to help those with eating disorders get the professional counseling they need.

1. Foster GD, Wadden TA, Vogt RA, et al. What is a reasonable weight loss? Patient's expectations and evaluations of obesity treatment outcomes. *J Consult Clin Psychol* 1997;65:79–85.
2. Polivy J, Herman CP. The false-hope syndrome: Unfulfilled expectations of self-change. *Psychol Sci* 2000;9:128–131.
3. Sears SR, Stanton AL. Expectancy-value constructs and expectancy violation as predictors of exercise adherence in previously sedentary women. *Health Psychol* 2001;20:326–333.

What Factors Affect Body Composition?

If you had taken exercise physiology in the 1980s, you would probably have learned that weight control was a simple matter of thermodynamics. People consume energy in food. They burn calories through resting metabolism, digestion, and physical activity. A pound of body fat is worth 3,500 calories. Create a 3,500 calorie deficit by decreasing energy intake and increasing energy expenditure, and a pound of fat should be lost. Simple.

Not quite. While the laws of thermodynamics do still apply to energy balance in humans, we have learned over the past several decades about many more factors that impact energy balance and body composition, and the complexity of losing and gaining weight. Some of the factors that athletes must take into consideration as they try to change body composition include the following.

GENETICS

For centuries scientists have observed enormous individual variation in body types, and in individuals' success at losing weight. Studies of twins have lead researchers to conclude that genetic predisposition is an important risk factor for the development of obesity (18–20). For some individuals and ethnic groups, genetic predisposition for obesity is extremely strong. Their "thrifty" genes allow them to capture every calorie they consume, and to efficiently store energy, primarily as fat, against future lean times. Unfortunately, in an environment where food is plentiful, these thrifty genes translate almost automatically into obesity. Athletes with a strong tendency to store body fat must be extra vigilant in developing healthful eating and exercise behaviors. They may also need to learn to be content with a stocky body type, and aspire to sports that require big, strong athletes.

ADOLESCENT DEVELOPMENT

The hormonal changes that bring about puberty have strong effects on body composition (21). Males and females both get bigger and stronger, and females tend to get fatter as they develop. Many boys like the changes they see in their bodies as they grow bigger and stronger, and start to look more athletic, while female athletes may dislike the extra fat they are putting on. It is easy to understand why eating disorders in females often begin in adolescence as girls resist the bodily changes nature imposes. If you coach middle or high school teams, you are well acquainted with adolescent changes in body composition. Admonishing girls to lose weight during this period is especially risky since self-esteem can be fairly fragile. Focus on healthy eating and exercise instead.

BIOCHEMISTRY

Adipose tissue used to be regarded as a fairly simple holding tank for extra calories. However, biochemists have recently discovered that this active tissue sends and receives chemical messages that regulate appetite, fat storage, and many other metabolic activities, and communicates extensively with other organs including the liver, muscle, bone, and appetite centers in the brain (22). For example, as fat stores dwindle, they release lower levels of a signaling chemical called leptin. Lower levels of leptin tell the brain we are hungry. While these messengers kept our ancestors from starvation in lean times by encouraging us to look for food, in today's environment they complicate our efforts to eat less and reduce body fat.

ENVIRONMENT

Our environment encourages overeating and discourages physical activity. You know this already! Food is everywhere. People must learn to make good food choices and to be vigilant about saying no to more food when they have had enough to eat. Yet people enjoy the taste of fat, sugar, and salt: three things we tend to get too much of in food.

Research suggests that larger portion sizes push people to overeat (23,24). If extra food is on our plates, we tend to eat more than we should (Fig. 10.4). In many fast-food restaurants, the more we eat, the better the bargain. Portion sizes in other restaurants have increased over the years as well. And many individual food items, such as candy bars, muffins, bagels, and sandwiches, have grown larger over the past 30 years.

Daily life for nonathletes requires less physical exertion than ever before. Children and adolescents can get by with very little exercise in school. A number of schools have limited activity opportunities at recess (or no recess) and have cut physical education programs. Many kids and teens spend their leisure time in sedentary pursuits, watching television and movies, and playing video and computer games. A majority of school-aged children get rides (bus or car) to school rather than riding their bicycles or walking. Thank goodness for sports and coaches!

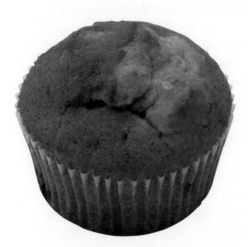

■ FIGURE 10.4 Portion size matters. Many muffins weigh almost 6 ounces, almost a full day's intake of grain equivalents for someone consuming 2,000 calories per day.

DOES THE COACHING PROFESSION CAUSE WEIGHT GAIN?

We have known many young coaches who experienced some weight gain as they made the transition from student athlete to coach. Of course, coaching, per se, does not cause weight gain, but if your activity level has decreased and you are still eating the same way you did as an athlete, you will experience an increase in body fat. This phenomenon is responsible for the mistaken belief that "muscle turns to fat" in retired athletes. You know that muscle tissue and fat tissue differ, and one kind of tissue will not "turn into" another. If you are less active your muscles may atrophy, so muscle loss occurs as you are gaining fat.

Coaches should model a healthful lifestyle for their athletes. Make time to be physically active, whether it is playing your old sport, other sports, walking, or working out. Eat a balanced diet. Get enough sleep. Enjoy life.

Does College Cause Weight Gain?

Many students do gain weight in college, especially during their first year—as did Kira, described at the beginning of this chapter. While people use the term "freshman fifteen" to describe college weight gain, the average weight gain is around 4 or 5 pounds (1). Even 4 or 5 pounds are a concern, particularly if they represent the beginning of the gradual increase in body fat that tends to occur in adults in North America. And some students do gain 10 or 20 pounds, or more, and plunge deeply into struggles with obesity and body image that may last several years or even a lifetime.

An increase in weight is not always bad, of course. Some students, especially young men, are still growing and filling out, and weight gain for them simply represents normal growth. The extra mass may be composed of muscle as well as fat, and may help in some sports. But most of the time, college weight gain is unwanted and interferes with athletic performance. Many factors influence how an athlete's body weight will respond to college life.

- College Environment: Students who leave home to go to college must adapt to a new environment and establish new habits. Life on a college campus is often marked by erratic schedules and regular opportunities to party. Some students adapt fairly quickly and establish a new routine that supports their ability to make the most of the academic and social challenges. The regular practice and competition schedule of athletics often assists students in developing a balanced routine. But other students have more difficulty self-regulating and settling into a healthful lifestyle. Changes in weight often represent the lifestyle a student develops. Some colleges and coaches do more than others to help students nurture healthful habits, but in the end it is usually up to the individual student to be sure he or she develops a healthful lifestyle.
- Activity Level: In season, most athletes get plenty of exercise. But some athletes slack off out of season. While students tend to walk from place to place, they also spend much of their time attending class, studying, reading, and writing—all sedentary activities. This lack of activity contributes to weight gain and also to feelings of stress.
- Stress: Many students encounter emotional challenges during the first year of college. First-year students often feel lonely and homesick, missing family and friends. The stress of difficult classes, roommate problems, and more demanding athletic teams can make the first year even more challenging. Feelings of stress often cause changes in appetite and eating behavior. Food is familiar and comforting, and can serve as a stand-in for missing family and friends.
- Fatigue: Fatigue increases hunger, as a lack of energy drives people to overeat. Students are notorious for skipping sleep and pulling all-nighters to complete assignments. A lack of time management and study skills, coupled with procrastination, increase the likelihood of sleep deprivation.
- Dieting: Ironically, students who try to lose weight by severely restricting food intake may end up gaining weight. Diets are often followed by periods of overeating as the dieter gives in to hunger and food cravings. Unfortunately, dieting behavior and more serious disordered eating behaviors are very common among college students, especially women.
- Social Eating: Most college social events involve food, from dining hall meals to campus parties. People are more likely to overeat in social settings, especially in all-you-can-eat dining halls where entrees are plentiful and dessert is served at every meal. Parties encourage excess alcohol consumption and snacking. Other students eat when bored, and snack as they study and work on assignments.

1. Graham MA, Jones AL. Freshman 15: Valid theory or harmful myth? *J Am Coll Health* 2002;50(4):171–174.

WEIGHT LOSS ADVICE FOR ATHLETES

Health professionals, teachers, coaches, and parents have expressed alarm at rising obesity rates in all segments of the population, including children and teens. In less than 30 years, the obesity rate for children and adolescents has doubled, and has tripled for children ages 6 to 11 (25). Much has been written about the probable short and long-term consequences of this obesity epidemic (26). Obesity increases the risk of developing type 2 diabetes, high blood cholesterol levels, high blood pressure, heart disease, and other health problems (27). Obesity increases the likelihood of emotional health problems for children as well, including low self-esteem, negative body image, and depression (26,28). Many overweight kids can attest to the observation that they are more likely than normal weight children to be the object of bullying and discrimination (28–30).

The number of overweight children, teens, and young adults you see on your teams will probably depend on your sport, age group, and competitive level. Many obese children learn to avoid physical activity, since it may be uncomfortable for them physically, and they may have unpleasant experiences in physical education and sport settings. Some sports are more welcoming than others, and less competitive leagues may accommodate less athletic people.

You have probably known some athletes who seemed overweight. You may have wondered why the athlete did not lose weight, or why the coach did not make the athlete trim down. Maybe you have some athletes on your team that seem a little heavier than desirable for peak performance. What should a coach do in this situation?

Coaching Athletes About Weight Control

If you have never struggled with body image or weight issues, you may wonder what the big deal is about a coach telling an athlete to lose some weight. Earlier in this chapter we discussed reasons why coaches should not measure body composition. The same issues arise regarding weight loss recommendations. You may think you are making recommendations in a kind, considerate fashion, but athletes can get quite defensive and upset about what they perceive to be criticisms. Your words may trigger an unwanted response, and you may inadvertently get wrapped up in an athlete's eating disorder issues.

The coach is a very powerful figure for many athletes, and, if you are lucky, your athletes will think highly of you and try to please you. Many people have a very hard time losing weight. If you suggest they lose some weight, they may go to extreme measures to do so, and be extremely disappointed if their weight control efforts do not work. Because some athletes have reported that their disordered eating started or worsened because of their coaches' suggestions to lose weight (31–33), several organizations, including the NCAA and the American College of Sports Medicine, have taken strong stands advising that coaches avoid telling an athlete to lose weight (16,34).

If you are very concerned about an athlete's body composition, you may approach your athletic trainer or team physician and get their advice. They may be able to talk to the athlete in a helpful and sensitive way, and give them some sound nutrition guidance.

FOCAL POINT

Where to Send Athletes for Sound Weight Control Advice

Counseling athletes safely and effectively about weight control takes a combination of scientific knowledge and good counseling skills. Many people market themselves as weight loss professionals, but lack adequate knowledge and training. Some people have the necessary certifications, but lack people skills or an understanding of the energy demands of an athlete's training. Ask around to find recommended professionals in your location.

(continues)

Where to Send Athletes for Sound Weight Control Advice *(continued)*

States regulate who is legally permitted to provide nutrition counseling, and define scope of practice in this area. You can find out more about your state regulations at Lifestyle Management Associates' Index of State Laws website (1). The following are the professions most likely to provide good weight control advice.

- Registered dietician—Registered dieticians have the initials "RD" after their names. A registered dietician is a nutrition professional who has fulfilled certain educational requirements, passed an exam, and maintains membership in the largest organization of nutrition professionals, the American Dietetic Association. To maintain their certification, members are required to fulfill continuing education requirements. To find an RD, go to the American Dietetic Association's website (2). You may also be able to find a registered dietician at your local hospital or sports medicine clinic, or look in the telephone book under dietitian or nutritionist.
- Nutritionist—Anyone may call him or herself a nutritionist. The terms nutritionist, certified nutritionist, and certified nutrition counselor are unregulated. If people call themselves nutritionists, check their certifications and educational background.
- Sports Nutritionist—This term may or may not refer to a qualified professional. Check certifications and educational background. Some RDs specialize in sports nutrition. Many belong to an organization called Sports Dietetics—USA (3).
- Athletic trainer—Your athletic trainers studied energy balance and weight control as part of their educational curriculum, and are accustomed to counseling athletes. Your ATs may or may not have time to work with individual athletes on weight control issues, but will probably know where to refer athletes for individualized counseling. Your ATs will also know where to refer athletes suspected to have eating disorders or other psychological problems, or athletes with nutrition-related health issues that require specialized counseling.
- Strength and conditioning coach—Certified strength and conditioning coaches usually study energy balance and weight control in their programs, and may provide good weight control advice to athletes.
- Health care providers—Doctors, nurses, physician's assistants, and nurse practitioners may or may not have studied nutrition as part of their medical education. Some may have experience working with patients on weight control, but most will probably refer patients to a registered dietician.

1. Lifestyle Management Associates. *Index of state laws*. Available online at http://lifestylemanagement.com/state_law_pages. Accessed August 30, 2007.
2. American Dietetic Association Website. Available online at http://www.eatright.org. Accessed August 30, 2007.
3. Sports, cardiovascular, and wellness nutritionists: A dietetic practice group of the American Dietetic Association. *Sports Dietetics—USA*. Available online at http:www.scandpg.org/sd_usa.php. Accessed August 30, 2007.

If athletes share with you that they are concerned about their weight, and ask advice on whether or not weight loss would be helpful, refer them to the medical team for evaluation. Be sure your response is helpful and respectful, and never make fun of your athletes who are worried about being overweight. Remind them that losing weight in season is not usually a good idea, although eating for peak performance is. They may just naturally lose a few pounds if they are more careful about food choices while consuming adequate calories, carbohydrates, and proteins.

Always maintain confidentiality regarding weight, body composition, and weight control issues. If an athlete has come to you with a weight-related concern, be sure not to share this with other members of the team. You can trust your medical team with the information, however, and they can help you reach athletes who are concerned.

Be sure to remind athletes who are working with a qualified professional to lose weight that performance, not weight, is the most important criterion. Measure performance regularly, just as you do for all of your athletes. If performance starts to decline, speak to the athlete and to the athletic trainer, and ask that weight loss efforts be adjusted so that they do not interfere with good health and competition.

FOCAL POINT

The Overweight Kids on Your Team

It is not always easy for coaches to relate to the overweight athletes on their teams. Sport is about physical accomplishment, and the most successful athletes spend hours training to achieve peak physical condition. Most athletic facilities are temples to the sleek physique or the buff, cut body builder look. Pictures of athletes adorn the walls. The students in the weight room have endless discussions about getting in shape and losing weight. Most of us live in a "lean" world. Many coaches and physical educators have had limited relationships with fat people. We have studied obesity as a disease state, and we are familiar with the treatment options, especially diet and exercise. But there our understanding stops and the problem relating to fat athletes begins, for fatness has a great deal of meaning beyond its association with health risks. We may have difficulty relating to the fat athletes on our team without patronizing or embarrassing them.

One of the qualities of fatness is high visibility. Being fat is not easy to hide. It's there, and it's judged (1). In our culture, we blame people for their fatness. It is considered a sign of moral weakness and a lack of self-discipline, the result of gluttony and sloth. How can she let herself go like this? I can't believe that fat man is eating ice cream.

Coaches should understand that it might not be easy to be the heaviest kid on the sports team. Coaches should conduct practices and contests in ways that show respect for all individuals on the team, including those who are overweight. Here are a few points to consider as you work with the overweight athletes on your team.

- A majority of people who try to lose weight are unsuccessful. Your athlete may be one of these. Researchers estimate that about 80% of overweight people who try to lose weight fail to keep it off for over a year (2). Assume weight is not changeable, and work from this assumption.
- Someone else has probably already told your overweight athletes they are overweight. Parents, other family members, teachers, doctors, and the media have probably transmitted this message. You don't need to mention it.
- Discuss performance, not weight. When an athlete is slow, it is tempting to say, "You would be faster if you lost some weight." Focus instead on training, good nutrition, and the factors you would discuss with all your other athletes.
- Evaluate injury symptoms, not weight. Fat people get tired of being told all their symptoms are related to their weight. Although some problems are caused or worsened by excess weight, your athlete still needs standard care. When your overweight athlete develops knee pain, send him to the athletic trainer or his health care provider, the same as you would for any other athlete on your team. Skip the lecture.
- Medical clearance procedures should be the same for all athletes. If your overweight athletes have made the team and are cleared to play, treat them like everyone else on the team.
- If overweight athletes try out for your team but fail to make the team, let them know how their performance fell short. Base your cuts on performance, not body composition.
- Promote an atmosphere of support and respect for all athletes on your team. Channel energy into challenging practices and building team spirit, and away from teasing. Do not tolerate bullying behavior.
- Prevent heat injury for all your athletes. Your athletes with extra weight have a harder time getting rid of heat since subcutaneous fat reduces heat exchange with the environment. If their heat tolerance is lower than others on the team, allow them to reduce activity level, drink plenty of fluids, and rest as necessary to prevent heat illnesses.

1. Teachman BA, Brownell KD. Implicit anti-fat bias among health professionals: is anyone immune? *Int J Obes* 2001:25:1525–1531.
2. Wing RR, Phelan S. Long-term weight loss maintenance. *Am J Clin Nutr* 2005;82(1):222S–225S.

Should You Adjust Practices to Help Athletes Burn More Fat?

Physical conditioning is probably one of your goals early in the season, especially if you work with athletes who do not train systematically out of season. Physical conditioning will help get your team ready for competition and prevent injury. Since you have limited practice time, you will want your conditioning program to be as sport-specific as possible, and improve the energy systems and skills most important to your sport, as discussed in Chapter 7.

Changing athletes' body composition is probably not feasible during the sport season. Exercise alone rarely causes a dramatic loss of fat, so your conditioning program will seldom lead to noticeable changes in body weight for your overweight athletes. Therefore, designing your practices to help athletes burn more fat may not be the best use of your practice time. Focus on performance goals for your team, not on body composition. Of course, the two sometimes go together. If your athletes need better endurance, endurance exercise will improve aerobic energy systems and burn calories in the process.

What about fat burning exercise? While low intensity exercise uses the greatest proportion of fat for fuel during exercise, this observation is irrelevant for weight control programs. At the end of the day, energy balance determines whether the body dips into fat stores for energy production. Low intensity exercise burns fewer calories per minute than high intensity exercise, so given limited time for physical conditioning, higher intensity exercise burns more calories and has a greater conditioning effect.

Should you give your overweight athletes some extra exercise, have them run a few more miles after practice? This is not a good idea, for the reasons given above, that exercise alone rarely leads to fat loss. Extra exercise may, however, lead to overtraining, reduced sports performance, and injury. Overweight athletes singled out for extra exercise may perceive the workouts as punitive or feel embarrassed.

FOCAL POINT

Overweight Athletes: What Can Coaches Do?

What can coaches do when they have obviously overweight athletes on their teams? Some days you feel you have to say something to someone, or do something to let your team know that being overweight hurts performance. Yet you cannot tell athletes to lose weight, you cannot put them on diets, you cannot measure body composition. What can you do?

- Invite a nutrition professional to speak with your team about sports nutrition. Hold this discussion early in your season during practice time. Require all athletes to attend.
- If athletes ask you questions about nutrition, endorse currently accepted guidelines.
- Refer athletes who ask for weight control advice to your athletic trainer, team physician, or to their health care providers.
- When you give your athletes out of season conditioning programs, encourage healthful eating as part of their training programs.
- Model healthful eating habits and a healthful lifestyle. Provide wholesome food during tournaments, while traveling, and at other team functions. Discourage overeating and empty calorie foods.
- If you work with children or adolescents, invite families to your sports nutrition presentation. If families help provide food for your team, tell them specifically what foods to send (and not to send).
- When you have concerns about specific athletes, speak to your athletic trainer or other member of your medical team.

What Diets Work Best for Athletes?

Although coaches do not perform weight loss counseling, they should still understand the basic principles of energy balance and weight control, since they will field questions from their athletes about these subjects. Coaches tell us that when they discuss sports nutrition with their teams, the topic that athletes are generally the most interested in, and ask the most questions about, is weight control.

VERY LOW-CALORIE DIETS DO NOT WORK

Many people still think "diet" when they decide they need to lose weight, especially very low-calorie diets, just like Kira in the example at the beginning of this chapter. Diets that severely restrict calories do cause rapid weight loss and, when the focus is on the scale rather than on body composition or performance, dieters appreciate the reward of watching the numbers on the scale go down.

But as you know, most of this fast weight loss is not fat loss. Rather, it is initially a loss of liver and muscle glycogen and water, as the body's carbohydrate stores are quickly depleted. If the diet continues for several weeks, some fat will be lost, but so will some muscle mass as well.

Coaches should discourage restrictive, very low-calorie dieting when the topic comes up. These diets generally do not lead to long-term weight loss. And because they do not provide enough calories to maintain good glycogen stores, they do not provide athletes with the energy they need for physical activity. Diets that eliminate or severely restrict carbohydrates are the worst, but any diet that provides too few calories will lead to glycogen depletion. Presumably your athletes should remain active throughout the year, even during the off-season, and very low-calorie diets do not support physical activity. Focal Point: Why We Think Diet is a Four Letter Word provides a summary of the reasons very low-calorie diets are ineffective for long-term fat loss, and even harmful for people who follow them.

FOCAL POINT

Why We Think Diet is a Four Letter Word

Restrictive, very low-calorie diets tend to be ineffective in producing long-term fat loss, and can even be harmful to the people who follow them. That is because these diets:

- Are difficult to stick to for very long. Because they do not provide enough calories, dieters experience hunger and strong food cravings that drive them to go off the diet, and even to overeat. For this reason, these diets can, ironically, result in weight gain rather than weight loss.
- Lead to a sense of failure. When people fail to lose weight on these diets, they feel bad, and blame themselves for a lack of self-control, rather than blaming the diet for being unrealistic.
- Do not address the causes of obesity. People gain weight because they consume more calories than they burn. A very low-calorie diet is only a short-term solution to a long-term problem. People must change the ways they eat and their levels of physical activity to maintain a weight loss.
- Teach dieters to ignore their feelings of hunger and satiety (feeling like you have eaten enough). They also teach people to ignore their appetites (what foods you feel like eating). This means after you have eaten the food prescribed by the diet, you may still feel like eating something else. Food becomes the enemy, and self-control becomes more difficult when you cannot eat foods you want to eat. More cravings develop, and make dieting more difficult. These diets do not help dieters develop a healthy relationship with food.
- Can lower resting metabolic rate. Dieters end up consuming fewer calories, but burning fewer calories as well, so weight loss stalls. Dieters may lose lean body mass, thus further reducing resting metabolic rate. Dieters also feel cold, tired, cranky, and even depressed as metabolic rate declines.

(continues)

Why We Think Diet is a Four Letter Word *(continued)*

- Lack adequate nutrition. Most very low-calorie diets urge dieters to take vitamin and mineral supplements. But dieters may still fail to consume adequate levels of certain nutrients. Poor nutrition can have long lasting, negative effects. For example, an inadequate calcium intake during adolescence and early adulthood may compromise bone density.
- Begin a life-long addiction to dieting and other dangerous weight control behaviors. Very restrictive diets may be a "gateway" behavior to other harmful practices, such as using diet pills, other drugs, and even to the development of eating disorders.

WEIGHT LOSS PROGRAMS FOR OBESE ATHLETES

Sound weight loss advice for athletes is similar to sound weight loss advice for everyone else, with the exception that athletes will need more calories to fuel a higher level of physical activity. In addition, athletes are usually encouraged to try to lose weight out of season, rather than in season, so that weight control efforts do not interfere with sports performance. This is especially true for obese athletes desiring to lose more than a few pounds of fat.

Dieticians working with athletes who need to lose weight begin with some sort of assessment. They will want to figure out why the athlete is overweight, so the cause of the obesity (such as overeating) can be addressed. The athlete may keep a record of what he eats for several days, where the food was eaten, and why he chose to eat. This food record can help uncover problems such as eating for emotional reasons (boredom, anger, stress, and loneliness, for example). It can also give the dietician information about the athlete's typical eating pattern, so that diet advice can be individualized to the athlete's food preferences. The dietician and athlete will also discuss weight loss goals (see From the Athletic Training Room: Helping Athletes Set Realistic Weight Loss Goals in this chapter).

The dietician will determine the athlete's daily calorie needs based on size and physical activity level, and then give the athlete dietary recommendations. These recommendations are often in the form of an Exchange Diet. The Exchange Diet was created by the American Dietetic Association and the American Diabetes Association as a flexible way to prescribe diet recommendations (35–37). The Exchange Diet divides foods into six groups (starch, meat/meat substitutes, fruit, vegetable, milk, and fat) and recommends how many servings of each group to eat throughout the day. A list of foods indicates which groups the food should be counted as. Portion sizes on each group list are roughly equivalent for calories. For example, on the starch list, ½ bagel is about the same number of calories as one slice of bread. The Exchange Diet can be adapted to most food preferences so athletes choose from foods to which they are accustomed. The Exchange Diet also educates athletes about food, and makes them more aware of what they are eating. If you are interested in learning more about Exchange Diets, you can find information in most nutrition textbooks (38). A good resource on diet planning for athletes using the Exchange Diet system may also be found at the Exercise Prescription on the Net website (39). Table 10.1 shows an example of an Exchange Diet Plan a dietician might recommend to an out of season athlete who would lose weight on a food intake of 2,000 calories a day, and the food choices an athlete might make using the plan.

Athletes working with nutrition professionals to lose weight can also track their calorie and nutrient intake using the mypyramid.gov website (40).

Some dieticians may simply ask an athlete to record a typical day's food intake, then go over it with him and suggest changes that would make the day's intake more nutritious and lower in calories. For example, simply reducing the number of soft drinks or switching from whole milk to skim milk can reduce daily calorie intake by several hundred calories.

What about commercial weight loss programs? Programs such as Weight Watchers that teach people how to eat a balanced diet are more highly recommended than programs that provide food or rely on meal replacement beverages. However, research shows that people can lose weight on just about any kind of program; it is keeping the weight off that is hard (41). Athletes must learn how to live with food.

TABLE 10.1 Sample Exchange Diet for 2,000 Calories

Dieticians commonly use some version of the Exchange Diet to give diet advice to their clients (1,2). This table gives an example of the food exchanges that might be recommended for a 2,000 calorie a day eating plan, and the foods an athlete might choose according to this plan.

Food Exchange Recommendations for 2,000 Calorie Plan

Food Group	Recommended Number of Exchanges
Starch	9
Vegetable	5
Fruit	4
Milk	3
Meat	6
Fat	7

Sample Food Group Recommendations for Meals and Snacks (2,000 Calorie Plan)

Meal	Starch	Veg	Fruit	Milk	Meat	Fat
Breakfast	2	–	1	1	–	–
Lunch	1	3	1	–	2	3
Snack	3	–	–	1	1	1
Dinner	2	2	1	1	3	2
Snack	1	–	1	–	–	1

Sample Menu Using Food Group Recommendations

Breakfast
½ cup lowfat granola (2 starch)
1 cup 1% milk (1 milk)
¾ cup fresh blueberries (1 fruit)

Lunch
2–3 cups tossed salad (greens, peppers, cucumbers, tomatoes, etc.) (2–3 vegetable)
2 oz tuna (2 meat)
1–2 T oil and vinegar dressing (3 fat)
4 fat-free whole grain crackers (1 starch)
1 small banana (1 fruit)

Snack (postexercise)
2 cups sports beverage (2 starch)
4 rice cakes (1 starch)
2 T peanut butter (1 meat, 1 fat)
1 cup skim milk (1 milk)

Dinner
3 oz broiled chicken (3 meat)
1 large baked potato with fat-free sour cream and salsa (2 starch)
1 cup steamed broccoli (1 veg)
1 cup steamed spinach (1 veg)
2 pats margarine or butter (2 fat)
1 cup cantaloupe cubes (1 fruit)
1 cup milk (1 milk)

Snack
1/3 cup lowfat frozen yogurt (1 starch, 0-1 fat)
1¼ cup whole strawberries (1 fruit)

Noncaloric beverages (e.g., coffee, tea, diet soda) and water may be consumed throughout the day.

1. Sizer F, Whitney E. *Nutrition: Concepts and Controversies.* Stamford, CT: Wadsworth, 2005.
2. Exercise Prescription on the Net (ExRx.net). Diet & Nutrition. Available online at http://www.exrx.net/nutrition.html. Accessed August 30, 2007.

LIFELONG WEIGHT CONTROL: WORK WITH YOUR BODY AND USE THE FORCE OF HABIT

Successful weight control programs work with, rather than against, your body. Weight that stays off is a byproduct of a healthy lifestyle that reduces the need to eat because of food cravings or emotional hunger. Successful weight control programs also help to create habits that support weight maintenance.

Most people find that restrictive eating guidelines lead to cravings for forbidden foods (42). Perhaps it is human nature to want what we cannot have. But the craving for forbidden foods may also be caused by changes in brain chemistry. If the brain thinks food is scarce, it may ramp up the drive to eat. Food restriction may also affect the levels and regulation of neurotransmitters, the chemical messengers that allow nerve cells to communicate with one another. For example, serotonin is one of the neurotransmitters that may play a role in food cravings, especially cravings for carbohydrates such as desserts, breads, pasta and fruit. Many physiological functions involve the release of serotonin, including mood, sleep onset, pain sensitivity, and blood pressure regulation. Many antidepressant medications relieve depression by increasing serotonin levels in the brain. Similarly, carbohydrate intake increases brain serotonin level, which may be why some people eat carbohydrate foods when stressed.

Research suggests that it is easiest to stick to new eating habits when you minimize hunger and food cravings. Suggestions for reducing hunger, food cravings, and emotional eating include the following:

- Eat breakfast, eat regularly, and do not skip meals. You are more likely to overeat when hungry. Hunger is especially likely to trigger overeating in the late afternoon. Consume regular meals and snacks that include small portions of protein foods for sustained energy.
- Listen to your body, including cues that tell you when you are hungry, what foods you feel like eating, and when you have had enough to eat.
- Enjoy your food, so you feel nourished rather than deprived. Avoid labeling foods as "forbidden"—you will just want them more. Enjoy small portions of foods you are craving, or low-calorie versions. Eat slowly and savor your food. Choose foods that are as delicious and satisfying as possible.
- Avoid fatigue. People experience more hunger and eat more when they are tired. When you are tired you may also feel more stressed.
- Manage stress. Stress is the leading cause of relapse in behavior change programs. When you feel bad, you do things to make yourself feel better—like eat (43,44). Instead, find other ways to soothe jangled nerves. Physical activity is a great stress reducer.
- Drink plenty of water. Thirst can be misinterpreted as hunger.
- Reduce food cues that trigger eating. When possible, avoid situations that cause overeating, or devise a better response. Mindless snacking while you watch television? Chew gum or choose more nutritious snacks. Watch less television.
- Address tendencies to overeat. If emotional overeating is a problem, find a qualified professional to help you create better ways to cope with stress.

Studies of successful losers have found that they tend to have several similarities in their strategies to maintain weight loss (41). People who have lost weight and kept it off for at least a year shape their environments and their habits to support their weight control efforts. Psychologists believe that self-control is a limited resource, even in the most self-disciplined of athletes (45,46). Using the force of habit reduces the need for will power, and increases the likelihood of success.

Athletes concerned with weight control must create eating habits that sustain a healthy body weight. Young people often live somewhat chaotic lives, with schedules that seem to change each day. As a coach, you can encourage your athletes to develop lifestyles that help them train and compete, and to create team habits that support peak performance. Coaches have shared with us ways they try to encourage their athletes to develop good eating habits and other positive lifestyle behaviors.

- Hold team discussions about the importance of good nutrition and adequate sleep, early in the season. Then check in to reinforce these topics from time to time.
- Discourage "pigging out" after competitions and tournaments. Celebratory eating (and drinking) can feature fun and a variety of food choices, but not unlimited volumes of food.
- Provide healthful snacks and meals when you eat as a team (see Chapter 9).
- Get team captains on board. Come up with team rituals that are positive, for example bagels, fruit, and yogurt on the bus home after a contest rather than stopping at the doughnut shop.
- Help your athletes see sport conditioning, including good sport nutrition, as a team effort. Social support enhances the likelihood of positive behavior change (47).
- Recommend positive, helpful books, articles, and websites, such as those listed in Focal Point: Helpful Resources for Successful Weight Control.

Helpful Resources for Successful Weight Control

When your athletes ask for recommendations for information on losing weight, here are some resources we recommend.

Book:

Clark N. *Nancy Clark's Sports Nutrition Guidebook.* Champaign, IL: Human Kinetics, 2003. This wonderful book contains a healthy serving of practical and sensible weight control advice, based in science but very readable.

Websites:

WIN: Weight Control Information Network. Available online at http://win.niddk.nih.gov

United States Department of Agriculture, MyPyramid. Available online at http://www.mypyramid.gov

Making Weight

Athletes who participate in wrestling, light weight rowing, power lifting, and boxing must weigh-in before competition at or below a set weight in order to compete. Ideally, athletes are not too far above their goal weight at the beginning of the season, so that the weight goal can be reached in a way that does not harm health or performance. Unfortunately, some athletes (with the support of their coaches) strive to achieve a weight their bodies were never meant to be, and end up resorting to dehydration to reach their goals. Dehydration may temporarily decrease weight, but it also impairs performance and puts athletes at risk for heat injury.

Achieving the lowest possible body weight in order to wrestle in the lowest possible weight class has been part of the sport of wrestling for many years. In 1997, the wrestling world was shaken when three previously healthy collegiate wrestlers, from three different states, died while working out in efforts to make weight through dehydration. In all three cases, the athletes were under direct supervision of athletic staff. All three deaths were attributed to hyperthermia and dehydration, as the athletes restricted food and fluid intake while working out in rubber suits to maximize sweating (48). To illustrate the severity of the dehydration, consider one of these cases. One athlete, a 19-year old man, had already gone from 233 lbs to 210 lbs during the previous 10 weeks. His goal was to reach the 195-lb weight class, however, so over a 12-hour period he tried to lose an additional 15 pounds. On November 6, 1997, from 3 p.m. to 11:30 p.m., he lost 9 lbs using the dehydration procedure described above, restricting food and fluid intake while exercising in a rubber suit. After a 2-hour break, he began exercising again at 1:45 a.m., on November 7. At 2:45 a.m., he stopped exercising due to extreme exhaustion. An hour later he experienced cardiorespiratory arrest (48).

These tragic and totally preventable deaths sparked efforts to reform weight cutting practices. Governing bodies such as the NCAA and the National Federation of High School Associations drafted rules and procedures to deter wrestlers from drastic weight cuts. Weight loss practices that lead to dehydration are prohibited, and if you are a wrestling coach, it is important for you to reinforce these rules, even though many of these behaviors were common practice among wrestlers not so long ago. Weight control measures that are no longer allowed include:

- Use of laxatives, emetics, and diuretics
- Excessive food and fluid restriction
- Self-induced vomiting
- Exercising in rooms hotter than 79°F (26°C)
- Using saunas and steam baths

- Vapor impermeable suits
- Artificial rehydration techniques, such as giving intravenous fluids between weigh-in and competition

Wrestlers participating in meets sponsored by the NCAA or NFHS must comply with weight certification programs that are designed to help each wrester establish a healthy wrestling weight at the beginning of the season (12,13). For high school athletes this weight is based on what the athlete would theoretically weigh at 7% body fat for males, 12% for females; for NCAA wrestlers, minimal weight is based on what the wrester would weigh at 5% body fat for males, 14% for females. If wrestlers are higher than minimal wrestling weight at the beginning of the season, they are limited in how much weight they can lose each week. For example, the NCAA wrestling rules allow a weekly weight loss of no more than 1.5% of body weight. Most wrestling programs include nutrition education for athletes, and for parents in the case of high school wrestlers, to help them achieve their wrestling weights with appropriate nutrition and exercise strategies. "Making weight" no longer means using dehydration to achieve a weight goal, but using good sports nutrition and exercise to lose weight slowly and safely.

We applaud the response of the Wrestling Coaches Association (17) and others to the harmful weight control practices that had become a routine part of the sport of wrestling. Research suggests that the rules are having the desired effect, with less weight fluctuations during the competitive season (49–51). Change happens slowly, however, and if you are coaching wrestling or other sports where weight cutting occurs, you will still see your share of harmful weight control behaviors, and must continuously work with athletes and athletic trainers to be sure recommended weight control procedures are followed. While the reforms seen in wrestling are substantial, even these better guidelines cannot prevent all problems. Wrestling coaches should still be aware of the following:

- Your athletes may still use prohibited weight loss behaviors to cut weight for their first weigh-in of the season, before they come under your care. Do what you can to discourage these practices.
- The NCAA allows athletes to lose 1.5% of body weight per week to achieve minimal weight. But this is actually a fairly rapid weight loss. Most doctors recommend only 1 to 2 pounds per week. A loss of 1.5% might be more than this for some athletes. Many athletes cannot achieve this rate of weight loss in a healthy way.
- Remember the range of error inherent in body composition estimates. The minimal weight established for a given athlete may not actually be achievable due to measurement error. And some people are simply unable to reach a very low body fat level.
- Competitions not governed by organizations which have implemented weight management rules still have wrestlers using a wide range of dangerous weight cutting behaviors (52). If you coach in this situation, we encourage you to work for better rules to protect your athletes from dehydration, hyperthermia, and potentially life-threatening situations.

GAINING WEIGHT

Some athletes may approach you with questions about how to gain weight. They might be thin, and want your advice on how to become more muscular and athletic looking. Or perhaps they play a position such as football lineman where bigger is better. Maybe you have even considered asking your scrawny linemen to chow down a little more to bulk up. How involved should the coach be with athletes who want to gain weight? When should you suggest to an athlete that he or she should gain weight?

Athletes Who Ask for Weight Gain Advice

Before handing your thin athletes a beefed up lifting and eating plan, first determine why the athlete is thin, and why he or she wants to gain weight. Your athlete may have an underlying medical condition that is responsible for the thinness, for example an imbalance in thyroid hormone levels. Some athletes have digestive system disorders, such as irritable bowel syndrome, that curb appetite and food intake. Be sure treatment for medical conditions has been addressed.

Why does the athlete want to gain weight? To enhance performance? Be sure your athletes' performance expectations are realistic for your sport. Is getting stronger and more muscular really going to help your soccer midfielder, or might extra weight training during the season compromise the aerobic endurance essential for this position? As a coach, you will not want your athletes to sacrifice sport performance to a weight gain program. Direct endurance athletes to postpone weight gain efforts until the sport season has ended.

Does the athlete want to gain weight to look better? It is normal for young people to want to look good. But some athletes may become obsessed with their appearance, and pursue a bodybuilding program to the exclusion of other interests. You may notice that they are exercising excessively and have become more interested in bodybuilding than in sport participation. They may show other signs of addiction, such as poor performance in school and exercising even when injured. If any of your athletes seem to fit this description, they should be referred to professional counseling.

Healthful Weight Gain

Most athletes want to gain muscle mass but not too much fat, although some athletes do not mind a little extra padding. But gaining too much fat can increase risk for obesity and obesity-related illness such as diabetes, hypertension, musculoskeletal problems, and heart disease. Coaches should encourage athletes to gain weight in ways that do not jeopardize future health. General weight gain advice includes the following (15,53).

- Analyze your current lifestyle. People with serious weight gain goals should work with a nutrition professional. The nutrition professional will probably have you record food intake and workouts for 3 or more days to get a picture of your lifestyle, and to figure out where changes can be made.
- Consider stress. Stress can interfere with digestive function and reduce appetite in some people. If you are having problems with stress, consult a counselor to address the issues causing stress. If available, a sports psychologist may be helpful.
- Increase resistance training. Resistance training stimulates weight gain in the form of lean body mass: muscle and bone rather than excess body fat. Athletes will want to condition in ways that enhance sport performance. A strength and conditioning coach may be able to help you design a challenging resistance training program that can enhance sport performance or be followed out of season.
- Consume protein and carbohydrate during recovery from exercise. Strength training stimulates muscle repair and growth. During recovery, your body replenishes muscle glycogen stores and rebuilds muscle fibers to make them bigger and stronger. Consuming some protein (about 6 to 20 g) along with some carbohydrate (at least 50 g) within half an hour following exercise allows recovery and muscle building metabolism to work in high gear (53). "Fast" carbohydrates that get into your blood stream quickly are best, for example fruit juice, sports beverages, sugar, or honey. If you are not hungry after a workout, consider a cool beverage such as a smoothie or shake. Some recovery sports beverages contain protein and carbohydrate.
- Allow time for full recovery following hard workouts. Muscle building requires adequate rest and recovery. Alternate hard and easy days, and include 1 rest day each week. If you strength train almost every day, alternate muscle groups.
- Eat more. To gain weight you must eat more calories. Take larger portions and add meals and snacks to your day. Think of snacks as small meals. You may need to plan ahead to be sure good food choices are available when you need to eat. Once you develop a routine, this task will be easier. If appetite is a problem, be sure to choose calorie-dense foods as much as possible. For example, choose chili or split pea soup rather than broth-based soups. Granola has more calories per bowl than puffy cereal. Healthful beverages such as smoothies are a great way to add calories.
- Be sure to consume some protein with each meal or snack. Weight gain supplements are not necessary—high protein foods such as meat, fish, eggs, and dairy products contain more amino acids at a lower cost than protein supplements. But if you have a poor appetite, meal replacement supplements can be helpful when consumed in addition to (rather than as a replacement for) your meals.

Should You Ever Recommend Weight Gain?

In the world of sport, size definitely matters. Many coaches want bigger athletes to take up more room on their teams. Bigger athletes make more intimidating linemen in football and goalies in ice hockey. More muscle means more powerful rowers, wrestlers, and throwers. Have you ever thought some of your athletes might be better with another ten or twenty pounds of body mass?

Remember that scientists no longer view fat tissue as a passive holding tank for extra calories. You cannot just temporarily expand adipose tissue without affecting the rest of the body. Rather, this metabolically active tissue interacts with other organs and influences neurochemicals that participate in many biochemical pathways. Extra fat tissue increases risk for many chronic illnesses (22).

If you are considering asking some of your athletes to gain weight, ask them to get fit instead. Make good sport nutrition and conditioning part of their training program, and they may gain weight, increasing lean body weight but not fat stores. Coaches should realize that overfeeding athletes to add fat weight, especially during adolescence and young adulthood, means increasing the size of individual fat cells, and in many cases also increasing the number of fat cells (22). Many athletes who overeat to acquire extra body weight in high school and college never lose the extra weight they gained. While fattening your athletes may help your team in the short run, in the long run extra body fat may fuel a lifelong struggle with obesity for overfed athletes.

PATHOGENIC WEIGHT CONTROL, DISORDERED EATING, AND EATING DISORDERS

Food, eating, weight, and body image can become problems; for some people, they become big problems. In this chapter we have already warned of the dangerous dehydration and hyperthermia that can result from harmful weight cutting practices. We have advised that very low-calorie dieting is ineffective and hurts athletic performance. We have cautioned you to avoid public weigh-ins and body composition checks, and making comments about weight. But despite your best efforts to encourage good sport nutrition and create a positive team culture, you may find yourself face to face with an athlete, or even a team, obsessed with food, appearance, and weight.

A full exploration of the causes and treatment of eating disorders is beyond the scope of this chapter, but this section will provide a brief overview of eating disorders and disordered eating behaviors, help you recognize their symptoms in your athletes, and make a plan for referring your eating disordered athletes for help should this need arise.

Problems with Food and Weight

Problems with food and weight range in severity from mild to life threatening. Many athletes have been known to occasionally follow crazy diets, take diet pills or laxatives, or exercise excessively. These practices occur widely in nonathletic populations as well, so it is no surprise to find them occurring in your athletes. All of these so-called pathogenic (harmful) weight control methods should be discouraged, and the coach should refer athletes trying to lose weight in harmful ways to a nutrition professional for sound weight control advice.

Athletes whose weight control behavior is not normal, but fails to meet the full criteria for classification as an eating disorder, may be referred to as having disordered eating. Disordered eating is a broad term with no exact definition, except to indicate that an athlete has mild to serious food and weight issues, and is practicing pathogenic weight control measures from time to time. Athletes with disordered eating may return to normal behavior once the sport season is over (think wrestlers). But sometimes the disordered eating evolves into the psychological obsession of full-blown eating disorders.

Clinical eating disorders are psychological illnesses that have clinical definitions devised by the American Psychiatric Association, to aid clinicians in diagnosis. We have drawn from the APA Diagnostic Manual (54) for the brief descriptions below (Table 10.2). Essentially, eating disorders are composed of three often overlapping behaviors: restricting, bingeing, and purging (Fig. 10.5). Some athletes may only restrict (anorexia nervosa), some may only binge (binge eating disorder), some may binge and purge (bu-

TABLE 10.2 Eating Disorders

Anorexia Nervosa

• Weight 15% or more below that expected for age, height, and sex, and a refusal to maintain normal body weight

• Intense fear of gaining weight

• Disturbances in the way one's body is evaluated, wanting to become even thinner although already very thin

• Denial of the seriousness of one's weight loss and behaviors

• Absence of at least three consecutive menstrual cycles (in females who have started their menstrual cycles)

Bulimia Nervosa

• Repeated episodes of binge eating

• Repeated episodes of purging behavior to prevent weight gain, including self-induced vomiting, misuse of laxatives, enemas, diuretics or other medications; fasting; or excessive exercise

• Episodes of bingeing and purging occurring at least twice a week for 3 months

• Disturbances in self-evaluation, with self-image being excessively influenced by body shape and weight

Binge-Eating Disorder

• Repeated episodes of binge eating, defined as eating larger than normal volumes of food in a discrete period of time, with a sense of lack of control over the eating behavior

• Three of the following characteristics: eating more rapidly than normal; eating until uncomfortably full; eating large amounts of food when not physically hungry; eating alone because of embarrassment about eating behavior; feeling guilty, disgusted, or depressed after bingeing

American Psychiatric Association. *Diagnostic and Statistical Manual*, 4th ed. Washington, DC: American Psychiatric Association, 2000.

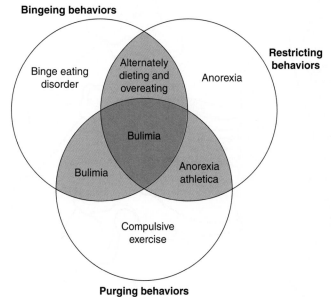

■ **FIGURE 10.5** Pathogenic weight control behaviors. Disordered eating and eating disorders may consist of numerous pathogenic weight control behavior patterns. Pathogenic weight control behaviors may be visualized as various combinations of several often overlapping behaviors, including restricting, bingeing, and purging. Examples of behaviors are given in each sector of the diagram above.

limia nervosa), and some may do all three at various times. Restricting, bingeing, and purging all have potentially negative health consequences.

Restricting calories can lead to many negative effects (55). The greater the weight loss below normal, the greater the health risks. Anorexia may result in dehydration and electrolyte imbalances, and damage to the heart muscle, all of which may lead to disturbances in heart rhythm and even heart attack and death. People with anorexia have very low resting heart rates and low blood pressure. They may experience fainting and seizures. Athletes diagnosed with anorexia may be medically disqualified from sport participation, since physical activity becomes too dangerous in their weakened state.

Bingeing can lead to a variety of gastrointestinal problems, and weight gain from the excessive intake of calories. Presumably continued weight gain in an athlete could cause a decline in performance and increased risk of injury.

The negative health effects of purging depend upon the purging behavior. Vomiting can cause conditions such as heartburn and acid reflux. It can also cause muscle weakness, electrolyte imbalances, and dehydration. Some people with bulimia experience disturbances in heart rhythm and damage to heart muscle, heart failure and even death.

Purging through dehydration, including all the behaviors listed above in the weight cutting section, lead to risk of electrolyte imbalances and hyperthermia. Medications used for purging calories all have negative side effects. Purging calories through excessive exercise can lead to overuse injuries.

The Female Athlete Triad: Long Term Health Risks Associated with Low Estrogen Levels

In women, estrogen levels fluctuate with the menstrual cycle. Menstrual disturbance is common in young women, including female athletes (56). When the cycle is absent, a condition known as amenorrhea, estrogen levels are usually very low. Irregular menstrual cycles may also be associated with lower than normal estrogen levels. Estrogen is an important anabolic hormone, and chronically low levels have been associated with low bone density, increased rates of bone loss, and increased risk for fracture and stress fractures in young women (Fig. 10.6). A syndrome known as the "female athlete triad" (the Triad) consists of three components: disordered eating, amenorrhea, and osteoporosis (34). Amenorrhea may be caused by disordered eating and low body weight, but high levels of physical activity, psychosocial stress, and other factors may also be involved. While athletics does not appear to be the primary cause of the Triad, the demands of athletic performance can intensify a young woman's desire to achieve an unrealistically thin physique (34).

Any of the three components of the Triad may have negative health consequences, and thus merit referral to a health professional. The more advanced any of the three components, the more difficult the treatment, and the more severe the consequences. For example, researchers have been particularly alarmed by the occurrence of hip fractures and compression fractures of the spine in some female athletes with prolonged disordered eating and amenorrhea (34). Thus, many sports medicine organizations have worked to alert coaches and other professionals working with athletes to recognize warning signs

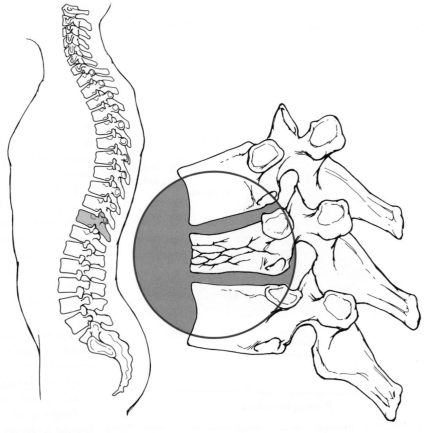

■ **FIGURE 10.6** Vertebral compression fracture. A vertebral compression fracture is one of the most serious symptoms of osteoporosis. They have been observed in young female athletes with severe amenorrhea and disordered eating. A vertebral compression fracture consists of a break in the bone of the vertebra. Vertebral compression fractures are painful, disfiguring, and difficult to treat.

of these disorders, and refer athletes for treatment as soon as possible to avoid long-term complications (8,34).

Which Athletes are at Risk for Developing Eating Disorders?

It is important to remember that, in general, the benefits of sports outweigh the risks, and that some studies have found participation in athletics may be somewhat protective against eating disorders in women (57,58). Nevertheless, coaches should be aware that all young people, including athletes and nonathletes, male and female, are at some risk of practicing pathogenic weight control measures and developing eating disorders. The clinical eating disorders are most likely to be found in females (90% of cases). However, because males are less likely to be suspected of developing eating disorders, they are less likely to be referred for treatment (59). As noted in the making weight section, rapid weight loss from dehydration is especially likely to be seen in wrestlers. In Chapter 11 you will learn that many athletes become preoccupied with building muscle. When this preoccupation becomes an obsession it is known as muscle dysmorphic disorder, which may eventually lead to exercise addiction and the use of substances such as steroids to aid in body building efforts (60). Substance abuse and pathogenic weight control often occur together in females as well as males (61).

Studies examining risk factors for the Triad suggest that up to 70% of young women, both athletes and nonathletes, are somewhat at risk (56). Athletes competing in "leanness" sports and nonathletes are at higher risk than females competing in nonleanness sports. "Leanness" sports include the following sport categories (34):

- Sports in which appearance contributes to score (figure skating, diving, gymnastics, dance)
- Sports that require revealing clothing for participation (swimming, diving, running, volleyball, dance, gymnastics)
- Sports in which a lower body weight enhances performance (distance running, cycling, Nordic skiing)
- Sports that use weight categories for participation (wrestling, light-weight rowing, some martial arts, horse racing)

Positive Focus: Primary Prevention of Eating Disorders

The most important thing coaches can do to prevent problems with food and weight from developing in their athletes is to promote a positive team culture. Your program should be focused on teaching sports skills, improving physical fitness, and encouraging good hydration and nutrition. You should model and encourage a good attitude, teamwork, character building, and safety (62). As discussed earlier in this chapter, you prevent eating disorders when you limit the focus on body composition and weight as keys to success.

What about education to prevent eating disorders? Should you invite someone in to give a lecture on the danger of eating disorders? Some research suggests that these educational approaches can backfire, and actually "teach" vulnerable young people pathogenic weight loss measures, and feed into obsessions with food and weight. While education sounds like a rational approach, addictions and obsessions are not rational, and do not respond to reasoning. They must be dealt with on an emotional level by a skilled medical team, not the coach. Keep your focus on promoting positive behaviors (Table 10.3), and refer troubled athletes to professional help.

Eating Disorders on Your Team

Despite your best efforts to create a positive team culture, you may find that one or more of your athletes are having problems with food and weight. Coaches may observe warning signs indicating the possibility of an eating disorder, or some of your athletes may come to you concerned about a teammate. Some of the warning signs that may indicate eating disorders are listed in Table 10.4. The more warning signs you observe, the more likely it is that your athlete has a problem.

TABLE 10.3   Eating Disorders Prevention: What the Coach Should Do and Not Do
There are many ways for a coach to promote a positive environment for training and competition.
What Coaches Should NOT Do:
• Have public weigh-ins or body composition checks
• Have frequent weigh-ins or body composition checks
• Talk about any athlete being fat or overweight
• Tell athletes they are fat or must lose weight
• Use fashion models as references for how athletes should look
• Use only elite athletes as role models for your athletes
What Coaches SHOULD Do:
• Stress good sport nutrition
• Stress adequate hydration
• Promote balanced lifestyle with training, rest, and good eating habits
• Discuss the athlete's fitness rather than body composition
• Use strong, healthy athletes as role models, especially ones your athletes can see and interact with on a regular basis
• Discuss the long-term benefits of exercise and good nutrition
• Choose uniforms that are as flattering as possible for all body types
• Limit time spent practicing in front of mirrors

American Academy of Pediatrics, Committee on Sports Medicine and Fitness. Promotion of healthy weight-control practices in young athletes. *Pediatrics* 2005;116(6):1557–1564.

Burney MW, Brehm BA. The female athlete triad. *JOPERD* 1998;69(9):43–45.

National Collegiate Athletic Association. NCAA Sports Medicine Handbook, 2006–2007. Available online at http://www.ncaa.org. Accessed February 29, 2008.

Sherman RT, Thompson RA, Dehass D, et al. NCAA Coaches Survey: The role of the coach in identifying and managing athletes with disordered eating. *Int J Eat Disord* 2005;13(5):447–466.

WHEN SHOULD YOU REFER?

If you have any suspicions that your athlete is trying to lose weight, using harmful weight control practices, or developing an eating disorder, make a point of talking to him or her in private to find out what is going on. Refer athletes who want to lose weight to a nutrition professional. Athletes with eating disorders will usually deny the problem. If your suspicions continue, refer them to your athletic trainer, their health care provider, a nutrition professional, and/or a counselor, depending on the nature of the problem. If in doubt, refer.

REFERRING AN ATHLETE

Most coaches report that telling an athlete to get help for a possible eating disorder is tricky business. Coaches often spend a quite a bit of time worrying about the situation, talking to their colleagues, and rereading this section of the textbook before confronting their troubled athlete. How do you tell an athlete you are concerned? Is it possible you might be wrong in your suspicions?

Every situation is different, just as every athlete is unique. The way you approach a referral situation depends a lot upon your relationship with that athlete: how long you have known him and how you think he will respond to your conversation. Here are some general suggestions on referring an athlete for professional help (3,63–65).

■ Take a team approach. Work with your school, athletic program, or other organization to refer athletes with eating disorders. Your school or organization should have guidelines and procedures in place for these referrals. If not, form a task force and create them. Be sure to involve all relevant staff members—athletic directors, athletic trainers, team physician, school nurse, and so forth—as appropriate

TABLE 10.4   Warning Signs that May Signal an Eating Disorder on Your Team
Signs of Anorexia
• Significant weight loss
• Withdrawal from team activities
• Avoiding situations where food is served
• Eating very small amounts of food, making excuses for not eating
• Wearing baggy clothes to hide thinness
• Low heart rate
• Dizziness, weakness
• Amenorrhea
• Excessive exercise (beyond exercise levels of the rest of your team)
• Recurrent overuse injuries
• Stress fractures
• Decline in athletic performance
Signs of Bulimia
• Disappearing after meals
• Frequent trips to the bathroom
• Secretive behavior to hide purging activities
• Dizziness, weakness
• Decline in athletic performance
• Swollen saliva glands, puffy cheeks
• Excessive exercise
• Frequent fluctuations in weight
• Depression
• Substance abuse
• Bloodshot eyes

Burney MW, Brehm BA. The female athlete triad. *Int J Eat Disord* 1998;69(9):43–45.
Clark N. *Nancy Clark's Sports Nutrition Guidebook*. Champaign, IL: Human Kinetics, 2003.
McArdle WD, Katch FI, Katch VL. *Sports & Exercise Nutrition*. Philadelphia: Lippincott Williams & Wilkins, 2005.

for your institution or organization. Once guidelines are in place, follow them. Communicate with others about athletes that concern you, and work with others to be consistent in your approach. Be sure to alert your supervisor if you have concerns, and have decided to confront a particular athlete.

■ Speak to your athlete in private. If necessary, you can still meet in a public place, but be out of earshot of others.

■ If your athlete is a minor, speak to the parents as well, on a separate occasion.

■ Open the conversation by expressing your concern. Say for example, "I am worried about you. I am wondering if you need some help."

■ Cite specific, observable behaviors to explain why you are concerned. "I have noticed you always skip occasions where we eat together. When we are traveling, you never eat with us, always saying you aren't hungry. In fact, I haven't seen you eat for 6 weeks. What's going on?"

■ If you have not observed anything out of the ordinary, but teammates have reported suspicious behavior, then be honest. "Some of your teammates have told me you go to the bathroom and vomit after meals." Do not name names, unless the teammates have given you permission.

■ Do not make references to thinness or weight loss. If you say, "I am worried because you have lost weight," or "You look too thin," they may take this as a sign of success! It is just what they want to hear.

- Give your athlete a chance to talk. Listen without interrupting. Be prepared for your athlete to deny the problem.

If you are still concerned, tell the athlete you would like her to meet with (fill in the blank). Give specific names, phone numbers, and procedures. Athletes with eating disorders may be more open to meeting with a nutrition professional or athletic trainer than a therapist. If you can get your athlete in to see one of them, they may help determine whether the athlete is at risk for an eating disorder, and help refer the athlete on for further help.

Male coaches have told us that referring female athletes with eating disorders can be very uncomfortable. When we asked them for advice to pass along to you, we got several suggestions. Some male coaches said they are always careful whenever they meet with individual female athletes for any reason, for fear of sexual harassment charges. They said they always leave the door open if such a meeting is necessary. Some coaches have a female assistant coach who is asked to be present at all meetings with individual students. Other male coaches ask a female staff member to be present, such as one of the female athletic trainers, or one of the female coaches. Unfortunately, having another person present at a referral discussion may make your athlete with a suspected eating disorder even more uncomfortable, defensive, and uncommunicative than usual, which is pretty bad. One male coach says he asks the player to stay after practice, then speaks with her in the "public" setting of the athletic field, where people are in view but cannot hear what they are discussing. One male coach asked us to remind you to keep a big box of tissues on hand if you are a male new to coaching girls and women. He has found that female athletes tend to cry more in his office than his male athletes.

TROUBLED ATHLETES AND TEAM DYNAMICS

You have referred your troubled athlete, and he or she is working with the athletic trainer, a health care provider, a dietician, and a therapist. Now what? If the athlete is still a member of your team, you may find your problems are still not over. Eating disorders are extremely difficult to treat. As a type of addictive behavior, eating disorders can take years to overcome.

Many coaches may get impatient, and be tempted to try to "talk some sense" into the eating disordered athlete. Some coaches have even gone so far as to schedule meals for the team to eat together to get an anorexic athlete to eat more. Some have tried meeting frequently with the troubled athlete and discussing recovery strategies. Your athlete with eating disorders may love all this attention, but your team will resent the diversion of your attention, and you may be in trouble for exceeding your scope of practice. Remember, you are a coach, not a therapist, and you have a whole team of athletes who deserve your attention.

You can keep your team up and running and help your troubled athlete the most by keeping things as normal as possible, and by not giving the troubled athlete extra attention. Here are some suggestions for working with athletes with eating disorders (3).

- Keep in touch with your athletic trainer and other members of your staff who are working with the athletes. Be sure the athletes are medically cleared to continue participating on your team.
- Do not get involved in discussions of weight and food with athletes with eating disorders. Do not give them advice about coping with eating disorders (with the exception of a referral). Do not ask them questions about food and weight ("What did you eat today?" "Did you have a good breakfast?").
- Do not force your athletes with eating problems to eat. They must take control of their problem; you cannot do it for them.
- On the other hand, do not ignore the situation. If you are still worried about your athlete, or you sense the situation is getting worse, talk to a member of your medical team. Be sure the professionals working with your athlete hear from you about your concerns.
- Encourage your athletes with eating disorders to participate fully in the life of the team. Try to keep them involved.
- Treat your troubled athletes with respect. Be firm but fair. Remember that the eating disordered behavior is probably out of their control, and that athletes with eating disorders are facing a long road to recovery. Be as supportive and as patient as possible.
- Do not expect change. Change comes slowly, and you will just be frustrated if you anticipate speedy improvements.
- Learn more about eating disorders. Good sources for you include the National Eating Disorders Association website (64) and the Something Fishy website on Eating Disorders (65). Keep in mind,

FOCAL POINT

Helping Troubled Athletes: Ideas that Didn't Work

Many athletes who have been on sport teams with an eating disordered teammate have shared their experiences with us. Here are two of their stories.

"When I was in college, one of my teammates (Division III Women's Soccer) had an eating disorder. Our coach had a speaker come to our team and give a presentation on eating disorders. It was so embarrassing. We all knew it was about the athlete with the eating disorder. We kept trying not to look at her, and pretend it was just an informational lecture. But we all knew what was going on."

"One of the players on my college (Division I Women's) softball team developed anorexia. Once the coach found out, she started making us all get together 2 hours before every game to have a meal together. We figured the coach was trying to get our anorexic teammate to eat. But most of us were furious! We didn't want a meal 2 hours before a game! Why should we all suffer just because one player was having problems?"

however, that referring people with eating disorders to a website can do more harm than good, as they may use the sites to "improve" their abilities to control food and weight. Chat rooms on the web can create opportunities to talk with other disturbed people and reinforce obsessive thoughts and behaviors. Let the therapists decide what information is best shared.

Sometimes young people "learn" disordered eating behaviors from each other. What can you do to prevent this from happening? All you can do is promote a positive team culture to the best of your abilities, keep your focus on peak performance, and try to nip emerging disordered eating in the bud. Refer athletes participating in pathogenic weight control to your athletic trainer or team physician. Continue to emphasize good training and sport nutrition. Meet with your team captains and get them on board your positive culture bandwagon. Talk to your athletic director, school medical staff, deans, and other appropriate personnel if you sense that disordered eating and eating disorders are becoming "contagious" and spreading on your team. Do not try to manage such a big problem yourself. Get help.

Remember to pat yourself on the back occasionally as you work to help troubled athletes. The athletes themselves, being young people, will probably ignore or resent you. Your reward will be in knowing that, as a coach, your influence is strong. While you may not see any progress during your time with a particular athlete, your efforts may still help turn a troubled person around in the future. They may even save a life.

SUMMARY

- Many athletes are able to lose or gain several pounds with a well-balanced weight control diet and appropriate exercise. However, much of a person's shape and size is outside of voluntary control.
- Body composition estimates are often more helpful than body weight in determining whether an athlete needs to gain or lose weight.
- Coaches should avoid administering body composition tests to their teams or to individual athletes, but refer athletes seeking weight control advice to an athletic trainer, strength and conditioning coach, exercise physiologist, or nutrition professional. These professionals can provide follow-up weight control counseling if testing indicates such a need. In some cases, especially wrestling, coaches may be required to assist with body composition assessment.
- Body composition is influenced by genetics, adolescent development, cellular biochemical signals, and the athlete's environment and behavior.
- Because some athletes have reported that their disordered eating started or worsened because of coaches' suggestions to lose weight, most professional organizations discourage coaches from telling athletes they need to lose weight.

- If you believe an athlete needs to lose weight, ask one of your athletic trainers or your team physician for advice, and for help talking to the athlete.
- Some athletes lose weight in season without compromising performance simply because they are burning more calories and eating better. But in general, weight loss programs should occur out of season so that they do not hurt performance.
- To lose weight, athletes must create a calorie deficit by consuming fewer calories than they expend.
- A majority of dieters end up regaining lost weight within 2 years. Successful weight loss programs teach athletes how to develop habits that support weight maintenance.
- In some sports, participation is based on body weight categories. Athletes who must make weight should set reasonable weight loss goals, and lose weight in safe ways that do not compromise athletic performance.
- Athletes who need to gain weight should aim to increase lean body mass rather than body fat mass. The best way to gain weight is to increase food intake, especially of foods high in nutritional content, and increase resistance training. Protein and carbohydrates should be consumed during recovery to facilitate muscle growth and repair. Since such training may interfere with sport performance for some athletes, it may be best to pursue weight gain programs out of season.
- Some athletes develop problems with food and weight. Pathogenic weight control behaviors include bingeing (consuming excessive calories at one sitting), restricting calorie intake to very low levels, and purging. Purging calories through use of diuretics, laxatives, and other drugs, or through vomiting or excessive exercise all have dangerous and sometimes lethal side effects.
- Low estrogen levels in women of childbearing age are associated with low bone density, and a failure to achieve adequate peak bone mass in young adulthood. In severe cases, athletes may develop osteoporosis and bone fractures.
- The most important thing coaches can do to prevent eating disorders from developing in their athletes is to promote a positive team culture.
- Coaches should be familiar with the signs of eating disorders, speak privately with athletes who may have an eating disorder, and follow the appropriate referral procedures for their organization. Coaches should work with the athletic trainer to be sure athletes with eating disorders are medically cleared to participate in sport practices and competitions.

References

1. Centers for Disease Control. *BMI—Body Mass Index*. Available online at http://www.cdc.gov/nccdphp/dnpa/bmi/index.htm. Accessed August 15, 2007.
2. Centers for Disease Control. *BMI—Body Mass Index: About BMI for Children and Teens*. Available online at http://www.cdc.gov/nccdphp/dnpa/bmi/childrens_BMI/about_childrens_BMI.htm. Accessed August 15, 2007.
3. McArdle WD, Katch FI, Katch VL. *Sports & Exercise Nutrition*. Philadelphia: Lippincott Williams & Wilkins, 2006.
4. American College of Sports Medicine. *ACSM's Guidelines for Exercise Testing and Prescription*. Philadelphia: Lippincott Williams & Wilkins, 2006.
5. Sopher AB, Thornton JC, Wang J, et al. Measurement of percentage of body fat in 411 children and adolescents: A comparison of dual-energy x-ray absorptiometry with a four-compartment model. *Pediatrics* 2004;113(5):1285–1290.
6. Clark RR, Bartok C, Sullivan JC, et al. Is leg-to-leg BIA valid for predicting minimum weight in wrestlers? *Med Sci Sports Exerc* 2005;37(6):1061–1068.
7. Kaminsky, LA. *ACSM's Resource Manual for Guidelines for Exercise Testing and Prescription*. Baltimore: Lippincott Williams & Wilkins, 2005.
8. National Collegiate Athletic Association. *NCAA Sports Medicine Handbook 2006–2007*. Available online at http://www.ncaa.org. Accessed February 29, 2008.
9. Clark RR, Bartok C, Sullivan JC, et al. Minimum weight prediction methods cross-validated by the four-component model. *Med Sci Sports Exerc* 2004;36(4):639–647.
10. Dixon CB, Deitrick RW, Pierce JR, et al. Evaluation of the BOD POD and leg-to-leg bioelectrical impedance analysis for estimating percent body fat in National Collegiate Athletic Association Division III collegiate wrestlers. *J Strength Cond Res* 2005;19(1):85–91.
11. Hetzler RK, Kimura IF, Haines K, et al. A comparison of bioelectrical impedance and skinfold measurements in determining minimum wrestling weights in high school wrestlers. *J Athl Train* 2006;41(1):46–51.
12. National Collegiate Athletic Association. *2006 NCAA Wrestling Rules and Interpretations*. Available online at http://www.ncaa.org/library/rules/2006/2006_wrestling_rules. Accessed February 29, 2008.
13. National Federation of State High School Associations. *Wrestling Sports/Rules Information*. Available online at http://www.nfhs.org/scriptcontent/va_Custom/vimdisplays/newspage.cfm?category_ID=36&Title=Wrestling%20Sports /Rules%20Information&ItemTitle=Item&ShowArchive=No&NewsHeader=WR&NewsFooter=WR_FOOT. Accessed February 29, 2008.

14. Bartok C, Schoeller DA, Randall CR, et al. The effect of dehydration on wrestling minimum weight assessment. *Med Sci Sports Exerc* 2004;36(1):160–167.
15. Clark N. *Nancy Clark's Sports Nutrition Guidebook*. Champaign, IL: Human Kinetics, 2003.
16. National Collegiate Athletic Association. *NCAA Nutrition and Performance Resource*. Available online at www.ncaa.org/nutritionandperformance. Accessed February 29, 2008.
17. National Wrestling Coaches Association. *NWCA Optimal Performance Calculator*. Available online at http://www.nwcaonline.com/nwcaonline/historical.aspx. Accessed February 29, 2008.
18. Malis C, Rasmussen EL, Poulsen P, et al. Total and regional fat distribution is strongly influenced by genetic factors in young and elderly twins. *Obes Res* 2005;13:2139–2145.
19. O'Rahilly S, Farooqi IS, Yeo GSH, et al. Minireview: Human obesity—Lessons from monogenic disorders. *Endocrinology* 2003;144(9):3757–3764.
20. Stunkard A, Foch T, Hrubec Z. A twin study of human obesity. *JAMA* 1986;256:51–54.
21. Mundt CA, Baxter-Jones ADG, Whiting SJ, et al. Relationships of activity and sugar drink intake on fat mass development in youths. *Med Sci Sports Exerc* 2006;38(7):1245–1254.
22. Evans RM, Barish GD, Wang Y-X. PPARs and the complex journey to obesity. *Nat Med* 2004;10:355–361.
23. Diliberti N, Bordi PL, Conklin MT, et al. Increased portion size leads to increased energy intake in a restaurant meal. *Obes Res* 2004;12:562–568.
24. Rolls BJ, Roe LA, Meengs JS, et al. Increasing the portion size of a sandwich increases energy intake. *J Am Diet Assoc* 2004;104:367–372.
25. Centers for Disease Control. Children and teens told by doctors that they were overweight – United States, 1999–2002. *MMWR Morb Mortal Wkly Rep* 2005;54(34):848–849.
26. American Academy of Pediatric. Prevention of pediatric overweight and obesity. *Pediatrics* 2003;112(2):424–430.
27. Thom R, Haase N, Rosamond W, et al. Heart disease and stroke statistics—2006 update: A report from the American Heart Association Statistics Committee and Stroke Statistics Subcommittee. *Circulation* 2006;113:85–151.
28. Ebbeling CB, Pawlak DB, Ludwig DS. Childhood obesity: Public health crisis, common sense cure. *Lancet* 2002;360:473–482.
29. Aronne LJ. Classification of obesity and assessment of obesity-related health risks. *Obes Res* 2002;10:105S–115S.
30. Zametkin AJ, Zoon CK, Klein HW, et al. Psychiatric aspects of child and adolescent obesity. *Focus* 2004;2:625–641.
31. Bechtel M, Pappu S. Starving for a win: ex-athlete with eating disorder successfully sues coach. *Sports Illustrated* 2004;100(14):17.
32. Jones RL. Slim bodies, eating disorders and the coach-athlete relationship. *Int Rev Soc Sport* 2005;40(3):377–391.
33. Kerr G, Berman E, De Souza MJ. Disordered eating in women's gymnastics: Perspectives of athletes, coaches, parents, and judges. *J App Sport Psych* 2006;18(1):28–43.
34. Otis CL, Drinkwater B, Johnson M, et al. American College of Sports Medicine Position Stand: The female athlete triad. *Med Sci Sports Exerc* 1997;29:i–ix.
35. American Dietetic Association Website. Available online at http://www.eatright.org. Accessed February 29, 2008.
36. Sports, cardiovascular and wellness nutritionists: A dietetic practice group of the American Dietetic Association. Sports Dietetics—USA. Available online at http:www.scandpg.org/sd_usa.php. Accessed February 29, 2008.
37. American Diabetes Association. Available online at www.diabetes.org/home.jsp. Accessed February 29, 2008.
38. Sizer F, Whitney E. *Nutrition: Concepts and Controversies*. Stamford, CT: Wadsworth, 2005.
39. ExRx.net (Exercise Prescription on the Net). Diet & Nutrition. Available online at http://www.extx.net/nutrition.html. Accessed August 30, 2006.
40. United States Department of Agriculture. MyPyramid.gov. Available online at http://mypyramid.gov. Accessed February 29, 2008.
41. Wing RR, Phelan S. Long-term weight loss maintenance. *Am J Clin Nutr* 2005;82(1):222S–225S.
42. Yanovski S. Sugar and fat: cravings and aversions. *J Nutr* 2003;133(3):835S–838S.
43. Giner-Sorolla R. Guilty pleasures and grim necessities: Affective attitudes in dilemmas of self-control. *J Pers Soc Psychol* 2001;80(2):206–221.
44. Vohs KD, Heatherton TF. Self-regulatory failure: A resource-depletion approach. *Psychol Sci* 2000;11(3):249–254.
45. Baumeister RF, Brattslavsky E, Muraven M, et al. Ego depletion: Is the active self a limited resource? *J Pers Soc Psychol* 1998;74(5):1252–1265.
46. Muraven M, Baumeister RF. Self-regulation and depletion of limited resources: Does self-control resemble a muscle? *J Pers Soc Psychol* 2001;80(2):206–221.
47. McAuley E, Blissmer B. Self-efficacy determinants and consequences of physical activity. *Exerc Sport Sci Rev* 2000;28:85–88.
48. Centers for Disease Control and Prevention. Hyperthermia and dehydration-related deaths associated with intentional rapid weight loss in three collegiate wrestlers—North Carolina, Wisconsin, and Michigan, November-December 1997. *MMWR Morb Mortal Wkly Rep* 1998;47(6):105–108.
49. Davis SE, Dwyer GB, Reed K, et al. Preliminary investigation: The impact of the NCAA Wrestling Weight Certification Program on weight cutting. *J Strength Cond Res* 2002;16(2):305–307.
50. Oppliger RA, Utter AC, Scott JR, et al. NCAA rule change improves weight loss among national championship wrestlers. *Med Sci Sports Exerc* 2006;38(5):963–970.
51. Ransone J, Hughes B. Body-weight fluctuation in collegiate wrestlers: Implications of the National Collegiate Athletic Association Weight-Certification Program. *J Athl Train* 39(2):162–165.

52. Alderman BL, Landers DM, Carlson J, et al. Factors related to rapid weight loss practices among international-style wrestlers. *Med Sci Sports Exerc* 2004;36(2):249–252.

53. Kleiner SM, Greenwood-Robinson M. *Power Eating*. Champaign, IL: Human Kinetics, 2001.

54. American Psychiatric Association. *Diagnostic and Statistical Manual*, 4th ed. Washington, DC: American Psychiatric Association, 2000.

55. American Dietetic Association. Position of the American Dietetic Association—Nutrition intervention in the treatment of anorexia nervosa, bulimia nervosa, and eating disorders not otherwise specified (EDNOS). *J Am Diet Assoc* 2001;101:810–819.

56. Torstveit MK, Sundgot-Borgen J. The female athlete triad: are elite athletes at increased risk? *Med Sci Sports Exerc* 2005;37(2): 184–193.

57. Bachner-Melman R, Zohar AH, Ebstein RP, et al. How anorexic-like are the symptom and personality profiles of aesthetic athletes? *Med Sci Sports Exerc* 2006;38(4):628–636.

58. DiBartolo PM, Shaffer C. A comparison of female college athletes and nonathletes: Eating disorder symptomatology and psychological well-being. *J Sport Exerc Psychol* 2002;24:33–41.

59. Baum A. Eating disorders in the male athlete. *Sport Med* 2006;3(1):1–6.

60. Goldberg L, MacKinnon DD, Elliot DL, et al. Preventing drug use and promoting health behaviors among adolescents: Results of the ATLAS Program. *Arch Pediatr Adolesc Med* 2000;154:332–338.

61. Elliot DL, Goldberg L, Moe EL, et al. Preventing substance use and disordered eating: Initial outcomes of the ATHENA (Athletes Targeting Healthy Exercise and Nutrition Alternatives) Program. *Arch Pediatr Adolesc Med* 2004;158(11):1043–1049.

62. American Academy of Pediatrics, Committee on Sports Medicine and Fitness. Promotion of healthy weight-control practices in young athletes. *Pediatrics* 2005;116(6):1557–1564.

63. Brehm BA. Addressing eating disorders. *Fitness Management* 2006;22(8):48.

64. National Eating Disorders Association. Available online at www.nationaleatingdisorders.org. Accessed February 29, 2008.

65. Something Fishy, a website on eating disorders. Available online at www.somethingfishy.org. Accessed February 29, 2008.

Health and Performance

Upon reading this chapter, the coach should be able to:

1. Understand the difference between colds and more serious respiratory infections, and decide whether athletes' symptoms warrant staying out of a practice or contest.

2. Understand how vigorous physical activity affects the immune system.

3. Give athletes sound advice on preventing illness, and staying healthy while traveling.

4. Understand what the coach can do to help prevent substance abuse among team members.

5. Refer an athlete with substance abuse problems to professional help.

6. Explain to athletes potential problems associated with performance enhancing supplements.

7. Discuss an athlete's asthma management plan and feel confident that you could respond to an asthma emergency should one arise.

8. Discuss an athlete's diabetes management plan and feel confident that you could respond to a blood sugar emergency (hypoglycemia or hyperglycemia) should one arise.

9. Understand that some therapeutic medications could cause a positive drug test and advise athletes accordingly.

Mara returned in the fall to her junior year of college. After working all summer, college was looking pretty good! Mara looked forward to seeing her friends again and, most of all, to returning to her seat on one of the varsity crew boats. She had made the team last year and enjoyed the sport's mix of camaraderie and hard work.

Fall workouts were often grueling, especially after a summer off, but Mara had good self-discipline and pretty soon she was no longer surprised when the alarm went off at 5 a.m. The first few weeks of school were fine, and Mara felt her strength returning. She was rowing well, and had a good chance at getting the stroke position in the second boat.

But only 2 weeks into the season Mara came down with a terrible cold. She worried that taking any time off would jeopardize her position on the team, so she kept attending workouts. She did not feel too bad once she was at practice, but would be exhausted later in the day. She had difficulty staying awake in her afternoon classes and trouble concentrating on her homework.

That cold lingered for 2 weeks. Mara was finally starting to feel a little better when she developed a second cold. She summoned the energy to keep up with workouts but started to fall behind in her schoolwork. After a week she developed a bad cough. Her coach sent her to health services, where the provider informed Mara she had bronchitis and needed rest.

Mara's cough lingered for over a month. Although she took several days off from practice and tried to rest as much as possible, she just could not seem to stay well for more than a few days. Her energy level and performance continued to decline. She was too sick to row in several regattas, and was eventually forced to agree with her doctor that she needed to take a break from rowing in order to get well.

Health and athletic performance go hand in hand. Health problems can compromise strength, endurance, speed, coordination, and alertness. Your athletes need to stay as healthy as possible so they can participate fully in every practice and be in top shape for important contests. Healthy athletes are less likely to sustain injuries due to fatigue and lack of concentration. Their reflexes are sharper and they make better decisions. As a coach, you will work with athletes who are coping with both acute and chronic illness. This chapter provides an overview of the most common health issues coaches are likely to encounter in their work.

We begin with a look at exercise, immunity, and the most frequent illness encountered on the playing field: the common cold. Every athlete gets sick from time to time, sick enough to miss practices and competitions. Athletes often seek advice from coaches regarding whether to attend practice or contests, and how to deal with a cold. Coaches sometimes need to decide whether to keep an athlete out of a practice or contest when an athlete shows up with a cold or other acute illness and wants to play.

One of the most frequent challenges you may face is getting athletes to take care of themselves to prevent upper respiratory tract infections and other illnesses from getting in the way of important competitions. Both coaches and teammates get frustrated with situations like Mara's, when an athlete can not stay healthy long enough to participate fully in the life of the team. Coaches can help educate athletes about the effects of training, overtraining, sleep, stress, nutrition, and other lifestyle factors on immune health.

If you are coaching young people, you will eventually face the issue of drug and alcohol use. If you coach in a high school or college setting, you may even be required by your school to apply sanctions to athletes charged with school drug rule violations and to participate in educational discussions with your athletes. Because drug use is such a pervasive and destructive force in many schools, coaches often feel the need to help their athletes address this problem. Players who get involved in drugs may end up on a path that hurts their health, along with both school and sport performance. Coaches sometimes lose good athletes to drug problems that might have been prevented with more intervention from the coach and teammates.

As a coach, you may also be called upon to work with athletes who have been cleared to play but have chronic health conditions such as asthma, diabetes, or seizure disorder. While athletes will generally manage these conditions without too much assistance, you should still be aware of warning signs that could indicate the need for intervention. You may also have athletes who cope with psychological disorders, including attention deficit disorders, and mood disorders such as anxiety and depression. While you will not be involved in the treatment of psychological disorders, these problems may interfere with an athlete's performance and benefit from your understanding and emotional support. Sometimes athletes have medication issues that impact their participation in practices and contests.

RESPIRATORY TRACT INFECTIONS

The respiratory system bears the brunt of the suffering when we catch a cold (or in reality, when a cold catches us!). We are all too familiar with the symptoms produced by the respiratory system in its attempt to eliminate a cold virus from the body: inflammation and excess mucus production. These in turn cause itchy, watery eyes; a stuffy, runny nose; sneezing; coughing; sore throat; and sometimes a low-grade fever.

Colds are referred to clinically as upper respiratory tract infections (URTIs). The upper respiratory tract includes the parts of the respiratory system in the head and neck: the nose and sinuses around the nose, and the throat, including the pharynx, larynx, and trachea (Fig. 11.1). URTIs are the most common infections, and are caused primarily by a wide variety of viruses, which is why health care providers are not supposed to prescribe antibiotics for the common cold (antibiotics only disable bacteria, not viruses).

We are susceptible to at least 200 different cold-causing viruses. As soon as the immune system learns to recognize and defend us from one virus, another comes along, and then another. This viral diversity creates quite a challenge for the immune system, so much so that most adults succumb to about two to four colds per year (1).

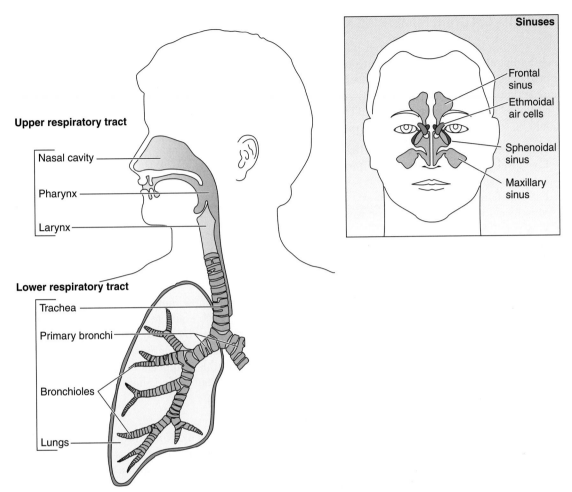

Upper respiratory tract
Nasal cavity
Pharynx
Larynx

Lower respiratory tract
Trachea
Primary bronchi
Bronchioles
Lungs

Sinuses
Frontal sinus
Ethmoidal air cells
Sphenoidal sinus
Maxillary sinus

■ **FIGURE 11.1** The respiratory tract. Colds are infections of the upper respiratory tract, which includes the nasal cavity, sinuses, pharynx, and larynx. The lower respiratory tract includes the lower airways (trachea, bronchi, and bronchioles) and the lungs. Bronchitis refers to infections in the bronchi. Pneumonia refers to infections in the lungs. (Modified from Willis MC, CMA-AC. *Medical Terminology: A Programmed Learning Approach to the Language of Health Care.* Baltimore: Lippincott Williams & Wilkins, 2002.)

Flu (influenza) viruses can also affect the respiratory system, but symptoms tend to be more widespread and more serious. The flu usually causes a high fever that lasts several days or more, extreme fatigue and pain in the muscles and joints. Athletes with the flu should definitely stay home and rest until their symptoms subside. It may take several days or even weeks before an athlete fully recovers from the flu (2).

Should I Come to Practice?

When your athletes ask whether or not they should come to practice when they have a cold, you have several factors to consider.

KEEPING YOUR TEAM HEALTHY

If you think the rest of your team has already been exposed to the cold that is going around the school, it probably will not hurt to let your athletes with a mild cold attend practices or competitions. Since teammates tend to be friends and see each other outside of practice, they have probably already been exposed to the cold germs. On the other hand, if you have an important competition in the near future and the rest of your athletes are healthy, you might consider encouraging sick athletes to stay home and rest. Even mild colds can interfere with energy level and performance. And sometimes athletes think they have a minor cold but may actually be coming down with a more serious illness, such as the flu.

IS IT JUST A COLD? OR SOMETHING MORE SERIOUS?

Many coaches let athletes practice or play if the symptoms are mild and only apparent in the head and neck. Symptoms only in these areas suggest the common cold. Symptoms that are systemic (such as fever) or below the neck (chest cough), or severe (a very sore throat) suggest that the illness may be something more serious such as the flu, bronchitis, or strep throat. The following symptoms suggest that your athlete's illness is more serious than a URTI, so they should be instructed to stay home from practice, and should be sent to see their health care provider (1,2,4):

- High fever (oral temperature over 102°F)
- Low fever (oral temperature over 100°F) that lasts more than 3 days
- Severe cough
- Extreme fatigue
- Muscle and joint aches, pains, and weakness
- Very sore throat with a fever
- Severe pain in ears, head, chest, or stomach
- Symptoms that last more than a week
- Breathing difficulties

You observe your athletes several hours each week, and get to know them pretty well. Most coaches can remember times when an athlete wanted to play but the coach could tell that the athlete was not healthy. The athlete may have looked or acted sicker than warranted by a cold. Maybe she looked sick, pale, and tired. Or she may not have been performing as well as usual. Sometimes medications taken for colds or other illnesses can interfere with performance. If your athlete appears to be sick, call her over and find out the details. Send her home, or let her sit out the workout if she is not feeling well.

GIVE SICK ATHLETES AN EASIER WORKOUT

Research suggests that a mild to moderate workout will not worsen a cold (5). However, a heavy workout can make a cold worse, or hasten its "progression" to something more serious, such as a sinus infection or bronchitis, perhaps by weakening the immune response. If you have athletes with a cold at practice, let them take it easy if you have scheduled a hard workout that day.

Can I Compete in the Contest?

If your athlete just has a cold, and you are pretty sure it is nothing more serious, he or she can usually play in a competition. Playing hard may increase the likelihood that cold symptoms will get worse, or that a secondary infection such as bronchitis may develop. However, sometimes athletes are willing to take that chance if the competition is an important one, and if they have some time to take it easy after the contest.

Do Cold Medicines Help?

Many over the counter medicines claim to help reduce URTI symptoms. Although these medications do not hasten recovery, they may provide temporary relief of symptoms such as nasal congestion. Many of these medicines have unpleasant side effects, however. Some (many antihistamines) make you sleepy, while others can interfere with sleep. Some, including those claiming to control cough, may have little efficacy (6). Athletes should not try a new medicine on the day of a competition, just in case side effects could interfere with performance. On the other hand, being unable to breathe can also interfere with performance, so athletes should use their best judgment.

Some ingredients in cold medicines, such as pseudoephedrine, are banned by the United States Anti-Doping Agency and other sport governing bodies such as the National Collegiate Athletic Association (7). If your athletes may be subject to drug testing, be sure they check the ingredients of their cold medicines against your organization's list of banned substances before consuming any medicine. (The list of banned substances for the NCAA can be accessed at http://www1.ncaa.org/membership/ed_outreach/health-safety/drug_testing/banned_drug_classes.pdf [7]. Information on substances banned by the U.S. Anti-doping Agency can be found at http://www.usantidoping.org/dro [8].)

THE ATHLETIC TRAINING ROOM

Exercise Training and the Immune System

While a moderate amount of exercise training appears to strengthen your immune response, too much exertion can weaken your defenses. Why the contradiction? In order to see how physical activity can either increase or decrease an athlete's chance of getting sick, it helps to have an understanding of the immune system and immunity.

Your body provides resistance to pathogens such as bacteria and viruses in many ways. Scientists classify the components of immune function into two basic categories that make this enormously complex system easier to understand: nonspecific and specific resistance.

Nonspecific resistance (also called innate immunity) provides immediate protection from a wide array of pathogens without targeting a specific microbe (Fig. 11.2). The skin and mucous membranes provide mechanical and chemical barriers that keep invaders out of your body. The acidity of your stomach kills many of the

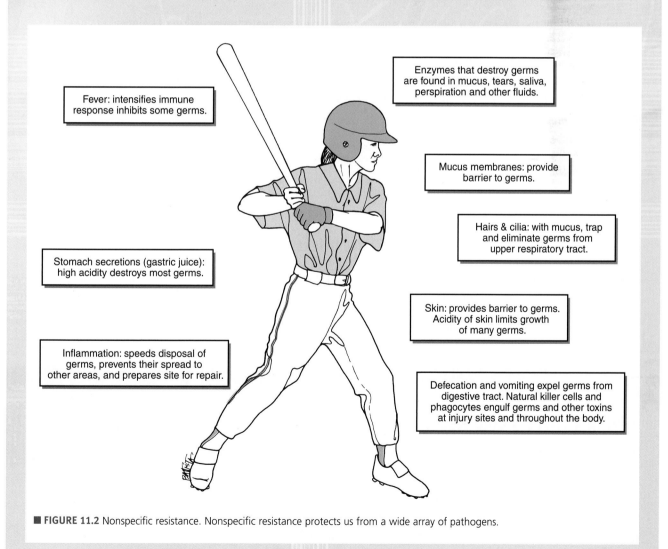

■ FIGURE 11.2 Nonspecific resistance. Nonspecific resistance protects us from a wide array of pathogens.

(continues)

Exercise Training and the Immune System *(continued)*

harmful microbes found in food. A fever may help to rev up the production of certain immune cells and inhibit the growth of some microbes. Inflammation helps to control the spread of microbes and other toxins at an injury site, and prevent the spread of infection. Special immune cells, such as natural killer cells and phagocytes (types of white blood cells), kill a variety of harmful invaders (1).

A good example of nonspecific resistance can be seen when you are suffering from a cold. Cold symptoms, including runny nose, cough, and fever, are not produced directly by the cold virus, but by the body's nonspecific defenses as they fight the virus.

Your body develops specific resistance in response to a specific pathogen. Specific resistance (also called acquired immunity) activates specific immune cells (B cells and T cells) that target a particular invader. After an encounter with certain pathogens, such as the chicken pox or measles virus, either through suffering from the illness or from exposure to a vaccine, your immune system retains a memory of the way that pathogen looks. When that invader next appears, the immune system recognizes the pathogen, and mounts a defense.

As usual, whether the effects of exercise are good or bad have to do with the question of balance. In general, regular physical activity strengthens both nonspecific and specific resistance. But too much exercise, especially prolonged exercise such as running a marathon, or suddenly increasing training volume, can decrease both nonspecific and specific resistance. Studies have observed less activity in several types of immune cells, including natural killer cells, phagocytes, and the B and T cells (2,3). This may explain why many athletes get sick after a big competition.

1 Tortora GJ, Grabowski SR. *Introduction to the Human Body*. New York: John Wiley & Sons, 2004.
2. Fleshner M. Physical activity and stress resistance: sympathetic nervous system adaptations prevent stress-induced immunosuppression. *Exerc Sport Sci Rev* 2005;33(3):120–126.
3. Gleeson M, Nieman DC, Pedersen BK. Exercise, nutrition and immune function. *J Sports Sci* 2004;22(1):115–126.

Preventing Respiratory Tract Infections

Athletes can reduce the number of colds and flu they catch each year in two ways. First, they can reduce the transmission of cold and flu germs by staying away from sick people and washing their hands frequently. Second, they can follow a healthful lifestyle to maximize the strength of the immune system. Give your athletes the guidelines from Focal Point: Giving Viruses a Cold Reception.

FOCAL POINT

Giving Viruses a Cold Reception

Exercise is good for you, but athletes who train hard sometimes catch more colds and have more sick days than their less-active friends. While moderate exercise can improve immune function, too much exercise can lead to an energy deficit that leaves the immune system run down and unable to fight the viruses that make you sick.

Is moderate not part of your vocabulary? To be the best, sometimes you have to train hard, and some sports require extreme levels of exertion. If this is you, then be sure to take extra measures to stay healthy so that you

(continues)

Giving Viruses a Cold Reception *(continued)*

do not lose training days or suffer poor performance because of sickness. Here is what you can do to stay as healthy as possible.

- Manage stress—Stress hormones are meant to help get you out of a tight situation by activating the fight or flight response. Great for sports performance! But stress hormones suppress the immune system, so chronic stress, like feeling overwhelmed by life day after day, hurts your immune function.
- Watch for symptoms of overtraining—Frequent illnesses and injuries are often indicators of overtraining. So are elevated resting heart rate, difficulty sleeping, fatigue, depression, and an unexplained decline in athletic performance. If you have symptoms of overtraining, talk to your coach. Train for shorter periods, cross train, and take more rest days.
- Get plenty of sleep—Try to get at least 8 hours of sleep a night. Sleep strengthens your immune system and allows muscles to heal after tough workouts.
- Avoid germs—Germs are everywhere, so adopt habits that will keep them out of your body. Avoid crowds as much as possible (without skipping school!) in the weeks preceding an important competition, and stay away from sick people. Wash hands often and well. Touching your nose or eyes gives cold germs an express ride to the home of their dreams: your mucus membranes, so keep your hands away from your eyes and nose.
- Pay attention to your diet—Athletes restricting calories or avoiding certain food groups are most at risk for nutritional deficiencies that can compromise immune health. Pay special attention to the following:
  - Adequate hydration keeps mucus membranes healthy, providing the best operating environment for patrolling immune cells.
  - Protein is what immune cells are made of. Athletes training at high levels need more protein than most people (about 0.6 to 0.8 grams of protein per pound of body weight, or 1.2 to 1.6 gm/kg body weight).
  - Carbohydrate consumed before and during exercise reduces the stress hormones that suppress immune response.
  - Many vitamins and minerals play important roles in the health of the immune system. If your diet is not always what it should be, a multivitamin and mineral supplement that supplies up to 100% of the RDA for most nutrients is a good idea.

Research indicates that cold viruses may be transmitted from the hands of an infected person to the hands of a susceptible person via a handshake, or simply when the susceptible person touches objects such as doorknobs, telephones, or cups that have been recently touched by the infected person. Viruses can survive on the skin for only a few hours and must reach the respiratory tract in order to invade the body. If all goes well for the virus, eventually the hand delivers the virus to its new home, the person's respiratory system, by touching the mucous membranes of the nose or the eyes (the virus can travel down the tear duct to the upper nose). Cold viruses may also be spread through the air when a sick person coughs or sneezes.

Given what we know about the transmission of cold viruses, the single best way to prevent colds is frequent hand-washing, especially when you are around people who have colds. Students have an especially high exposure to the cold and flu viruses, and should wash hands frequently, washing each time for at least 20 seconds with warm water and soap. It is best to avoid sharing objects such as telephones, keyboards, drinking glasses, and towels with people who have colds, and to try not to touch the nose or eyes. People with colds should cough and sneeze into facial tissues and then throw the tissues away.

Athletes are more vulnerable to respiratory infections following strenuous exercise. But they can maximize the health of their immune systems by cultivating a balanced lifestyle. Athletes should try to get at least 8 hours of sleep each night, eat well, drink plenty of water, and manage stress. Hopefully none of your athletes smoke, but if so, cold prevention is yet another good reason to quit.

Staying Healthy on the Road

Athletes' chances of coming down with a cold or the flu increase when they travel. They are exposed to more new germs along with the stress of traveling. Crowded airports and train and bus stations are teaming with germs, and the dry air on airplanes and in hotels reduces the effectiveness of nasal passages in keeping out bacteria and viruses. Do your best to follow the guidelines for preventing colds presented in this chapter. Encourage your athletes to be as vigilant as possible about washing their hands frequently, eating well, and getting enough rest. Give your athletes guidance for coping with jet lag (Focal Point: Overcoming Jet Lag).

If you are traveling in areas where water and/or food may cause gastrointestinal infections, be sure your athletes have access to clean water and well-cooked food. Teach them which foods to avoid, such as raw fruits and vegetables. More information on preventing traveler's diarrhea can be found on the Centers for Disease Control website (9).

OTHER INFECTIONS

Respiratory infections are not the only infections you may encounter as a coach. You may be confronted with athletes who have a "stomach bug" or other gastrointestinal infection. Coaches who work with contact sports such as wrestling, boxing, and martial arts should be especially aware of skin infections, since

FOCAL POINT

Overcoming Jet Lag

We live in a world whose natural cycles reflect the rhythm of day and night. Over evolutionary time animals, including humans, have adapted to the 24-hour cycle of light and dark. All of our physiological functions are governed by this 24-hour cycle, known as the circadian ("about a day") rhythm. Everything from bowel function and body temperature to mental alertness and reaction time fluctuates in this 24-hour pattern (1).

What happens when your athletes change time zones and lose or gain a few hours, or several hours? Pull an all-nighter, or travel half way around the world? Only in very recent history have our bodies had to adapt to sudden changes in the light-dark cycle. Some people seem to adapt to such changes more easily than others, but almost everyone experiences a feeling of being out of sync when their circadian cycles are suddenly disrupted.

Symptoms of jet lag can be worsened by the stress that accompanies travel. Noisy accommodations, too much caffeine and alcohol, restaurant dining, and frantic schedules can disrupt the body's normal routine. Travel delays, bad weather, and health problems can add insult to injury.

If your team must cross several time zones, try to arrive at your competition location as many days in advance of your event as possible. Your athletes will perform better if they have a few days to adjust to the time change (2).

The best way to reset your internal clock is to get back into a daily schedule as soon as possible. Regular physical activity and exposure to daylight can help an athlete (and coach!) recover more quickly from jet lag.

Early morning workouts will help athletes move "back" in time, if they need to wake up earlier than usual. Afternoon or evening workouts will help athletes stay up later. But any "daytime" exercise gives your internal clock the message, "It's daytime now, and I am active and alert"(2).

1. Rajaratnam SM, Arendt J. Health in a 24-h society. *Lancet* 2001;358:999–1005.
2. Waterhouse J, Nevill A, Carvalho S, et al. Identifying some determinants of "jet lag" and its symptoms: a study of athletes and other travelers. *Br J Sports Med* 2002;36:54–61.

many of these are very contagious, and spread easily with the close body contact involved in these sports. Lastly, you may learn that one of your athletes has a blood-borne infection such as HIV or Hepatitis B, and want more information on how a coach should accommodate athletes with these chronic infections.

Gastrointestinal Infections

Gastrointestinal (GI) infections are marked by GI symptoms that may include one or more of the following: stomach and abdominal cramps, vomiting, and diarrhea. These infections may be caused by a multitude of viruses, bacteria, and parasites (10).

Unfortunately, these symptoms may also be caused by stress and stress-related disorders such as irritable bowel syndrome. They may also result from food intolerances, such as lactose intolerance. Your athlete will probably be able to tell whether symptoms are unusual, or just a routine round of diarrhea commonly experienced due to nerves, that often happens before an important contest.

If your athlete is experiencing more than nerves, GI symptoms will probably keep him out of practice or competition, since symptoms will interfere with performance. Send him home until symptoms have been gone for at least 24 hours. What if you are traveling? Allow your athlete to rest.

WHEN DO GI SYMPTOMS SIGNAL AN EMERGENCY?

If you are traveling, and the athlete is in your care for several days, you may wonder whether you should send your athlete home or look for emergency medical care. The following symptoms suggest that your athlete needs immediate medical attention:

- Severe abdominal pain, especially pain in the lower right abdomen
- Fever greater than 101°F
- Severe nausea
- Vomiting with head injury
- Severe headache, sleepiness, or lethargy
- Signs of dehydration
- Blood in the vomit or stools (blood may be black or red)

IS IT FOOD POISONING?

Food poisoning is caused by bacteria from foods, usually from improper handling and poor sanitation. Symptoms include nausea, vomiting, stomach and abdominal cramps, and diarrhea. Symptoms may begin anywhere from a few hours to 2 days after consuming the tainted food. You might suspect food poisoning if several athletes develop GI symptoms after consuming the same food. Unless symptoms are severe, most health care providers recommend that food poisoning must simply run its course (11).

RECOMMENDATIONS FOR RECOVERY FROM MILD GI INFECTIONS

Most GI infections will clear up quickly on their own. Athletes with symptoms that persist longer than a few days should seek medical advice.

Athletes with mild diarrhea should avoid food for several hours, until symptoms improve. They should drink fluids such as water and sports drinks to prevent dehydration. Once they start to feel better, they should consume small amounts of bland foods such as bananas, applesauce, rice, crackers, and dry toast (10).

Skin Infections

Skin infections may be caused by bacteria, viruses, fungus, and parasites. Coaches must be concerned about skin infections for two reasons. First, the infection itself may be transmitted to other athletes. And second, an open sore increases risk of transmission of blood-borne infections such as the hepatitis B virus.

Athletes with skin infections should be examined by a qualified health care provider and cleared for participation. Some chronic skin conditions, such as psoriasis, are not contagious, although if the skin has open sores, that athlete will be at increased risk of acquiring blood-borne pathogens in sports that have a high degree of body contact.

Coaches of contact sports such as wrestling and boxing must be extremely vigilant about skin infections. These infections may be transmitted directly from one athlete to another, or via exercise surfaces, towels, and equipment. The NCAA Injury Surveillance System reports that skin infections are the cause of at least 15% of the practice time loss in college wrestling (12).

You can help your athletes reduce risk of skin infections by teaching them about infection control measures and good hygiene. Surfaces of mats and equipment that comes into contact with players' skin should be disinfected regularly. Athletes should shower after activity, and not share towels, razors, brushes, combs, protective gear, or water bottles.

Blood-borne Infections

Blood-borne infections such as HIV and hepatitis B and C can be transmitted through exposure to contaminated blood, but that risk of transmission can be reduced by following standard precautions. These precautions are important for both you and your athletes. Up to half of all people infected with blood-borne pathogens do not know they harbor an infection, and people who know they are infected are protected by medical confidentiality (12). They are not required to tell you, the coach, their teammates, or their opponents that they have an infection. Standard precautions treat everyone equally and prevent viruses from spreading. The importance of following standard precautions when dealing with blood and other body fluids is also discussed in Chapter 16.

SHOULD ALL ATHLETES BE TESTED FOR BLOOD-BORNE INFECTIONS?

In the Joint Position Statement of the American Medical Society for Sports Medicine (AMSSM) and the American Academy of Sports Medicine (AASM) (13) mandatory HIV testing is not recommended. The NCAA also does not recommend mandatory testing (12). These organizations state that testing is not justified for medical reasons for participation and that such testing would not prevent infection, promote health, or be easily implemented. Voluntary testing should be recommended to any athlete who has been exposed to a blood-borne pathogen.

HOW CAN INFECTED ATHLETES GET MEDICAL CLEARANCE TO PARTICIPATE?

Athletes infected with HIV or hepatitis viruses are only cleared to play if they are asymptomatic. While they may carry the virus in their blood, they are otherwise healthy, and capable of participating in sports training and competition. When symptoms such as fever or swollen liver are present, these athletes will not be cleared.

The risk of blood-borne virus transmission during sports is extremely low (14–16). The one exception is for HBV transmission during sports such as wrestling that involve sustained contact between athletes with the risk of bleeding. The NCAA Sportsmedicine Handbook suggests that athletes with HBV should not participate in wrestling (12).

RECOMMENDATIONS FOR TRAINING AN INFECTED ATHLETE

While infected athletes are not required to share their medical histories with their coaches, some athletes may choose to tell you that they are HIV or HBV positive. In this case, you would be expected to keep this information confidential. This athlete may have special guidelines for sport participation that are shared with you. Follow medical recommendations for such an athlete, just as you would for an athlete with any chronic disorder, such as asthma or diabetes. If an athlete has been cleared to play, you can assume that he or she can participate fully in practices and competitions (16).

SUBSTANCE ABUSE AND SPORTS

Like most things in life, the influence of sport on the lives of young people can be good or bad, or some mixture of both. Participation in sport offers a majority of children, teens, and young adults a wealth of positive experiences (Focal Point: Sports Teams as Positive Peer Pressure). For many, participation helps to promote a healthful lifestyle and may even protect to some extent against involvement in problem behaviors, such as smoking tobacco, smoking marijuana, and abusing alcohol and other drugs (17,18). But for some young people and even adults, participation may increase opportunities for substance abuse or promote other unhealthy behaviors such as harmful weight control practices (19–21).

What Does Substance Abuse Have to do with Coaching?

Many coaches would prefer to turn a blind eye to substance abuse issues, and confine their work with athletes to performance during sports practice and competitions. This is rarely possible, however, for three reasons. First, you probably will not be able to avoid substance abuse issues. Alcohol and drug problems are pervasive among adolescents and young adults. If you are working with this age group, at some point in time you will probably be drawn into issues regarding alcohol and drug use among students at your institution, as well as players on your team.

Second, coaches face legal repercussions if they condone illegal drug use or the consumption of alcohol by minors. Whether you agree with the laws or not is irrelevant, and you may lose your job, indeed your coaching career, if you fail to work within your institution's guidelines regarding substance abuse.

Third, substance abuse interferes with athletic performance, not to mention life in general. While some adolescents and young adults will experiment with alcohol and drugs with few negative effects, others may develop problems with addiction, mood disorders such as depression, and delinquent behaviors. We must all work together to help young people find enjoyable and fulfilling activities (like sports!) that build character and self-discipline, and give young people the skills they need to create a meaningful life. At some point in your coaching career, you may even be called upon to provide the "tough love" that forces an athlete to confront the fact that he or she is developing an addiction, is in trouble, and should seek help.

Team Culture

Many factors influence whether sport promotes or protects athletes from substance abuse. The biggest influence is the team culture. For example, if your team leaders throw drinking parties after contests, the other athletes will probably join in. If your team leaders model eating healthfully and going to bed early to maximize performance at a competition the next day, the rest of the team will hopefully follow suit.

FOCAL POINT

Sports Teams as Positive Peer Pressure

Peer pressure from team mates can reinforce both positive and negative behaviors. One of the best stories we heard came from a college basketball player recounting his experience on his high school team.

"I thank my basketball coach and my teammates for my success in high school and college. I attended a large public high school in Brooklyn, NY. We lived in a rough neighborhood, and there were lots of drugs and alcohol at my school. But if you wanted to play sports, you had to sign a pledge not to use substances. My coach took this very seriously. We were a great team, and he didn't want any of us to lose our eligibility, either because of drugs or academics. He also didn't want us to get kicked out of school, quit school, or flunk out. We all had to attend study hall after school, before practice, so we kept up with our work. We all helped each other, too. We went everywhere together. If one player looked like he was going to get into trouble, like get into a fight, or have a drink or something, we would all get him out of the situation as fast as possible."

Coaches exert a strong influence on player behavior and team culture. Coaches must model good attitudes and set clear guidelines regarding substance use. They can convey the belief that substance use is unhealthy and interferes with training and peak performance. They can work with team leaders to develop a healthy, supportive team culture. They can promote the idea that productive practices, well-structured workouts, adequate rest and recovery, and good nutrition are the best vehicles to peak experiences and peak performance.

Several researchers have studied the elements associated with positive team cultures and positive sport experiences. Recently, sport psychologist Donald Siegel reviewed the characteristics of youth sport programs most strongly associated with positive outcomes.[18] According to his analysis, sport programs were more likely to encourage positive behaviors when they included the following components:

- Physical and psychological safety: Athletes feel free from threat of physical and psychological harassment or teasing.
- Structure, stability, and predictability: Rules are clear, age appropriate, and consistently and fairly enforced.
- Positive youth-adult mentoring relationships: Athletes feel respected by the coaches, and they care what the coach thinks and expects of them, so they work harder to achieve goals.
- Inclusion and a sense of belonging: Individuals feel they are important members of the team.
- Reinforcement of positive values and behavior: Siegel gives as an example former UCLA basketball coach John Wooden. In addition to his excellent coaching on the court, Wooden required his players to pick up towels and soap in the locker room, show respect to managers, and wear jackets and ties when traveling (22).
- Creation of meaningful experiences: These can be in or out of sport, including community service, and help build participants' self-confidence and sense of purpose.

Work with Your Institution: Prevention, Referral, and Enforcement

If you coach in a school setting, your school probably already has well-articulated rules regarding alcohol and drug use by athletes. Other organizations, such as community recreation and sports programs, may have policies in place as well. If you coach outside of an institution, your sport governing body may have guidelines in these areas. Be sure you understand the policies you are supposed to follow. If there are no policies, you should develop your own, especially if you work with minors. A clear policy set forth at the beginning of the season will make your enforcement decisions easier should problems arise.

If you work with minors, you must promote a no alcohol policy for legal reasons. If you work with players of legal drinking age, your regulations can be more sport-oriented: drinking should be limited before practices and contests because it interferes with training and performance. Ask your athletes to help make the rules, so it is their policy, created for the success of the team. One NCAA Division III women's basketball coach told us how she and her team established guidelines for alcohol use. "On our team, we work with the athletes to set rules around alcohol use. Half the team is over 21, so are of legal drinking age. The team usually adopts the '24/48 hour rule': no alcohol 24 hours before practice or 48 hours before a game. Because we practice or play almost daily, my captains told me there was only one night of drinking this past season."

AN OUNCE OF PREVENTION

If you coach at a college or high school, you may be required, along with all the other coaches, to provide preventive education about substance abuse. You may be asked to schedule an educational session during practice time early in the season, or at the beginning of the year. Your athletic director or athletic trainer may be in charge of these efforts. At some high schools, the guidance counselors are involved. An expert in alcohol and drug education for your age group, or trained peer educators, should lead the discussion, rather than the coach, if possible. Unless you have special training in this area, your athletes may know more than you and sense your discomfort with the topics. Workshops that engage participants in discussion and role play and work to address the causes of alcohol and drug use in athletes appear to be more effective than preachy lectures (23).

Many health educators have asked the question: does preventive education work? Or is it a waste of valuable practice time? Or could it even make the situation worse, increasing the incidence of problem behaviors? Research on educational programs aimed at preventing substance use and eating disorders show that information-giving strategies are generally ineffective. In some cases, these interventions have even been associated with an *increase* in substance abuse (24,25) or eating disorders (26), perhaps by normalizing the behavior or providing information that inadvertently promotes the behavior.

So if talking about substance abuse does not prevent it, what does? Some research suggests that the best defense (against substance abuse and other negative behaviors) is a good offense: creating a team culture that teaches and reinforces positive behaviors. If you work with teens, and are interested in building a holistic sports experience for your athletes that not only focuses on sport, but also on improving lifestyle and life skills as vehicles to peak performance (and school success), you can learn more about the ele-

FOCAL POINT

Sport Plus Programs

Several interesting programs have used sport as a vehicle to promote school success and life skills, and to prevent negative behaviors in participants. We introduce three here which have achieved noteworthy success. If you are interested in developing a similar focus for your team, you might be interested in finding out more about these programs. (Sources on each of these programs is listed below.)

1. Phyllis A. Jones, a girl's basketball coach at an inner city school in Pittsburgh, developed her program to address the most common reasons her athletes quit playing: lack of interest, academic ineligibility, and unplanned pregnancy. In addition to developing sports skills, her program included a prepractice study hall, mentoring components to help the girls develop long-term goals and deal with personal issues, and group activities to promote positive group support. When Jones' team was compared to a similar team who received basketball coaching only and a control group that did not play basketball, researchers found that Jones' team had a higher GPA (3.09 vs. 2.46 and 2.30) (1). In addition, significantly more players from Jones' team went on to attend college (95% vs 40% and 50%).

2. The Adolescent Training and Learning to Avoid Steroids Program (ATLAS) studied 31 high school football teams, half of which received extra activities designed to prevent substance, including steroid, use (2). Extra activities included classroom and exercise sessions led by peer educators (including team leaders), coaches, and strength coaches. Groups receiving the intervention had less intention to use steroids, and 1 year later had less substance use (including alcohol) than control teams. You can find more information about this program online at http://www.ohsu.edu/hpsm/atlas.html.

3. The Athletes Targeting Healthy Exercise and Nutrition Alternatives (ATHENA) Program is the sister program to the ATLAS program above. Researchers in this program studied 40 girls sports teams, including cheerleading, half of whom received the intervention curriculum (3). The curriculum included eight weekly sessions (45 minutes) incorporated into team practices that focused on healthy sport nutrition, effective exercise training, depression prevention, and substance abuse and eating disorders prevention. Discussions were scripted by the investigators, but led by team leaders. Athletes receiving the intervention reported less current use of diet pills and substances, and less intention to use substances or participate in harmful weight reduction behaviors in the future. The ATHENA program research is described in more detail online at http://www.ohsu.edu/hpsm/athena.html.

1. Jones DF, Jones PA. Model for success: the impact of a grant-funded program on an inner-city girls' basketball program. *J Phys Ed Rec Dance* 2002;73(5):22–25.
2. Goldberg L, MacKinnon DP, Elliot DL et al. The adolescents training and learning to avoid steroids program: preventing drug use and promoting health behaviors. *Arch Pediatr Adolesc Med* 2000;154(4):332–338.
3. Elliot DL, Goldberg L, Moe EL et al. Preventing substance use and disordered eating: initial outcomes of the ATHENA (athletes targeting healthy exercise and nutrition alternatives) program. *Arch Pediatr Adolesc Med* 2004;258(11):1043–1049.

ments that prevent substance abuse and other problem behaviors, and help build successful programs (Focal Point: Sport Plus Programs). While sport alone does not always protect teens from harmful behaviors, sport programs can be structured in ways that promote positive behaviors along with training for peak performance.

REFERRAL: REACH OUT TO HELP ATHLETES IN TROUBLE

You may have noticed that athletes often go to their coaches when they are in trouble. (Maybe you even went to one of your coaches when you were having difficulties as a teen or young adult.) You, the coach, spend more time with them than almost any other adult in their lives, except for family members. You are the "trusted adult" they might turn to when they do not know what to do, someone who can really make a difference in their lives.

But athletes who need help with a substance abuse problem will rarely approach you with a concern. It is more likely that they will attract your attention by not showing up or showing up late for practices and competitions, or arriving under the influence. Their school work may begin to suffer. Some of the most common signs of a substance abuse problem include the following (27,28):

- Changes in appearance, especially looking more tired or less focused than usual. Athlete may look less healthy or sloppier, taking less care of personal appearance.
- Emotional changes that appear to have no cause, such as more irritability, anger, depression, or moodiness.
- Problems in school, including more lateness, absences, or a decline in grades.
- Problems with sports, such as decline in performance, more absences, more illness, weight loss, or decreased motivation.
- Change in attitude toward you, the coach. Athlete may avoid you or respond to criticism more defensively.

Most of the items on this list are common in adolescents, and may be due to any number of problems unrelated to substance abuse or sport. But if several of these items begin to appear, keep your eyes open for more concrete evidence of a problem. You might smell alcohol on the athlete's breath or clothes, or teammates may tell you that this athlete is getting drunk or using drugs at parties. You can find more information on substance abuse at the websites listed in Focal Point: Finding More Information about Drugs and Drug Use Patterns.

If teammates have expressed concern, and you have observed some of the changes listed above, you should make time to speak with your athlete and share your concern. Review the guidelines for sharing concerns about eating disorders in the previous chapter. The principles are the same for sharing concerns about substance abuse.

FOCAL POINT

Finding More Information about Drugs and Drug Use Patterns

If you are interested in finding out more about drugs and drug use patterns in the United States, you can find a great deal of excellent information from several websites, including the following.

1. Monitoring the Future: Results online at http://monitoringthefuture.org.
2. Youth Risk Behavior Surveillance System, a school survey that collects responses from high school students on a variety of risky behaviors. Available online http://www.cdc.gov/nccdphp/dash/yrbs/index.htm.
3. The National Survey on Drug Use and Health, available online at http://www.drugabusestatistics.samhsa.gov.
4. The National Institute on Drug Abuse has statistics and helpful fact sheets online at http://drugabuse.gov.

- Speak to your athlete in private. Schedule a time when you will not be interrupted.
- Express your concern. Let your athlete know you are worried, and that you care about him or her as a member of your team, and as a person.
- Cite specific, objective, observable behaviors that concern you. "You missed 3 practices in the last 2 weeks," or "Your times are 7 seconds slower than they were 6 weeks ago."
- Give the athlete a chance to respond. If he or she talks, listen without interrupting.
- Take some time to think over your response, in terms of consequences for the athlete, especially if new information has been divulged by the athlete in this conversation. You do not need to deliver a punishment immediately. You may say or do something you regret if you act hastily. It is okay to let your athlete know you need some time to think the matter over if a response from you is required.
- Refer the athlete to a counselor if you are concerned. Even if the athlete is not using substances, but admits to being depressed or having family problems, suggest counseling to help with these issues. If the athlete will not talk to you, you can still express concern and refer him or her to counseling. "I don't know what's wrong, but you seem angry all the time. I'd like to see you talk to the guidance counselor tomorrow."
- Let the athlete know he or she has your support. Express confidence in their ability to deal with the situation in a positive fashion. Share your expectations for what they are supposed to do now.

After you meet with your athlete, you may still need to decide on your response. If there is solid evidence that the athlete is abusing substances (e.g., you catch him or her in the act), follow your institution's protocols for referral and/or sanctions. Work with your school's judicial board or other system for dealing with these issues. If your athlete is a minor, you should notify the parents if the athlete has violated any rules, or if you think the athlete needs outside support, such as counseling.

You should not have to make these decisions alone. Talk to your athletic director, athletic trainers, or other colleagues to make a plan that follows institutional protocols and will be most helpful to your athlete and your team.

ENFORCING SANCTIONS

Coaches must work with their institutions and follow the guidelines of their sport governing bodies to enforce rules regarding penalties for substance use by their athletes. This will probably be out of your hands, and you and the athlete will be given instructions from the administration regarding in which practices and/or competitions the athlete may not participate. Obviously, rules must be enforced as clearly and fairly as possible.

If you are not affiliated with an organization and must enforce your own regulations, do so fairly. Talk to other coaches of the teams in your league if you need help making decisions about an athlete's behavior.

One of the most difficult decisions that coaches occasionally face is whether to suspend an athlete from the team. In institutional settings, this decision may be out of your hands, although you may still be involved as part of the group making such decisions. An athlete with a substance abuse problem usually benefits from continued team and coach support as he or she works to address the problem behavior, unless the sport environment somehow makes the behavior worse. On the other hand, an athlete who fails to respond to repeated warnings and sanctions may need a stronger consequence to "get the message" that substance abuse will not be tolerated. Other athletes on the team also need to see that team rules are enforced, even for athletes who are team captains or other valuable players. Suspension is generally a more effective consequence for the athlete who has repeatedly broken the rules than permanently cutting him or her from the team, since suspension holds out the hope of rejoining the team at a later date, which may motivate the athlete to overcome problem behaviors.

Performance Enhancing Drugs

Winning is the basic idea behind sport competition. Athletes and coaches spend endless hours in training, striving for peak performance and a competitive advantage. It is not surprising that drugs and supplements which promise to enhance performance are extremely attractive to athletes, as well as to their athletic trainers and coaches.

Performance enhancing drugs include prescription and illicit drugs taken specifically to improve sports performance. These drugs may improve performance through a wide variety of channels. Some work by increasing endurance, strength, speed or power; or by altering body composition, either by building muscle or decreasing fat. Some drugs claim to enhance performance by increasing alertness and energy level, or by reducing pain. Examples of performance enhancing drugs include the steroid family of substances, human growth hormone, erythropoietin (along with red blood cell transfusions, or blood doping) and amphetamines (including caffeine, Dexedrine, Adderall, Ritalin, and other drugs prescribed for attention deficit disorder, and illicit amphetamines and stimulants such as MDMA [ecstasy] and cocaine).

The U.S. Centers for Disease Control and Prevention's surveys suggest that in 2005 approximately 4% of high school students had taken steroid pills or shots at least once in their life (29). Other surveys place the estimate on steroid use by high school students to be somewhere between 3% and 9% (30). The NCAA estimates that approximately 1% of college student-athletes currently use steroids (12), although use varies widely with the type of sport and division. While steroid use has dropped slightly over the past few years, amphetamine use has risen slightly (29). For more information on drug use in the United States, see the resources listed in Focal Point: Finding More Information about Drugs and Drug Use Patterns.

Unless you have been living on another planet, you already know that use of performance enhancing drugs by Olympic, professional, collegiate, and high school athletes has attracted enormous media attention over the years. Educational institutions and sport governing bodies have unequivocally condemned the use of performance enhancing drugs by athletes. Professional organizations, such as the National Athletic Training Associating, the American College of Sports Medicine and the National Strength and Conditioning Association have likewise mandated that its members promote drug-free sport participation (32–34).

Objections to performance enhancing drugs are based on several factors (34).

- Use of performance enhancing drugs is unfair. Many argue that sport should be based on the notion of "fair play." The use of performance enhancing drugs gives certain athletes an unfair advantage, and so is morally and ethically wrong.
- Use of performance enhancing drugs undermines the idea that extensive training, good coaching, and sound nutrition are the respected ways to athletic excellence and peak performance.
- Use of performance enhancing drugs has many negative health effects for athletes. These drugs are often taken at very high doses, increasing the likelihood of negative side effects.
- Use of performance enhancing drugs is illegal, according to most institutions and sport governing bodies. As a coach, you must promote drug-free participation for your athletes because that is part of your job, and so that your athletes do not get disqualified because of a positive drug test.

Performance Enhancing Supplements

Performance enhancing supplements are dietary supplements that claim to enhance sport performance. Because dietary supplements are derived from natural substances, are legal, and are available over the counter, people assume they are safe. Many athletes use supplements, and may ask for your opinion about them. Your advice on supplement use will be a little more complicated than your advice on drug use ("Just say no"). Some supplements, such as the standard, one-a-day multivitamin complex, are safe when used as directed. Others have ingredients whose long-term safety has not been determined. Some supplements may even contain ingredients banned by sport governing bodies, and have even led to cases of athletes being disqualified because they tested positive for these substances on a drug test. Supplements are regulated very loosely in the United States (Focal Point: Dietary Supplement Regulation in the United States).

SUPPLEMENT USE IN CHILDREN AND TEENS

A mother of a 10th grade soccer player told us this story. "I am worried that my son's sport program is turning him into a drug addict. I thought participating in sports would be good for him, keep him busy after school, build character, and all that. He's 16, and so many of his friends are getting into trouble with

FOCAL POINT

Dietary Supplement Regulation in the United States

In the United States, dietary supplements are regulated by the Food and Drug Administration (FDA), a division of the Department of Health and Human Services (Fig. 11.3). The Center for Food Safety and Applied Nutrition (CFSAN) is the branch of the FDA that works with food and dietary supplements. You can find a lot of good information on supplements and their regulation at their website, www.cfsan.fda.gov.

Whenever you read about supplement regulation, you will see references to DSHEA. Congress passed the Dietary Supplement Health and Education Act (DSHEA) in 1994. This Act allows manufacturers to market many products as "dietary supplements" rather than as drugs. To qualify as a "dietary supplement" the product must contain one or more of the following substances: "a vitamin; a mineral; an herb or other botanical; an amino acid; a dietary substance for use by man to supplement the diet by increasing the total dietary intake (e.g., enzymes or tissues from organs or glands); a concentrate, metabolite, constituent or extract" of the above (1).

The DSHEA mandates that manufacturers of dietary supplements must be sure that their products are safe before they are sold. However, supplements do not need approval before being sold, nor do manufacturers need to submit any studies to the FDA before marketing a new product. The FDA does not need to look at a product unless it receives enough complaints about it. When a questionable product comes to the FDA's attention, the FDA must show that the dietary supplement is unsafe before it can remove the product from the marketplace.

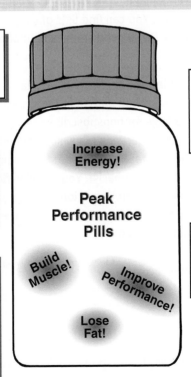

■ **FIGURE 11.3** Dietary supplement regulation in the U.S. Dietary supplement manufacturers are allowed a great deal of freedom in the manufacture and marketing of their products. Products do not have to show safety or efficacy, although if the FDA can demonstrate evidence that a product is harmful, it may be withdrawn from the market.

(continues)

Dietary Supplement Regulation in the United States *(continued)*

The DSHEA does not mandate that dietary supplements be effective. If a product is shown to be ineffective, the FDA need not require that the product be removed. However, if many complaints are received, action may be taken by the Federal Trade Commission (FTC), which may investigate fraudulent advertising.

Some sports nutrition and weight loss products, such as sports drinks and bars, fall into the category of food, not supplements. Both foods and supplements are subject to labeling requirements of the Nutrition Labeling Education Act of 1990 (NLEA). The NLEA prohibits labels from claiming that a product or its ingredients help to treat or prevent disease, except for certain health claims allowed by the FDA. Since sports performance is not a disease, statements claiming to improve sport performance are allowable without proof that the claim is true. Just check out dietary supplements on the web and you will find this principle in action! Marketing and labels for these products are often misleading and deceptive.

Many supplements can be harmful to your health. Even vitamins and minerals can be toxic at high doses. Most vitamin and mineral supplements contain safe levels of nutrients, but some consumers may get the same vitamin in different preparations. For example, someone may take a multi, then something for the eyes, something for the immune system, and something to enhance athletic performance. Each may contain zinc and vitamin A, both of which may be toxic at high doses.

Some supplements on the market are known to be risky. For example, supplements with kava, comfrey, and chaparral have been associated with liver damage. Ephedra use has been linked to a number of deaths, especially when taken in high doses with caffeine. You can find lists of supplements to avoid at the FDA website, www.cfsan.fda.gov/%7Edms/ds-warn.html. Other good sources of information about dietary supplements include:

1. National Institutes of Health, Office of Dietary Supplements. Available online at ods.od.nih.gov.
2. ConsumerLab.com tests products and lists those that meet their specifications. Subscribers get full reports, but some good information is also available for nonsubscribers. Available online at www.consumerlab.com.
3. The Natural Pharmacist provides detailed reports on many supplement ingredients, based on reports in peer-reviewed journals. You can access The Natural Pharmacist at the commercial site www.iherb.com. Under "health links" you can click on The Natural Pharmacist. You can also find good information in the German Commission E Monographs in the same health links section.
4. The National Council Against Health Fraud has a helpful website that includes good information on supplement fraud. Available online at www.quackwatch.org.

1. U.S. Food and Drug Administration. *Center for Food Safety and Applied Nutrition. Dietary Supplement Health and Education Act of 1994.* Available online at www.cfsan.fda.gov/~dms/dietsupp.html. Accessed March 3, 2008.

alcohol and drugs. I hoped that playing sports would give him healthy peak experiences! Well, there he was yesterday in the kitchen, mixing up his sports recovery drink. I never thought much about it, but lately he is taking a lot of supplements. So I finally read the label—and couldn't believe it! Hormones, caffeine, a million chemicals I can't even begin to pronounce. I thought the product was just a protein shake. How did this stuff get into my house?"

In general, performance-enhancing supplements should be off-limits to children and teens for several reasons. First, many supplements, especially the weight loss, muscle building supplements, may contain ingredients that are harmful to young people, such as prohormones and amphetamines. If not immediately harmful, the long-term effects are unknown, especially for young, growing bodies. Even creatine, widely used by many high school athletes, has no long-term studies of its safety or efficacy in adults or children.

Second, the use of legal performance-enhancing substances by teens has been linked to later use of illegal substances, such as steroids (30,34). Adolescents may develop a performance-enhancing, weight-control, getting-built focus that gets out of control very quickly.

Lastly, promoting the use of substances detracts from what we are trying to teach young people, that the most productive path to performance enhancement lies in self-discipline and hard work: a well-designed training program, good coaching, attending every practice or workout, good nutrition, and sufficient rest and recovery. Popping pills to give you a competitive edge should not be part of the youth sport picture.

CAN COACHES RECOMMEND DIETARY SUPPLEMENTS TO ADULT ATHLETES?

Most sport-related organizations admit that whether or not coaches should recommend dietary supplements to their athletes is controversial. On the one hand, it is beyond our scope of practice to give nutrition advice, beyond the basic recommendations for a standard healthful diet. On the other hand, many coaches do recommend recovery beverages that contain carbohydrate and protein to speed muscle healing and glycogen resynthesis. We might have our endurance athletes consuming gels and sports bars to keep blood sugar up. How about a protein shake for your athletes who are trying to gain weight? A little creatine for your power athletes? As you can see, supplement use can be a slippery slope. We urge you to err on the side of caution, and refrain from directly recommending supplement use to your athletes. For most athletes, supplement use does not offer much advantage. When your athletes have questions about supplement use, refer them to your athletic trainer or sports nutritionist.

The NCAA urges caution for athletes contemplating supplement use, stating that "(m)any nutritional/dietary supplements contain NCAA banned substances. In addition, the U.S. Food and Drug Administration (FDA) does not strictly regulate the supplement industry; therefore purity and safety of nutritional dietary supplements cannot be guaranteed. Impure supplements may lead to a positive NCAA drug test. The use of supplements is at the student-athlete's own risk. Student-athletes should contact their institution's team physician or athletic trainer for further information" (7).

ATHLETES WITH SPECIAL HEALTH NEEDS: WHAT THE COACH SHOULD KNOW

As a coach, you will probably find athletes on your team who are coping with chronic health challenges that run the gamut from somewhat annoying to potentially life threatening. Be sure that every one of your athletes follows your organization's protocols for medical clearance and waivers for participation. Athletes whose chronic health problems, such as asthma and diabetes, are well controlled may be cleared for participation, and often make fine athletes. This section gives you the information you need to understand these common health problems, offer support to your athletes as they manage their conditions, and recognize and respond to potential emergency situations. This section will also give you a sense of how the coach works with athletes with chronic health problems, so when you have athletes with a problem not covered here you will have a general idea of the coach's responsibilities.

Athletes with Asthma

Asthma is a chronic disorder of the lower airways, the bronchi and the bronchioles, characterized by recurring periods of breathing difficulty. During an asthma attack the airways become inflamed and swollen, and produce excess mucus. The small muscles in the airways contract, causing the passages to narrow or even close, a condition called bronchoconstriction (Fig. 11.4). Asthma symptoms include difficulty breathing, wheezing, and coughing (Focal Point: Out of Shape? Or Exercise-induced Asthma?) . Asthma attacks range in severity from very mild to life-threatening.

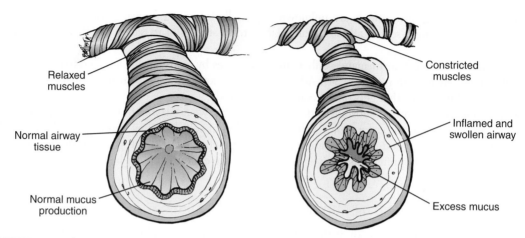

■ **FIGURE 11.4** Asthma airway changes. With asthma, the muscles of the bronchial tubes constrict, reducing the diameter of the airways. In addition, the airways become inflamed and swollen, and extra mucus is produced, which further narrows the airways.

FOCAL POINT

Out of Shape? Or Exercise-induced Asthma?

Sometimes coaches are the first to recognize exercise-induced asthma (EIA) symptoms in their athletes. You may notice a player who gets more out of breath than peers who seem to be in comparable physical condition, or whose breathing takes much longer than normal to recover to resting levels following a workout. People often fail to realize they have exercise-induced asthma because the symptoms mimic the normal fatigue and breathlessness associated with intense exercise.

The most common symptoms of EIA include the following. These may be experienced either during or after exercise, or both:

- Shortness of breath — your athlete may still feel breathless up to 10 minutes after exercise
- Chest tightness
- Excess mucus production during exercise
- Wheezing, a whistling or rasping sound during breathing
- Cough, feeling a need to clear your airways

Less common symptoms include:

- Excessive fatigue with exercise, feeling out of shape at workloads that should not elicit such fatigue
- Lower performance than would be expected with current training levels
- Sore throat with exercise
- Headache
- Stomach cramps

If you suspect your athlete has EIA, he should be evaluated by his health care provider. EIA can be confirmed with a lung function test, comparing resting values with the values recorded after a breathing challenge test.

No one knows why some people develop asthma and become hyperreactive to the substances and conditions that trigger bronchoconstriction. Asthma prevalence has risen dramatically in the past 20 years in North America, and some researchers blame chemicals found in air pollution (35). Outdoor air pollutants that commonly trigger asthma include ozone, sulfur dioxide, and nitrous dioxide. The most common source of indoor air pollution is tobacco smoke. Other common asthma triggers include allergens such as pollen, house dust mites, pet dander, cockroach allergens, and mold. Food allergens such as peanuts, tree nuts, and soy beans can trigger asthma. Aspirin, emotional stress, cold air, and respiratory viruses are common asthma triggers (3). Chlorine and bromine byproducts in indoor swimming pool air trigger asthma in some swimmers.

Ninety percent of people with chronic asthma experience bronchoconstriction during exercise. But about 10% of people with normal lung function at rest experience bronchoconstriction only during or following exercise (36). The term exercise-induced bronchospasm (EIB) commonly refers to bronchoconstriction with exercise in people with or without chronic asthma (36), although the two conditions may be somewhat different (37). Some researchers suggest that EIB without chronic asthma does not always involve as much inflammation as other forms of asthma (37).

Exercise-induced asthma appears to be more common in athletes than in the general population. Studies of athletes have reported EIB rates ranging from 11% to 50% (37,38). The highest rates of asthma have generally come from studies of athletes who exercise in a cold environment. Rates of 35% have been reported in figure skaters (39) and ice hockey players (40). (Some researchers have suggested that poor air quality in ice skating rinks may be a contributing factor in some cases.) The highest EIA rates, up to 50%, have been found in cross-country skiers (41).

Why is the EIB rate higher in athletes? Researchers are not sure. Some suggest that large volumes of exercise, especially in cold air, may somehow lead to physiological changes in the airways that make them more likely to constrict during exercise (42), but not all research supports this notion (38). Or perhaps EIB is simply diagnosed more frequently in athletes because they exercise.

Asthma is such a common condition that it is easy to become complacent about the risk it entails. But any condition that causes difficulty breathing should be taken very seriously. Although most asthma attacks respond well to medication, every year many people are rushed to the hospital with breathing difficulties resulting from asthma. Some people, including athletes, even die from asthma attacks. Almost 5,000 asthma deaths occur in the United States each year (43). One study of asthma deaths in recreational and competitive athletes reported that asthma was the main cause of death in 61 cases between 1993 and 2000 (44). Fifty-one percent (18 athletes) of the competitive athletes had their fatal event while participating in their sport, 14 during practice, and 4 during competitions (44).

Despite these sobering statistics, it is important to remember that supervised physical activity has been linked to better asthma management and quality of life in people with asthma (45). Given the high prevalence of asthma, coaches must be prepared to work with athletes with this disorder, and to provide a safe and supportive atmosphere for them. Athletes whose asthma is well-controlled can work just as hard as the other members of your team and may be some of your best performers. Athletes with chronic asthma usually anticipate having breathing difficulties with exercise, and are usually well-prepared with their rescue inhalers and asthma action plan. Unless they are newly diagnosed or new to exercise, they are probably quite adept at recognizing the onset of asthma symptoms and will self-medicate effectively.

Coaches should:

- understand what asthma is and how it is diagnosed.
- be sure an athlete with asthma has received medical clearance to participate.
- offer to read and discuss an athlete's asthma management plan.
- be sure athletes with asthma always have access to their medications.
- refer athletes back to their health care providers if asthma is not well controlled.
- know when an athlete should receive emergency care for an asthma attack.
- know when athletes may return to play after an asthma attack.

Coaches whose athletes are subject to drug-testing should be sure athletes who are using asthma medication comply with all governing body regulations regarding documentation of the drugs' medical necessity. (The Standard Therapeutic Use Exemption [TUE] Form can be found on the United States Anti-Doping Agency website, www.usantidoping.org.)

FROM THE ATHLETIC TRAINING ROOM

Peak Flow Values

People with asthma (and their health care providers) monitor airway restriction by measuring how well they can forcefully exhale. They use a spirometer to measure peak flow value, also known as forced expiratory volume (FEV). You may see the abbreviation "FEV1" on their charts. This refers to the volume of air that can be forcefully exhaled in 1 second. When bronchoconstriction occurs, less air is moved with a forceful exhalation.

You may see some athletes using spirometers to monitor the severity of their asthma and the efficacy of their medications. Optimal peak flow values vary from person to person, and are largely a function of the person's lung volume and body size.

People with asthma learn what a normal value is for them when their asthma is well controlled. Their providers may even recommend medication dosages based on spirometry tests: larger or more frequent doses for poorer scores.

HOW IS ASTHMA DIAGNOSED?

Asthma is usually diagnosed when a person complains of breathing difficulties or a chronic cough. The health care provider will consider many factors in making the diagnosis and ruling out other health problems. The most objective test for asthma is performed with an instrument called a spirometer (see From the Athletic Training Room: Peak Flow Values).

The patient exhales as forcefully as possible into the spirometer, which measures the volume of exhaled air. Lower than normal scores, or changes in these values following a breathing challenge such as exercise, indicate airway narrowing.

Athletes who exhibit normal spirometry values in the provider's office but complain of symptoms indicative of EIB may be given an inhaler to use before exercise. If this medication resolves symptoms, the athlete may not be asked to perform an exercise or other breathing challenge test, but may simply be instructed to continue to use the inhaler before exercise (46). However, when a definitive diagnosis is required, or when the inhaler is not always effective in controlling EIB symptoms, more extensive testing is recommended.

MEDICAL CLEARANCE

Athletes with asthma are almost always cleared to exercise, as long as their condition is well-controlled with medication. If you see an asthma diagnosis on the preparticipation physical paperwork, ask your athlete about her asthma management. Are symptoms generally well-controlled? If she still seems to have questions about managing her asthma, encourage her to continue working with her provider so that she is clear on her asthma management plan, and so that optimal control is achieved. Offer to discuss the asthma management plan with the athlete or her parents, if the athlete is young.

READING AN ASTHMA MANAGEMENT PLAN

Athletes with asthma must work closely with their health care providers to come up with an asthma management plan that works. This may involve several visits to the provider and good record keeping on the part of athletes and/or their parents (if athletes are young). The goal of asthma management is to reduce inflammation and airway responsiveness. While many excellent medications have been developed for the treatment of asthma, it may take several months to adjust dosages and types of medications to achieve maximum asthma control. Most people with asthma take some sort of medication to reduce inflammation and another medication to help open the airways. The asthma management plan should contain concrete instructions regarding timing and dosage of all medications in relation to sports practices and contests.

Finding More Information on Asthma

If you would like to find out more about asthma, the following organizations have very helpful websites:

American Academy of Allergy, Asthma and Immunology. www.aaaai.org.

American College of Allergy, Asthma and Immunology. www.acaai.org.

American Lung Association. www.lungusa.com.

National Heart, Lung, and Blood Institute. www.nhlbi.nih.gov.

USA Swimming created a report on asthma for swim coaches, but most of the information is relevant to coaches of other sports as well. The web address for this document, *Managing Asthma—A Comprehensive Guide for Swim Coaches*, is www.usaswimming.org/USASWeb/_Rainbow/Science%20&%20Technology%20Research%20Grants/f33d55eb-3d5b-443c-b779-e9e1dfdbc1cb/Asthma-A%20Comprehensive%20Guide%2004%20Nov%2029.pdf.

When your athletes share their plans with you, you should pay special attention to what they do when they feel the asthma symptoms may be becoming more serious. If they have had asthma emergencies before, discuss with them their strategies for coping with an emergency, and what that might mean for you. If you have any questions, discuss the situation with the athlete, your athletic trainers, and/or the parents, if the athlete is a minor. You may also learn more about asthma from the websites listed in Focal Point: Finding More Information on Asthma.

ACCESS TO MEDICATION

All athletes who have been diagnosed with asthma or prescribed an inhaler must have easy access to their rescue inhaler or other prescribed medication at every practice or contest. Be sure your athletes with asthma understand that if they forget their medication, they will not be allowed to practice or compete. You do not want to find yourself in a situation where an athlete is having an asthma attack with no medication available for treatment.

CAN A COACH TELL IF AN ATHLETE IS USING THE RESCUE INHALER TOO OFTEN?

Some coaches wonder if an athlete's asthma is not well-controlled when they see that athlete repeatedly using an inhaler during exercise. In general, an athlete will take two puffs of an albuterol inhaler before exercise. This dose should be sufficient for 2 to 3 hours. You will probably become familiar with how frequently your athletes with asthma use their inhalers before and during practices and contests. If you notice an athlete using an inhaler more frequently than normal, you should ask if he is doing all right. Advise the athlete to check in with the athletic trainer or other health care advisor if the asthma appears to be becoming more problematic (37,47).

WHEN ASTHMA BECOMES A MEDICAL EMERGENCY

Talk to your athletes with asthma (or their parents, if they are young) about what they do, and what you should do, if and when an asthma attack strikes. Have a plan in place to deal with an asthma emergency should one arise. It is generally not possible for the coach to recognize an oncoming asthma attack, although the athlete with asthma may recognize a worsening of symptoms. By the time your athlete tells you he is having difficulty breathing, the attack may be in full swing.

The following guidelines are very general. Use guidelines specific to your athlete if available.

Responding to an Asthma Attack

1. Stay calm.
2. Administer the rescue inhaler, using the spacer for more effective dosing (Fig. 11.5).
3. Call the athletic trainer on duty, if one is available.
4. Call 911 if you are not sure the athlete will be OK. Most athletes with asthma can tell you if their symptoms are "normal" for them and will probably respond to medication, or if their symptoms feel out of control. If in doubt, call 911.
5. Move your athlete to a safe, quiet location.
6. Monitor symptoms. Call 911 if symptoms do not improve as quickly as you or your athlete thinks they should.

RETURN TO PLAY

Asthma symptoms and response to medication vary greatly from one athlete to another, so, unfortunately for the decision maker, there are no hard and fast guidelines regarding when an athlete may return to play after experiencing asthma symptoms (48). In general, an athlete whose symptoms have been controlled by medication may return to play once he or she is feeling back to normal. An athlete who has had serious breathing difficulties to the point of alarming you should probably rest for the remainder of the practice or contest. If you have another event later that day, the athlete can probably participate if symptoms are well controlled, unless the asthma is being triggered by something that continues to pose a risk, such as a serious respiratory infection.

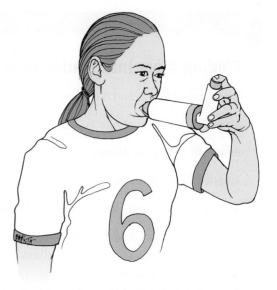

■ **FIGURE 11.5** Asthma inhaler with spacer. Asthma medication is often delivered to the airways with an inhaler. The inhaler ejects the medicine into a spacer, which allows for more effective administration of the medication.

Athletes With Diabetes

Diabetes is a chronic disorder of blood glucose regulation. People with type 1 diabetes are unable to make insulin, a hormone that helps blood glucose enter the body's cells. This is the type of diabetes seen most often in children, adolescents, and young adults. Approximately one in 400 to 600 people under 20 years old have type 1 diabetes (49). Type 2 diabetes occurs when the body's cells become insensitive to insulin and is usually secondary to obesity. Type 2 diabetes is more often seen in adults than in children, although the incidence in children is rising with the increasing incidence of obesity (49). Young athletes with type 2 diabetes often manage their condition with diet, weight loss, and physical activity, and may not require medications until the condition becomes more advanced. (In advanced stages, the ability of the pancreas to make insulin may decline.) Type 1 diabetes must be managed with medication (insulin), along with diet and exercise, and has a much higher potential for adverse reactions, especially high or low blood sugar, during practice and contests. This section will focus primarily on type 1 diabetes.

BLOOD GLUCOSE CONTROL

Normally, the body regulates blood glucose level with exquisite control (Fig. 11.6). When blood glucose levels decline, hormones, including glucagon and epinephrine, signal the liver to make more glucose from glycogen or certain amino acids. Blood sugar returns to normal, and all of the body's cells are happy. If blood sugar gets too high, the pancreas releases the hormone insulin which signals the body's cells to take up more glucose, and get the glucose out of the blood and into storage. If the cells do not require the extra glucose for immediate fuel, they will convert the glucose to glycogen or fat (50,51).

When the body cannot make insulin, insulin must be supplied via injections or an insulin pump. People with diabetes learn to think like a pancreas, and administer insulin when it is most needed, such as before a meal. People with diabetes may check their blood glucose levels several times a day and adjust their meals, exercise, and insulin medications accordingly.

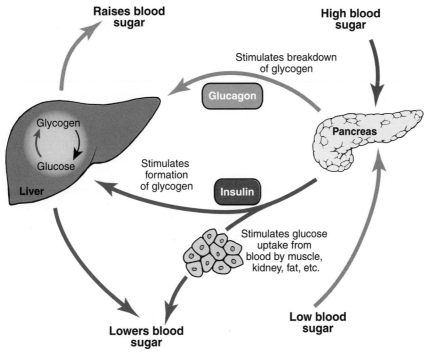

■ **FIGURE 11.6** Blood glucose regulation. Blood glucose is regulated by two hormones secreted by the pancreas. When blood sugar is too high, the pancreas releases insulin, which acts on cells to take up glucose from the bloodstream, thus lowering blood glucose level. When blood sugar falls too low, the pancreas releases glucagon which stimulates the liver to break down glycogen, and release glucose into the blood stream.

Learning to live with diabetes is often very challenging since it requires constant awareness. Young people who are newly diagnosed usually spend several weeks or longer working with their diabetes management team, often including their parents and other family members, to figure out how to keep blood sugar at a healthy level. A parent may closely monitor a young athlete, and even be present during practices and contests to help the child monitor his or her blood sugar. Older children and adolescents may manage pretty well on their own. They should be very familiar with the signs of hypo- and hyperglycemia and know how to respond before blood glucose reaches dangerous levels (52). Most young athletes with type 1 diabetes learn to manage very well, and can participate fully in practices and competitions (53).

When blood glucose is not well regulated, either hypoglycemia (low blood sugar) or hyperglycemia (high blood glucose) may result. Both produce symptoms in their early stages that your athlete must learn to recognize and treat before the condition worsens. Low blood sugar causes shakiness, weakness, dizziness, confusion, hunger, and headache. If blood sugar falls too low, the athlete may lose consciousness or, in extreme cases, experience a seizure. High blood sugar causes an increase in urine output, as the kidneys desperately try to lower blood sugar. The athlete will urinate more, feel more thirsty than usual, feel very tired, and may have blurry vision. If blood glucose level gets too high, the athlete may lose consciousness (54) (see Table 11.1, Symptoms of Hypoglycemia and Hyperglycemia).

Physical activity is good for people with diabetes, but the extra blood sugar demands require adjustment to the diabetes management plan. Physical activity can lead to either hypo- or hyperglycemia.

Hypoglycemia results when insulin is present, the muscles have been using the blood glucose to fuel contraction, but there is an inadequate supply of glucose. This may result from inadequate carbohydrate intake or from depleted glycogen stores, or both. When physical activity seems to be causing hypoglycemia, people with diabetes may need to work with their diabetes management team to lower insulin dosage or increase carbohydrate intake before exercise.

Hyperglycemia results when insulin levels are not adequate. There is glucose in the blood, but it is not getting into the cells fast enough. In this case, insulin dosages may need to be raised to help the cells get the glucose they need.

TABLE 11.1   Symptoms of Hypoglycemia and Hyperglycemia
Hypoglycemia
• Tired
• Dizzy or lightheaded
• Shaky, anxious
• Sweating
• Hungry
• Confused, having difficulty concentrating
• Headache
Hyperglycemia
• Excess urine production (having to pee more than usual)
• Very thirsty
• Very tired
• Blurry vision
• Nausea and vomiting

Kidshealth.org. *Sports, Exercise and Diabetes.* Available online at http://kidshealth.org/teen/managing_diabetes/living/sports_diabetes.html. Accessed March 3, 2008

Coaches do not have the training or the time to be major players in the diabetes management team. But you should be able to do the following:

- understand what diabetes is
- be sure an athlete with diabetes has received medical clearance to participate
- offer to read and discuss an athlete's diabetes management plan
- allow athletes with diabetes access to their snacks and medications, even if the athlete must temporarily come out of a practice or competition
- refer athletes back to their health care providers if diabetes is not well controlled
- know when an athlete should receive emergency care for hypo- or hyperglycemia

EMERGENCY RESPONSE TO DIABETES SYMPTOMS

If your athlete shows symptoms of fatigue (beyond those expected for the given level of exertion) or disorientation, or any of the other symptoms listed in Table 11.1, call the athlete out of practice or competition and ask him how he is feeling. Call your athletic trainer if one is available. The trick with treating diabetes symptoms is distinguishing between high and low blood sugar, and normal exertional fatigue. High blood sugar requires additional insulin, while low blood sugar requires quick fuel (for example, juice, candy, or sugar) and sometimes glucagon injections. Give the wrong substance, and you quickly make the condition worse.

Hypoglycemia is the more common problem (55). Your athletes will almost always know whether they are experiencing hypo- or hyperglycemia. Nevertheless, they should test their blood sugar. If blood sugar is low, they should eat their quickly absorbed carbohydrate, wait 15 or 20 minutes, then test blood sugar again. If it is still low, they should eat some more. Some athletes with diabetes may give themselves glucagon injections to raise blood sugar. If blood sugar is too high, your athlete should take insulin. Keep your athlete out of play until symptoms are resolved and blood sugar returns to normal.

You or your athletic trainer should ask the athlete about prior food intake and medication dosage to have the information available for medical personnel should the blood sugar emergency worsen and should the athlete lose consciousness. (If there is no athletic trainer on the scene, you should record the information.) If symptoms do not respond to treatment, or appear to worsen, consult your athletic trainer (if available) or call emergency services. If your athlete loses consciousness before you can determine whether they have hypo- or hyperglycemia, call emergency services immediately, and treat for shock.

Athletes with Attention Deficit, Hyperactivity, and Mood Disorders

It is beyond the scope of this book to cover in detail the many attention deficit, hyperactivity, and mood disorders (such as depression and anxiety disorders) you may encounter among your athletes. As with the other health issues presented in this chapter, athletes whose conditions are well controlled can make great athletes, and, indeed, benefit greatly from participation in sports. In general, the coach will have no involvement in the treatment of these disorders, and may not even need to be aware that they exist, unless special management is required. Presumably, in such cases you will work with parents or administrators, and receive the necessary information and advice from them.

If your athletes are subject to drug testing, and are on medication for attention deficit or mood disorders, they should complete any necessary paperwork for your governing body, since some of these drugs, especially amphetamines, are banned substances, and could result in a positive drug test.

Other Chronic Health Issues

Through the years, you will no doubt work with athletes who are coping with other chronic health issues not covered in this text. Your athletic trainer and other medical personnel at your institution will usually give you good support and advice. If the athlete is a minor, parents may be very helpful. Your primary concern is to clarify your role, as coach. This is generally limited to ensuring that athletes have access to necessary treatments, such as medications, during their time with you, and understanding what constitutes an emergency that requires calling emergency services.

Sport participation can help build self-confidence and improve quality of life for athletes with health problems. You may find that the self-discipline they have acquired from coping with these challenges makes them some of your hardest workers and most devoted players.

SUMMARY

- Colds are infections of the upper respiratory tract and can interfere with athletic performance. Athletes with colds should be encouraged to rest, although research suggests that mild to moderate exercise will not worsen a cold if symptoms are not severe and are "above the neck."
- Athletes with more serious symptoms, such as fever; cough; extreme fatigue; muscle and joint pain; or pain in the ears, head, chest, or stomach should not attend practice or contests, and should see their health care providers.
- Athletes can reduce the number of colds and other respiratory infections they catch by limiting their exposure to germs (and especially by washing their hands frequently) and by strengthening their immune systems with adequate rest and good nutrition.
- Athletes with gastrointestinal symptoms should be allowed to rest. Athletes reporting severe abdominal pain; fever; severe nausea; severe headache, sleepiness, or lethargy; or blood in the vomit or stools should receive immediate medical attention.
- Athletes with skin infections or blood-borne infections such as HIV or hepatitis B should not participate in contact sports such as wrestling or boxing. Otherwise, these athletes may participate in sport if they have received medical clearance.
- Coaches should set and communicate clear guidelines regarding substance (including alcohol, performance-enhancing drugs, and other drugs) abuse, and convey the idea that substance abuse is unhealthy and interferes with training and peak performance. Coaches should work with team leaders to develop a healthy, supportive team culture that discourages substance abuse.
- If a coach has evidence that an athlete may be abusing substances, he or she should arrange a meeting with the athlete and discuss the evidence, referring the athlete for counseling if the athlete appears to have a substance abuse problem, or other emotional health problems.
- Coaches must work with their institutions to enforce sanctions in a clear and fair manner.
- Coaches should discourage the use of performance-enhancing dietary supplements, since long-term safety has not been determined for most of these substances. In addition, because dietary supplements are only loosely regulated, they may contain banned substances that will result in a positive drug test.

- Asthma is a disorder of the lower airways (bronchi and bronchioles), characterized by recurring periods of breathing difficulty. Exercise-induced asthma is common in athletes.
- Coaches should be sure athletes with asthma always have access to their medications. Coaches should know when an athlete should receive emergency care for an asthma attack.
- Diabetes is a chronic disorder of blood glucose regulation. Both type 1 and type 2 diabetes are managed with some combination of diet, exercise, and/or medication. Type 1 diabetes has a much higher potential for adverse reactions, including high or low blood sugar.
- Coaches should be sure athletes with diabetes have access to their medications and snacks, and should know what to do when an athlete is experiencing a blood sugar emergency.
- Athletes taking medications for attention deficit, hyperactivity, or mood disorders may need to complete paperwork granting them permission to use medication even though the medicine contains banned substances.

References

1. American Lung Association. *Cold and Flu Guidelines*. August 2005. Available online at http://www.lungusa.org/site/pp.asp?c=dvLUK9O0E&b=23161. Accessed March 3, 2008.
2. Centers for Disease Control and Prevention (CDC). *Seasonal Flu*. Available online at http://www.cdc.gov/flu/ (updated weekly). Accessed March 3, 2008.
3. National Institute of Allergy and Infectious Diseases. *US Department of Health and Human Services*. Available online at http://www.niaid.nih.gov. Accessed March 2006.
4. Centers for Disease Control and Prevention (CDC). *Questions and Answers: Cold versus Flu*. Available online at http://www.cdc.gov/flu/about/qa/coldflu.htm. Accessed January 8, 2004.
5. Weidner TG, Cranston T, Schurr T, et al. The effect of exercise training on the severity and duration of a viral upper respiratory illness. *Med Sci Sports Exerc* 1998;30(11):1578–1583.
6. Irwin RS, Baumann MH, Bolser DC, et al. Diagnosis and management of cough executive summary: American College of Chest Physicians evidence-based clinical practice guidelines. *Chest* 2006;129:1S–23S.
7. National Collegiate Athletic Association. *NCAA Banned Drug Classes*. Available oline at http://www1.ncaa.org/membership/ed_outreach/health-safety/drug_testing/banned_drug_classes.pdf. Accessed May 10, 2006..
8. United States Anti-doping Agency. *Drug Reference Online*. Available online at http://www.usantidoping.org/dro. Accessed May 10, 2006.
9. Centers for Disease Control. *Safe Food and Water*. Available online at http://wwwn.cdc.gov/travel/contentSafeFoodWater.aspx. Accessed August 7, 2007.
10. Centers for Disease Control. *Viral Gastroenteritis*. Available online at http://www.cdc.gov/ncidod/dvrd/revb/gastro/faq.htm. Accessed March 3, 2008.
11. Gateway to Government Food Safety Information. Available online at www.FoodSafety.gov. Accessed March 3, 2008.
12. National Collegiate Athletic Association. *NCAA Sports Medicine Handbook 2005–2006*. Available online at http://www.ncaa.org/health-safety. Accessed March 3, 2008.
13. American Medical Society for Sports Medicine and American Academy of Sports Medicine. Human immunodeficiency virus (HIV) and other blood-borne pathogens in sports: joint position statement. *Am J Sports Med* 1995;23:510–514.
14. American Academy of Pediatrics. Human immunodeficiency virus and other blood-borne viral pathogens in the athletic setting. *Pediatrics* 1999;104:1400–1403.
15. Dorman JM. Contagious diseases in competitive sport: What are the risks? *J Am Coll Health* 2000;49:105–109.
16. Kordi R, Wallace WA. Blood-borne infections in sport: risks of transmission, methods of prevention, and recommendations for hepatitis B vaccination. *Br J Sports Med* 2004;38:678–684.
17. Beedy JP, Zierk T. Lessons from the field: Taking a proactive approach to developing character through sports. In: Terry, JP. *CYD Anthology*. Sudbury, MA: Institute for Just Communities, 2002:113–119.
18. Siegel D. Re-conceptualizing and recreating youth sports in Boston. Report written for the Barr Foundation, Boston, MA, 2002. Available online at http://www.barrfoundation.org/resources/resources_show.htm?doc_id=239284. Accessed May 7, 2006.
19. Aaron DJ, Dearwater SR, Anderson R, et al. Physical activity and the initiation of high-risk health behavior in adolescents. *Med Sci Sports Exerc* 1995;27:1639–1642.
20. Kokotailo PK. Substance use and other health risk behaviors in collegiate athletes. *Clin J Sport Med* 1996;6:183–189.
21. Shields DL, Bredemeier BJ. *Character Development and Physical Activity*. Champaign, IL: Human Kinetics, 1995.
22. Walton, GM. *Beyond Winning: The Timeless Wisdom of Great Philosopher Coaches*. Champaign, IL: Human Kinetics, 1992.
23. Komro KA, Toomey TL. *Strategies to Prevent Underage Drinking*. National Institute on Alcohol Abuse and Alcoholism. Available online at http://pubs.niaaa.nih.gov/publications/arh26-1/5-14.htm. Accessed March 5, 2006.
24. Hanson D. The effectiveness of alcohol and drug education. *J Alcohol Drug Educ* 1982;27:1–13.
25. Moskowitz J. The primary prevention of alcohol problems: a critical review of the research literature. *J Stud Alcohol* 1989;50:54–88.

26. Mann T, Nolen-Hoeksema S, et al. Are two interventions worse than none? Joint primary and secondary prevention of eating disorders in college females. *Health Psychol* 1997;16(3):215–225.

27. Greydanus DE, Patel DR. The adolescent and substance abuse: Current concepts. *Curr Probl Pediatr Adolesc Health Care* 2005;35(3):78–98.

28. Martens R. *Successful Coaching*. Champaign, IL: Human Kinetics, 2004.

29. Centers for Disease Control. *Youth Risk Behavior Survey—United States, 2005*. Morbidity and Mortality Weekly Report 2006; 55(SS-5):1–108. Available online at www.cdc.gov/Healthyyouth/yrbs/index.htm. Accessed March 3, 2008.

30. Metzl JD. Anabolic steroids and the pediatric community. *Pediatrics* 2005;116(6):1542.

31. American College of Sports Medicine. *ACSM Position Stand: The Use of Anabolic-Androgenic Steroids in Sports*. Available online at http://www.acsm-msse.org/pt/pt-core/template-journal/msse/media/0587.pdf. Accessed June 2, 2006.

32. National Athletic Trainers' Association. *National Athletic Trainers' Association Official Statement on Steroids & Performance Enhancing Substances*. Available online at http://www.nata.org/publicinformation/docs/steroidstatement.pdf. Accessed June 2, 2006.

33. National Strength and Conditioning Association. *NSCA Position Statements: Anabolic-androgenic Steroid Use by Athletes*. Available online at http://www.nsca-lift.org/Publications/posstatements.shtml#steroid. Accessed June 2, 2006.

34. American Academy of Pediatrics. Use of performance-enhancing substances. *Pediatrics* 2005;115(4):1103–1107.

35. Thurston JD, Bates DV. Air pollution as an underappreciated cause of asthma symptoms. *JAMA* 2003;290(14):1915–1917.

36. Storms WW. Review of exercise-induced asthma. *Med Sci Sports Exerc* 2003;35(9):1464–1470.

37. Parsons JP, Mastronarde JG. Exercise-induced bronchoconstriction in athletes. *Chest* 2005;128(6):3966–3975.

38. Parsons JP, Kaeding C, Phillips G, et al. Prevalence of exercise-induced bronchospasm in a cohort of varsity college athletes. *Med Sci Sports Exerc* 2007;39(9):1487–1492.

39. Mannix ET, Farber MO, Palange P, et al. Exercise-induced asthma in figure skaters. *Chest* 1996;109:312–315.

40. Leuppi JD, Kuhn M, Comminot C, et al. High prevalence of bronchial hyperresponsiveness and asthma in ice hockey players. *Eur Respir J* 1998;12:13–16.

41. Wilbur RL, Rundell KW, Szmedra L, et al. Incidence of exercise-induced bronchospasm in Olympic winter sport athletes. *Med Sci Sports Exerc* 2000;32:732–737.

42. Karjalainen EM, Laitinen A, Sue-Chu M, et al. Evidence of airway inflammation and remodeling in ski athletes with and without bronchial hyperresponsiveness to methacholine. *Am J Respir Crit Care Med* 2000;161:2086–2091.

43. National Heart Lung and Blood Institute. *National Asthma Education and Prevention Program*. Available online at http://www.nhlbi.gov/about/naepp/naep_pd.htm. Accessed March 3, 2008.

44. Becker JM, Rogers J, Rossini G, et al. Asthma deaths during sports: report of a 7-year experience. *J Allergy Clin Immunol* 2004; 113(2):264–267.

45. Fanelli A, Barros Cabral AL, Neder JA, et al. Exercise training on disease control and quality of life in asthmatic children. *Med Sci Sports Exerc* 2007;39(9):1474–1489.

46. Boyajian-O'Neill L, Cardone D, Dexter W, et al. Determining clearance during the preparticipation evaluation. *The Physician and Sportsmedicine*, 2004;32(11). Available online at http://www.physsportsmed.com/issues/2004/1104/ppe.htm. Accessed March 3, 2008.

47. USA Swimming. *Managing Asthma—A Comprehensive Guide for Swim Coaches*. April 2004. Available online at www.usaswimming.org/USASWeb/_Rainbow/Science%20&%20Technology%20Research%20Grants/f33d55eb-3d5b-443c-b779-e9e1dfdbc1cb/Asthma-A%20Comprehensive%20Guide%202004%20Nov%2029.pdf. Accessed March 3, 2008.

48. Allen TW. Return to play following exercise-induced bronchoconstriction. *Clin J Sports Med* 2005;15(6):421–425.

49. American Diabetes Association. *National Diabetes Fact Sheet*, 2005. Available online at http://www.diabetes.org/uedocuments/NationalDiabetesFactSheetRev.pdf. Accessed March 3, 2008.

50. Camacho RC, Galassetti P, David SN, et al. Glucoregulation during and after exercise in health and insulin-dependent diabetes. *Exerc Sport Sci Rev* 2005;33(1):17–23.

51. Tortora GJ, Grabowski SR. *Introduction to the Human Body*. New York: John Wiley & Sons, 2004.

52. Draznin MB. Type 1 diabetes and sports participation: Strategies for training and competing safely. *Phys Sportsmed* 2000; 28(12):49–56.

53. Guelfi KJ, Jones TW, Fournier PA. Intermittent high-intensity exercise does not increase the risk of early postexercise hypoglycemia in individuals with type 1 diabetes. *Diabetes Care* 2005;28:416–418.

54. Kidshealth.org. *Sports, Exercise and Diabetes*. Available online at http://kidshealth.org/teen/managing_diabetes/living/sports_diabetes.html. Accessed March 3, 2008.

55. American Diabetes Association. *Type 1 Diabetes: Conditions and Treatment*. Available online at http://www.diabetes.org/type-1-diabetes/hypoglycemia.jsp. Accessed March 3, 2008.

SPORTS INJURIES

Basic Principles of Treatment and Rehabilitation

Upon reading this chapter, the coach should be able to:

1. Discuss the role of the coach in the rehabilitation process.

2. Describe the components of the musculoskeletal system that are commonly injured.

3. Differentiate between acute and chronic injuries.

4. Discuss the primary components of injury management and the healing process.

5. Describe common uses of therapeutic modalities in the rehabilitation process.

6. Explain methods that can be used to achieve the goal of injury rehabilitation.

7. Discuss the criteria used to determine when an athlete is ready to return to play and competition.

Sylvie was the youngest of five children with four older brothers who were high school basketball stars. As long as she could remember she was playing basketball with her brothers, whether on their driveway court, in the park, or during family vacations. While she was as talented as her brothers, she did not play on her high school team. As the youngest child she was always compared to her older brothers in the classroom. She did not want to live up to the expectations she thought would be put on her on the basketball team and she was tired of living in their shadows. She continued to play at home with her brothers and played recreationally whenever she had an opportunity.

She never lost her love of the game and after she started her first year of college at a Division III school, she approached the basketball coach and asked to try out for the team. Away at college she had no footsteps to fill and she came to the team without anyone having any expectations of her. Her talent was quickly recognized and she soon became one of the starting players.

Midway through her first season she was playing in a very aggressive game against the rival team. Coming down from a rebound she was knocked off balance by an opposing player. As she landed her right foot came down on the foot of another player and she sustained an injury to her ankle. She was helped off the court and examined by the athletic trainer who determined she had a probable grade II ankle sprain. Her foot and ankle were wrapped with an elastic bandage and ice was placed on her ankle as she laid back and elevated her foot.

Prior to going home that evening the athletic trainer placed a brace on her foot and she was instructed in the use of crutches to help unweight her right ankle. She was also instructed to continue to use ice repeatedly for 10 minutes at a time until she returned to the training room the next day.

Athletes and coaches often regard ankle sprains as a trivial injury and do not always appreciate the consequence of recurrent injury and chronic disability if the athlete returns to play before rehabilitation is completed. Now that Sylvie has returned to competitive play, she does not want to be on the sidelines. What does she need to do to fully rehabilitate her ankle so she will not continue to have repeat injuries? How will you know when she is ready to practice and compete again?

Physicians, athletic trainers, and physical therapists are the members of the sports medicine team who have the primary responsibility in the treatment and rehabilitation of injured athletes. However, coaches are the

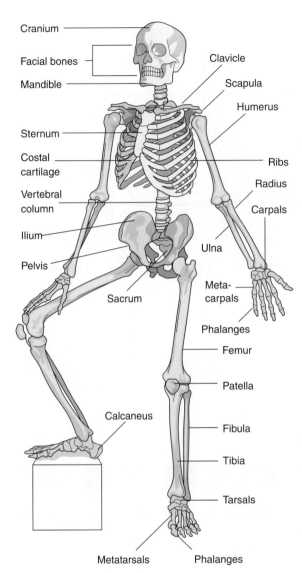

Cranium

Facial bones

Mandible

Clavicle

Scapula

Humerus

Sternum

Costal cartilage

Ribs

Radius

Vertebral column

Carpals

Ilium

Ulna

Pelvis

Meta-carpals

Sacrum

Phalanges

Femur

Patella

Calcaneus

Fibula

Tibia

Tarsals

Metatarsals

Phalanges

■ **FIGURE 12.1** Anterior view showing major bones of the skeleton. The axial skeleton is shown in color and the rest of the bones form the appendicular skeleton. (Reprinted from Cohen BJ, Wood DL. *Memmler's the Human Body in Health and Disease*, 9th ed. Philadelphia: Lippincott Williams & Wilkins, 2000.)

most knowledgeable in terms of the physical requirements of the sports they coach. They can play an important role in ensuring that rehabilitation has returned the athlete to pre-injury status. Knowledge of common injuries and how they are treated can help the coach better understand the limitations imposed during the rehabilitation process as well as what the athlete may still be able to do during the recovery process.

Athletic injuries occur due to trauma or overuse. Following an injury, rehabilitation is necessary to return the athlete to play at a fitness level that is the same or greater than before the injury. Injuries to the musculoskeletal system are common in sports.

THE MUSCULOSKELETAL SYSTEM

The musculoskeletal system consists of several structures that can be injured during athletic activities.

Bones

Bones are the skeletal foundation that provides shape, support, and protection of internal organs. The bones of the head, neck, and trunk form the axial skeleton and the bones of the limbs form the appendicular skeleton (Fig. 12.1).

Joints

Joints are formed by the articulation of two adjacent bones. The synovial joint is the most common type and provides free movement between the bones of almost all limb joints. These joints are held together by the joint capsule and ligaments. The synovial cavity (joint cavity) is filled with synovial fluid (a lubricating substance) and lined with a synovial membrane (Fig. 12.2). Cartilage and tendons are also associated with joints and some joints have adjacent bursa.

Ligaments

Ligaments are fibrous tissue that reinforce the joint capsule and connect the adjacent bones that form the joint (Fig. 12.2).

Cartilage

Cartilage is a connective tissue that is found on the articulating surface of bones and provides shock absorption and reduces friction between the adjacent bones (Fig. 12.2).

Muscles

Skeletal muscles are made of contractile tissue and most connect to bones by means of a tendon. These muscles allow movement of the skeletal structures. The muscle fiber is the structural unit of skeletal muscles. Bundles of muscle fibers form a fascicle. Each muscle is composed of multiple fascicles that are held together with connective tissue (Fig. 12.3).

Tendons

Tendons are fibrous connective tissues that attach the muscle to bone (Fig. 12.3).

Bursae

Bursae are fluid filled sacs that are typically located between muscles or tendons and an underlying bone and serve to reduce friction where one structure moves over another. Figure 12.4 illustrates the location of bursae around the knee joint.

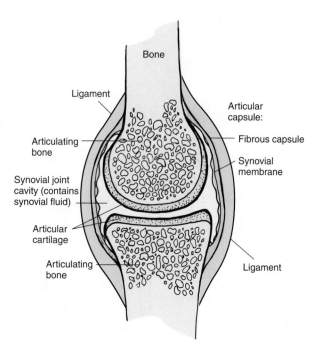

■ **FIGURE 12.2** Typical synovial joint. (Modified from Oatis CA. *Kinesiology—The Mechanics and Pathomechanics of Human Movement.* Baltimore: Lippincott Williams & Wilkins, 2004.)

ACUTE INJURIES

Acute injuries are the result of a sudden trauma. While in sports they occur most commonly in musculoskeletal structures they can also occur in nervous tissue and the internal organs. The following are among the more common musculoskeletal injuries seen in sports.

Contusions

A contusion is a bruise and is the result of a direct blow to muscles, bones or organs. The blow results in damage to the tissue with bleeding and accumulation of fluids. There is often pain, swelling, and discoloration and with deep contusions there can be loss of function. A contusion to a vital organ can be life-threatening.

Muscle Strains

While contusions are an example of extrinsic injury, muscles strains are an intrinsic injury in that they are damaged by their own power. Strains can occur to the muscle belly, the tendon, or the junction where the muscle and tendon meet. They are a stretching or tearing injury in which the fibers of the muscle or tendon are torn. Muscle strains often occur in two-joint muscles such as the quadriceps, hamstrings, and gastrocnemius. These muscles cross and act on two different joints. The quadriceps and hamstrings both act on the knee and hip and the gastrocnemius acts on the ankle and knee.

Strains are classified by the amount of tissue damage (Fig. 12.5).

Grade I—mild with only a few fibers stretched or torn.
Grade II—moderate with more fibers torn.
Grade III—severe with a complete rupture of the muscle belly, complete separation of the muscle and tendon or the tendon being torn from the bone.

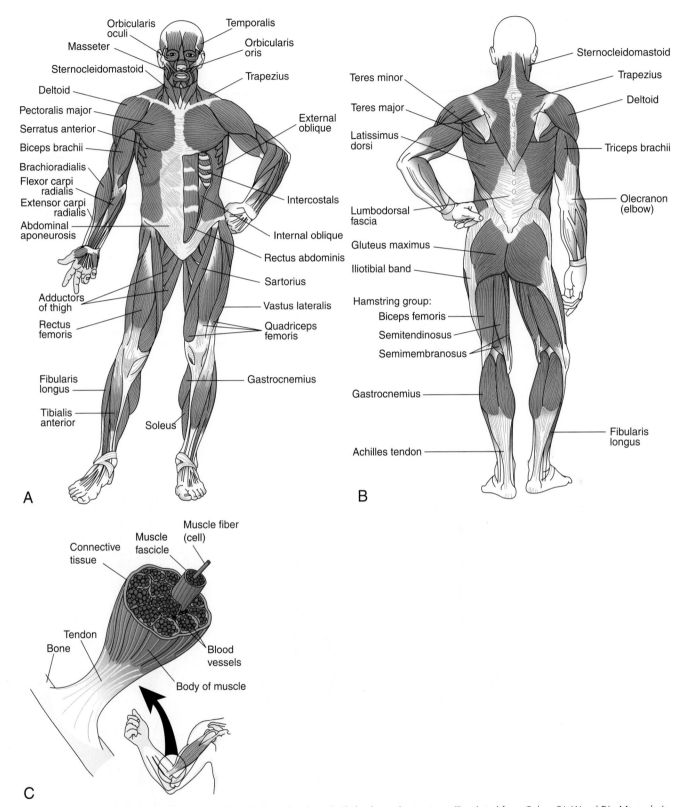

■ **FIGURE 12.3 A.** Superficial muscles, anterior view. **B.** Posterior view. **C.** Skeletal muscle structure. (Reprinted from Cohen BJ, Wood DL. *Memmler's the Human Body in Health and Disease*, 9th ed. Philadelphia: Lippincott Williams & Wilkins, 2000.)

Ligament Sprains

While a strain is an injury to a muscle, a sprain is a stretching or tearing injury of a ligament and depending on the severity can cause disruption of a joint (Fig. 12.6).

Grade I—stretching of the ligament and possibly some torn fibers.
Grade II—moderate tearing of the fibers.
Grade III—complete tear of the ligament.

Depending on the degree of injury, there will be various amounts of instability in the joint along with pain, swelling, and loss of joint function.

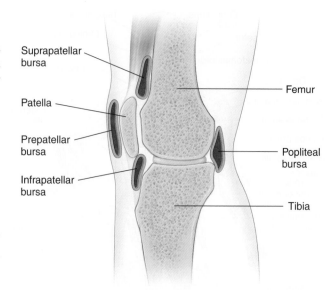

■ **FIGURE 12.4** Location of bursae of the knee joint. (Reprinted from Premkumar K. *The Massage Connection Anatomy & Physiology*. Baltimore: Lippincott Williams & Wilkins, 2004).

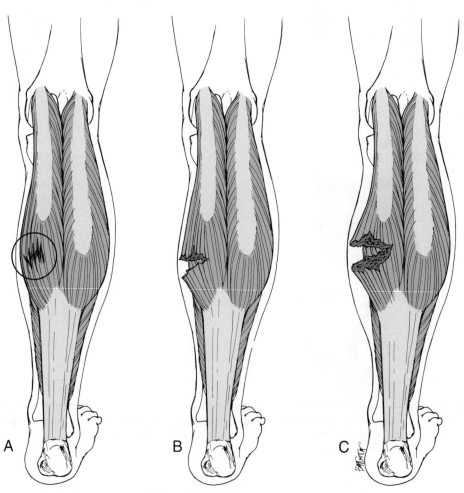

■ **FIGURE 12.5** Muscle strains. **A.** Grade I. **B.** Grade II. **C.** Grade III.

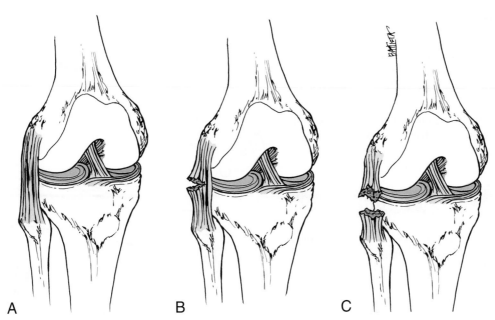

■ **FIGURE 12.6** Ligament sprains. **A.** Grade I. **B.** Grade II. **C.** Grade III.

Dislocations

A dislocation is when a bone is moved out of its normal joint position. If a bone "pops" out of place and "pops" back in on its own, this is called a subluxation. A dislocated bone should be repositioned or "reduced" by a physician. Dislocations and subluxations can injure the surrounding joint tissues such as the ligaments and cartilage. Nerve and blood vessel damage is also possible.

Fractures

A fracture occurs when a bone is compressed, twisted, or struck and the force is greater than the bone can withstand. There are several types of fractures which include: closed, open, avulsion, and stress. A closed fracture is a simple fracture in which the bone is broken, but the skin is intact. In an open fracture or compound fracture the broken bone has pierced the skin. In an avulsion fracture a fragment of bone has pulled away with the ligament or tendon that was attached to the bone (Fig. 12.7). Stress fractures are discussed below with chronic injuries.

FOCAL POINT

Growth Plate Fractures

Growth plate fractures can be a concern in young athletes whose bones have not yet reached their full growth potential. Growth plate fractures are also known as epiphyseal fractures. These fractures are important to recognize and treat appropriately to prevent permanent growth damage. Bone growth stops when the cells at the growth plate stop dividing and this can occur with some types of fractures of the growth plate. Appropriate care by an orthopedic specialist is essential if a growth plate fracture is suspected (1).

1. Brukner P, Khan K. *Clinical Sports Medicine*, 3rd ed. North Ryde, New South Wales: McGraw-Hill Australia, 2007.

Nerve Injuries

Nerves provide innervation to muscles so they can contract. Injury to a nerve can occur anywhere along its path and particularly where its movement is restricted. Injuries can occur through trauma or overuse conditions caused by friction, compression, or stretch.

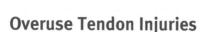

CHRONIC INJURIES

Chronic injuries are those that occur over time as opposed to a single traumatic incident. They can be caused by overuse or repeated friction, blows, or overstretching. Chronic injuries affect various structures of the musculoskeletal system. They can occur when there are imbalances in muscle strength or flexibility or when an athlete overtrains. Sometimes the term chronic refers to the length of time since onset of symptoms with chronic injuries being those present for at least 2 weeks (1).

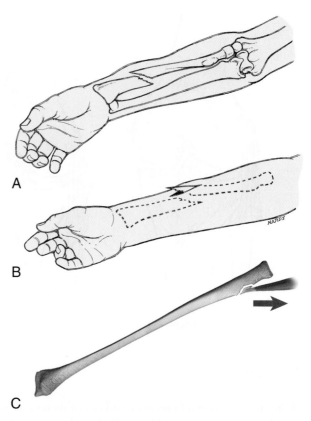

■ **FIGURE 12.7** Fractures. **A.** Closed. **B.** Open. **C.** Avulsion. (Figures A and B, Neil O. Hardy, Westpoint, CT; Figure C, LifeART Image ©2007 Lippincott Williams & Wilkins. All rights reserved.)

Overuse Tendon Injuries

Tendinitis is a frequently diagnosed chronic injury. Tendons can become irritated with repeated overuse or overstretching, especially if there are biomechanical irregularities and weak or tight muscles. Tendinitis means inflammation of a tendon. Other names are used depending on the location and type of tendon injury. Tendinosis is when there is degeneration of the tendon fibers. Tenosynovitis is the term for inflammation of the synovial sheath that covers many tendons.

While tendinitis has been a commonly used term related to chronic tendon injuries, the term tendinopathy is preferred as a general descriptor of tendon conditions arising from overuse (2). In chronic tendon injuries acute inflammation may not be present making tendinitis a misnomer (3,4).

Chronic Muscle Strains

A chronic strain can occur when a muscle is repeatedly overworked or overstretched. Unlike an acute strain, such as occurs suddenly when sprinting, a chronic strain develops over a period of weeks to months. Recurrent injuries may be the result of inadequate rehabilitation following the initial injury (5,6).

Bursitis

Bursitis is an inflammation caused by repeated pressure or irritation. Often the irritation occurs as a result of repeated rubbing of a tendon against the bursa. Figure 12.8 illustrates joints where bursitis is common.

Osteoarthritis

Osteoarthritis is a chronic bone injury that typically occurs from wear over many years. It can also develop in a few years following a traumatic injury such as joint dislocation.

Stress Fractures

A stress fracture is a microscopic or hairline break in a bone generally caused by repetitive activity in high impact sports or high velocity activities. Running is an example of a high impact activity and pitching is a high velocity activity that can lead to stress fractures.

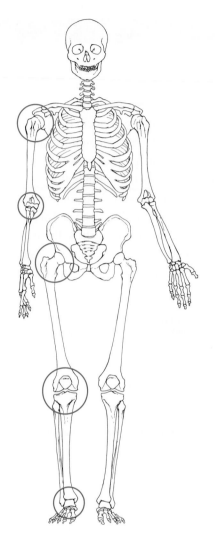

■ **FIGURE 12.8** Joints where bursitis commonly occurs. (Reprinted from Premkumar K. *The Massage Connection Anatomy & Physiology*. Baltimore: Lippincott Williams & Wilkins, 2004).

INJURY MANAGEMENT

While each type of injury has its own unique aspects, there are some common principles that apply to the immediate care and rehabilitation of most injuries. Acute injuries are usually accompanied by swelling which is due to bleeding and fluid accumulation at the site of the injury. When the swelling is controlled or minimized, the injury can be less painful and there will be less limitation of motion. Swelling can be controlled by the application of the RICE principle: rest, ice, compression and elevation (Fig. 12.9). The term PRICE is also used in the management of acute injuries with the "P" representing protection.

Protection

The injured area can be protected from further insult by immobilization. This is especially important when there is a fracture or joint instability. Slings, splints, casts, braces, and immobilizers are often used to limit movement. When an injured athlete must be moved from the playing field protection is also important to prevent any further damage.

Short periods of immobilization are also beneficial for muscle injuries. Protecting the muscle from movement for a few days allows for scar tissue to form at the sight of injury (7). This can help prevent reinjury.

Rest

Rest is a relative term. It does not mean that the athlete lounges about without any activity. Rest implies that stress to the injured area is reduced to promote the healing process. Only the injured area needs to rest, not the entire body. The athlete can continue with general exercise while the injury is healing as long as the activity is not painful to the injured area. Ways to impose rest include the use of splints, casts, crutches, or other devices.

Crutches can provide a means of both protection and rest for an injury to the lower limb. Crutches allow the athlete to limit the amount of weight placed on the injured limb. With crutches the athlete can completely unweight the limb and progressively bear more weight as pain decreases and healing takes place. While athletes are often reluctant to use crutches, whenever they are limping because of an injury they should be encouraged to use crutches to maintain a more normal gait pattern. Prolonged limping can result in compensatory changes in normal structures that adapt to the altered gait pattern and the new gait pattern can become habit.

FROM THE ATHLETIC TRAINING ROOM

NSAID Use

The use of nonsteroidal anti-inflammatory drugs (NSAIDs) has become a routine practice for many athletes following muscle injuries or soreness. The generic drug ibuprofen (trade names include Motrin and Advil) is an example of a commonly used NSAID. Aspirin is also an NSAID. While the common gastrointestinal side-effects are well known, there are other side effects of the drugs that seem to be less known and remain controversial. According to some reports, these drugs should not be used for all musculoskeletal injuries (1–8). While they may be helpful in treating some inflammatory conditions such as bursitis and when there is soft-tissue impingement, they could have a deleterious effect on tissue healing for other injuries or routine muscle soreness. For muscle and ligament injuries where swelling and inflammation are present and for tendon injuries where there is impingement, short-term use of NSAIDs is still advocated (6). When inflammation is not present their use may not be warranted. Further well controlled research studies are needed to better define the benefits and risks of these medications.

1. Mishra DK, Fridén J, Schmitz MC, et al. Anti-inflammatory medication after muscle injury. *J Bone Joint Surg* 1995;77-A:1510–1519.
2. Trappe TA, White F, Lambert CP, et al. Effect of ibuprofen and acetaminophen on postexercise muscle protein synthesis. *Am J Physiol Endocrinol Metab* 2002;282:E551–E556.
3. Stovitz SD, Johnson RJ. NSAIDs and musculoskeletal treatment: What is the clinical evidence? *Phys Sportsmed* 2003;31:35–40.
4. Bondesen BA, Mills ST, Kegley KM, et al. The COX-2 pathway is essential during early stages of skeletal muscle regeneration. *Am J Physiol Cell Physiol* 2004;287:C475–C483.
5. Scott A, Khan KM, Roberts CR, et al. What do we mean by the term "inflammation?" A contemporary basic science update for sports medicine. *Br J Sports Med* 2004;38:372–380.
6. Paoloni JA, Orchard JW. The use of therapeutic medications for soft-tissue injuries in sports medicine. *Med J Aust* 2005;183:384–388.
7. McAnulty S, McAnulty L, Nieman D, et al. Effect of NSAID on muscle injury and oxidative stress. *Int J Sports Med* 2007;28:909–915.
8. Mackey AL, Kjaer M, Dandanell S, et al. The influence of anti-inflammatory medication on exercise-induced myogenic precursor cell response in humans. *J Appl Physiol* 2007;103:425–431.

Ice

Ice is used to help control pain and to constrict blood vessels in order to limit bleeding in the tissue and control the inflammatory response. Ice can be applied in many ways. Common forms include ice bags, commercial ice packs, and ice massage. Premade ice cups are needed for ice massage. Water is frozen in containers and the block of ice is slowly rubbed over the injured area. Frozen bags of peas also make good ice packs, and can be reused multiple times. Just be sure that bag is not served at dinner! More on the application of ice can be found later in the chapter in the section on therapeutic modalities.

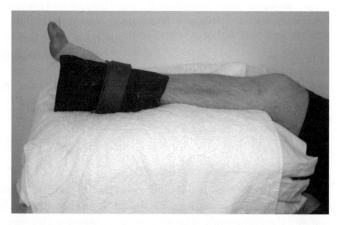

■ **FIGURE 12.9** ICE - ice, compression and elevation to help control swelling.

Compression

Compression is used to apply pressure to the injured area to limit swelling and bleeding. This is most commonly done by using elastic bandages. The bandage is applied in a circular, overlapping pattern starting at the toes or fingers and wrapping up the limb towards the torso. The circular pattern is on a slight diagonal. Starting at the distal portion of the limb is important. For example, if the knee is injured and you only wrap the knee, the area between the knee and ankle can swell because the bandage will limit fluids flowing from the lower limb back to the trunk.

Elevation

To help manage swelling and prevent fluid from accumulating in the injured limb, the part should be elevated higher than the heart as much as possible. The elevation can be accomplished by resting the affected limb on pillows.

THE HEALING PROCESS

When tissue is damaged by injury, new tissue must form to replace it. Most tissue damaged in athletic injuries is not able to completely repair and is replaced by scar tissue. Our skin and bones, however, are able to heal with the same type of tissue that was damaged. There are three phases to the healing process (8). While specific durations are associated with each phase, they can overlap and vary by individual.

Inflammatory Phase

Within minutes of an injury occurring an acute inflammatory response begins. This is a normal tissue response and is usually beneficial in protecting the injured area and to help with healing. The acute inflammatory response can localize the extent of the injured area and help rid the site of body waste products from the initial trauma. There are five clinical manifestations of inflammation, as listed below (9). They can serve to remind the athlete of the injury and prevent the athlete from returning too quickly and causing a reinjury. Often with injury there is bleeding from disruption of small blood vessels which can result in the formation of a hematoma which is a localized mass formed from the pooled blood within the tissues. The initial treatment using the RICE principle is aimed at controlling the swelling and bleeding to minimize the magnitude of the hematoma so the healing process can begin sooner. The inflammatory response lasts from about 1 to 7 days post injury.

FROM THE ATHLETIC TRAINING ROOM

Clinical Manifestations of Inflammation

- Redness
- Warmth
- Swelling
- Pain
- Loss of function

These are all signs and symptoms of acute inflammation and when present, an athlete should be receiving medical care for the injury and active participation in practice or competition may not be indicated.

Proliferative Phase

After the dead tissue from the injury site is cleared away by internal processes, new collagen tissue begins to form. Collagen is the main protein in the structures in the musculoskeletal system. By the fourth or fifth day following injury there is new collagen in the injured area. However, the new collagen takes several weeks before it is mature and has the same tensile strength as normal tissue. Care must be taken to prevent reinjury during this repair phase that typically lasts from 7 to 21 days postinjury.

Maturation Phase

During this phase major changes occur to the newly formed tissue. When it is first formed the new tissue is relatively unorganized with the fibers randomly arranged. During this phase the fibers become organized and the strength of the scar tissue increases. The maturation process can take a year or longer or may be complete in 3 weeks, depending on the nature of the injury.

Healing Time Frames

Healing time depends on the type of injury, location and severity. Tissues do not all heal at the same rate. The healing time for bone depends on the athlete's age, fracture site, type of fracture, and the blood supply to the bone (10). A fractured bone may be placed in a cast for 3 to 8 weeks (depending on whether it is a large or small bone) and may not be completely healed when the cast is removed. Remodeling of the bone continues after the cast is removed. A mild hamstring muscle strain might heal in 10 days to 3 weeks and a severe one may take 2 to 6 months to heal (11). A ligament injury may take 6 to 12 months to heal (10). The time frame for a nerve injury to heal depends on the type of damage. A mild injury, such as a slight pressure or pull on a nerve, can be repaired in a few days or weeks. If a nerve is pinched, crushed or subjected to prolonged pressure the nerve heals at a rate of 1 mm/day or 3 cm/month (10). It needs to heal from where it originates in the spinal cord to the site of injury. That means if the injury is in the foot, the time to heal would be based on the distance from the spinal cord to the foot. With the most severe type of nerve injuries there is no regeneration resulting in a permanent loss of function to the muscles innervated by the injured nerve.

THERAPEUTIC MODALITIES

Therapeutic modalities are widely used in sports medicine to break the pain spasm cycle and promote healing. There are many ways to categorize the various modalities, but we are primarily interested here in the heat and cold modalities. Electrical modalities are also widely used in sports medicine. The primary effects of these modalities are to:

FROM THE ATHLETIC TRAINING ROOM

Pain-Spasm Cycle

Pain and muscle spasm often occur following musculoskeletal injuries. Muscle spasm is a protective mechanism to help prevent further injury to the traumatized area. The muscle spasm is an involuntary muscle contraction used as an attempt to splint the damaged region. The muscle spasm causes increased pressure on nerve endings and results in more pain. The increased pain triggers further muscle spasms. Thus, the name pain-spasm cycle is used. Treatment is aimed at breaking the cycle.

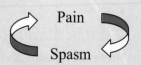

- modify inflammation and healing
- relieve pain
- alter collagen extensibility

Therapeutic modalities are not a new invention, but have been used for centuries. The ancient Greeks and Romans had bathhouses with steam rooms and pools. As early as the 1st century AD, torpedo fish were used as an electrical treatment for headaches and gout (12).

The information presented here is for the coach to be aware of the therapeutic modalities that are commonly used by athletic trainers and physical therapists. In the absence of these health care professionals, a coach may choose to use ice with an injured athlete. Each state has laws that govern the use of therapeutic modalities and many modalities can only be administered by licensed health care professionals. The coach must not administer any modalities for which a license is required.

Cryotherapy

Cryotherapy is a term that applies to the therapeutic use of any cold modality. As mentioned earlier in the chapter, cold packs, ice bags, and ice massage are common forms and are used to control inflammation, pain and edema (swelling).

EFFECTS OF COLD

The use of cold has hemodynamic, neuromuscular and metabolic effects (13). When cold is applied there is an initial decrease in blood flow due to vasoconstriction (constricting of the blood vessels). If applied for a long time it results in an increase in blood flow. That is why repeated short applications are most effective. Cold application also results in decreased nerve conduction velocity and an increased pain threshold. That is the reason it can be an effective analgesic. Cold application results in a decreased metabolic rate.

PRECAUTIONS

While we tend to think of ice as a harmless substance, it can cause harm. Adverse effects have included frostbite, tissue death, nerve damage and unwanted vasodilation. Some individuals have cold hypersensitivity and will develop a skin rash and others have intolerance to cold and experience severe pain or numbness. Cryotherapy should not be used with those individuals. It should also not be used over a regenerating peripheral nerve. If applied for long periods over superficial nerves there is a risk of nerve damage. In a recent survey of athletic trainers the most common complications associated with cryotherapy were allergic reactions, burns, and intolerance/pain (14).

Coaches need to be aware that in addition to controlling swelling and reducing pain, cold treatments can impair proprioception, reflex activity and motor function. Athletes may be more susceptible to injury for up to 30 minutes following cryotherapy (15). In a recent study, proprioception and throwing accuracy were decreased following 20 minutes of cryotherapy with an ice bag applied to the throwing shoulder (16). Applying ice prior to activity may not always be in the athlete's best interest.

APPLICATION

When using cold packs a layer of toweling should be placed between the pack and the skin. With ice massage the ice is applied directly to the skin, but is constantly moving. During treatment the skin should be checked for an adverse reaction and if present the ice should be removed. Ice packs may be most effective when applied repeatedly for 10 minutes at a time (15). The repeated applications help to decrease the muscle temperature without causing damage to the skin. Ice massage is typically done for about 5 to 10 minutes or until analgesia is achieved (13).

While each athlete may have a slightly different response to cryotherapy, the typical sequence is to first feel intense cold at the start of application. That sensation is often followed by burning which can be followed by aching. The final and desired response is analgesia and a sensation of numbness.

Thermotherapy

Thermotherapy is a term used to describe the therapeutic use of heat modalities. Using hot packs is the most common form of heat therapy. Heat is used to control pain, increase soft tissue extensibility, increase circulation, and accelerate healing.

EFFECTS OF HEAT

The use of heat also has hemodynamic, neuromuscular, and metabolic effects (13). Heat causes vasodilation which increases circulation to the area. It also results in increased nerve conduction velocity as well as an increase in the pain threshold. Heat application increases the metabolic rate. With the exception of increasing the pain threshold, the effects of heat are the opposite of the effects of cold. Heat can also help decrease joint stiffness and increase muscle flexibility.

PRECAUTIONS

Heat should not be used when there is an acute injury or inflammation, recent or potential hemorrhage, or impaired sensation. Caution must be used when placing heat over an open wound and when a counterirritant (topical pain reliever such as Biofreeze, Polar Freeze, or Icy Hot) has recently been applied. Burns are the primary adverse effects of heat. In the athletic training room when moist hot packs are used, multiple layers of towels must be placed between the hot pack and skin and the skin must be checked often for adverse effects.

APPLICATION

Moist hot packs are commonly used for superficial heat in the athletic training room. They come in various shapes and sizes and are kept warm in thermostatically controlled hot pack containers. As mentioned above, multiple layers of toweling or hot pack covers must be used to prevent burns. Other common methods of applying superficial heat include warm whirlpools, showers, and baths.

Ultrasound

Ultrasound can be used as a form of deep heat or as a means to promote tissue healing. As a heating modality, ultrasound can penetrate a greater distance into the tissues than hot packs. It can also be used for nonthermal effects. Ultrasound can increase the rate of some metabolic functions such as increasing cell membrane permeability, macrophage responsiveness, and protein synthesis. These nonthermal effects are thought to help speed the healing process.

Electrical Stimulation

Various forms of electrical stimulation are used in the athletic training room and rehabilitation facilities. The type of unit that is used to deliver the stimulation depends on the purpose of the treatment. There are three broad categories for which electrical stimulation is used. It can be used for strengthening muscles, controlling pain, and promoting tissue healing.

Heat Versus Cold

Athletes often question when they should use heat versus cold and, if they are using cold, when they can switch to using heat. During the acute phase of the injury cryotherapy should be used to control the swelling and pain. Cold is generally used for a minimum of 72 hours following the injury. Because heat increases blood flow to the area, the use of heat too soon can increase swelling. When in doubt, continue to use cold. Switching to heat may be safe when there is no longer active swelling and the injury is not tender to touch.

FROM THE ATHLETIC TRAINING ROOM

Important Components of the Rehabilitation Program:

- Immediate first aid to control swelling
- Reduce/control pain
- Protect healing tissue
- Restore normal range of motion to affected region
- Restore or increase muscular strength, endurance and power
- Neuromuscular re-education
- Sport specific functional progression
- Maintain cardiovascular fitness

THE GOAL OF REHABILITATION AND HOW TO ACHIEVE IT

The primary goal of rehabilitation is to return the athlete to participation as quickly and safely as possible and to return the athlete to the same or higher level of competition as before the injury. To accomplish this goal there are several components to an optimum rehabilitation program. These components, along with the initial recovery phase, can be viewed as a progressive rehabilitation program (Fig. 12.10).

Control Swelling, Reduce/Control Pain and Protect Healing Tissue

These components have been discussed above in the injury management and therapeutic modalities sections.

Restore Normal Range of Motion to Affected Region

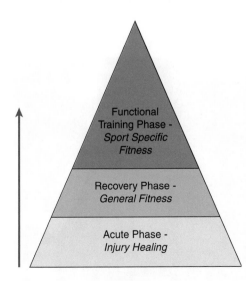

Injuries to joint structures and surrounding muscles can result in a loss of motion. The motion can be limited by swelling or pain. When motion is limited for a prolonged period of time adaptive shortening can occur in the joint structures. Whenever possible, early mobilization should occur to maintain or restore normal joint range of motion and promote optimal tissue healing. While immobilization for a few days following a muscle injury is beneficial for appropriate scar formation, prolonged immobilization is detrimental (17).

Active or passive range of motion exercises should be done within the athlete's pain-free limits. With active range of motion exercise the athlete moves the joint through the available pain-free range and progressively tries to move further into the restricted range. With passive or assisted range of motion exercise gravity, the athlete's other limb, or another person helps move the joint through the available pain-free range (Fig. 12.11).

■ **FIGURE 12.10** Phases of progressive rehabilitation.

Restore or Increase Muscular Strength, Endurance and Power

Following injury and disuse, muscles can atrophy rapidly. Restoring strength, endurance, and power are essential to return the athlete to pre-injury status. The three primary types of exercise are isometric, isotonic, and isokinetic and they can be done in an open or closed chain. In an open chain exercise the distal segment of the limb is free to move and is not fixed to any surface. Knee extension sitting on a weight machine is an example of an open chain exercise. The foot is free to move (Fig. 12.12). In a closed chain exercise the distal segment is fixed and

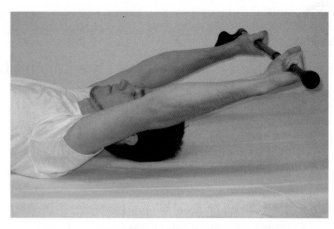

■ **FIGURE 12.11** Assisted range of motion: the athlete uses the cane and the uninvolved limb to help move the injured limb through the available range of motion.

maintains contact with the adjacent surface. The leg press is an example of a closed chain exercise (Fig. 12.13).

ISOMETRIC EXERCISE

An isometric exercise is one in which the muscle contracts, but there is no associated joint movement. Isometric exercises are often the first exercises used following an injury and can be started as soon as the athlete is able to perform them without pain. When the injury is to the muscle, isometric exercise should be done within pain-free limits prior to the initiation of other exercise and are typically started on day 3 to 5 following the muscle injury (17). Isometric exercises can be done while a limb is still immobilized. They are also used when resistance training through the full range of motion is not possible.

Isometric exercise can prevent muscle atrophy and can help reduce swelling by a pumping action that can remove accumulated fluid. Typically the exercises are held for 5 seconds with a 10 second rest between each contraction for a total of 10 repetitions and are repeated frequently throughout the day. Quad sets is an example of an isometric exercise. The quadriceps muscle is contracted without movement of the knee.

Multiple angle isometric exercise should be used whenever possible. Strength is gained specific to the angle the joint is in during the exercise with an overflow of about 20 degrees on either side of the angle (18). For example, if using isometric exercise to strengthen the quadriceps muscle, the exercise should be performed with the knee bent to 90 degrees as well as with the knee straight and several angles in between.

ISOTONIC EXERCISE

An isotonic exercise is one in which the joint moves through the range of motion against a constant resistance. Isotonic exercise can be done using free weights or machines. Exercises that use both concentric and eccentric contractions should be used in the rehabilitation program.

- concentric—a shortening contraction. The muscle fibers shorten bringing the proximal and distal attachments of the muscle closer together.
- eccentric—a lengthening contraction. With an eccentric contraction the muscle fibers lengthen under tension and the proximal and distal attachments

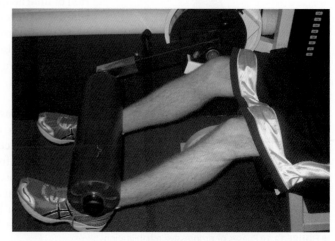

■ **FIGURE 12.12** Open chain exercise—knee extension.

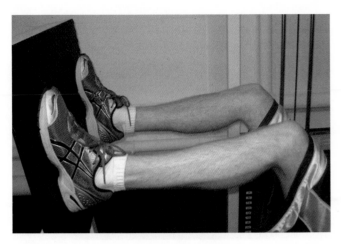

■ **FIGURE 12.13** Closed chain exercise—leg press.

move further apart. Eccentric exercises are used when movement is controlled against gravity.

When performing a biceps curl with a dumbbell, the weight is lifted with a concentric contraction as the elbow flexes. An eccentric contraction allows the same muscles to lengthen under tension to return the dumbbell to the starting position. The eccentric contraction allows a controlled decent of the weight that otherwise gravity would control (Fig. 12.14).

Eccentric exercise can result in delayed onset muscle soreness (DOMS). Any exercise with a large component of eccentric contractions should start at a very low level and progress gradually to a higher intensity and volume. This applies to both rehabilitation and training.

Machines with variable resistance provide a variation of isotonic exercise. With these machines, such as those made by Nautilus or Cybex, the weight is constant, but the resistance varies throughout the range of motion. More resistance is applied in the part of the range where the muscle is strongest and less resistance in the part of the range where the muscle is weakest thereby providing maximal resistance throughout the range of motion. Unlike the isokinetic machines described below, the speed is not held constant.

ISOKINETIC EXERCISE

Isokinetic exercise is performed on an exercise machine that allows a fixed speed of movement with a variable and accommodating resistance that provides maximal resistance throughout the range of motion. The velocity is set at a predetermined rate and the resistance varies to match the force generated by the athlete at every point in the range of motion. Isokinetic exercise machines, such as the KinCom or Biodex, allow for movement at velocities that are much greater than those used in isotonic exercise and more closely match velocities in athletic performance. Isokinetic machines can also be used to test whether muscle strength has been fully regained in determining readiness for return to play.

RESTORING MUSCLE ENDURANCE

Muscle endurance is the ability of the muscle to sustain a contraction or perform repeated contractions. Endurance conditioning should occur along with the strengthening program. While high load with low repetition exercise is ideal for gaining strength, low load with high repetition exercise is used to increase muscle endurance.

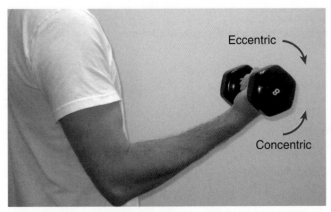

Eccentric

Concentric

■ **FIGURE 12.14** A concentric contraction is used to lift the dumbbell and an eccentric contraction is used to lower it while controlling against the force of gravity.

RESTORING MUSCLE POWER

Muscle power is the rate at which a muscle works and reflects how quickly muscle force is generated. Sports that require explosive strength need to include muscle power training in the later stages of the rehabilitation program. The training should be sport specific and can include fast speed isotonic or isokinetic exercise, functional exercises at increased speed, and plyometric exercise.

Neuromuscular Re-education

Neuromuscular re-education encompasses several areas of the rehabilitation program that relate to coordination of movement patterns, balance, and proprioception (19). The nervous system controls movement and, following injury, both the nervous system and muscles must be addressed in the rehabilitation program.

While the larger muscles in the body are responsible for movement, many smaller muscles provide joint stability and coordinated movement. Some injuries can be the result of faulty coordination of these muscles. Whether the cause or consequence of the injury, rehabilitation programs should include motor re-education of any faulty movement patterns with the emphasis on establishing joint stability prior to global strengthening.

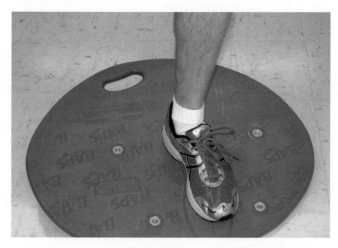

■ **FIGURE 12.15** Use of a rocker board in rehabilitation helps address proprioceptive deficits often seen following lower extremity injuries.

Balance and proprioception training are also part of neuromuscular re-education. Proprioception refers to the nerve impulses that originate in the joints, muscles, and tendons and relay information to the central nervous system about joint position, motion, and pressure. Injuries can cause damage to the nerve endings which may result in impaired balance, decreased coordination and an altered position sense. Impaired proprioception commonly occurs with lower limb injuries.

Standing on one leg is a simple proprioceptive exercise. Adding an unstable surface such as a rocker board adds increased challenge. Balancing on the rocker board should start on two feet and progress to one (Fig. 12.15). Exercises on a mini-trampoline present further challenges.

Sport Specific Functional Progression

The primary purpose of the rehabilitation program is to restore normal function so the athlete can return to competition. The functional progression of activities is designed to return the athlete to a specific sport. Sports skills are broken down into component parts and the athlete progressively reacquires the skills within physical tolerance (20). Careful attention should be paid to the correct form and technique. Below is an example of a progression of functional exercises for an athlete returning to running following a lower extremity injury.

- Walking
- Jogging
  - start with jog/walk and progressively increase jog time and decrease walk time
- Running
  - increase pace intermittently during the run
- Sprinting
  - progressively increase sprint distance
- Agility drills
  - 45 degree zigzag (progressively increasing speed)
  - run a square (forwards, sideways, backwards, sideways)
  - carioca (grapevine)

Maintain Cardiovascular Fitness

Maintaining cardiovascular fitness while recovering from a musculoskeletal injury is especially important for endurance athletes. An athlete should be able to return to play following rehabilitation for the injury with a level of cardiovascular fitness that is similar to the level before the injury. The coach can substitute alternative activities that allow for maintenance of the fitness level without compromising the injured structure. When there is an injury to the lower limb that requires limited weight-bearing, cycling, swimming, or water exercises can be used to maintain cardiovascular fitness. However, cardiovascular fitness is dependent on both the central mechanisms in the heart and lungs as well as those in the muscle tissues. Only when the same muscles that are used in the sport can be used in the substitute activity can cardiovascular fitness be maintained at the same sport specific level. With some injuries in the initial stages of rehabilitation the muscles used in the sport may not be able to be used in an alternative fitness activity.

CRITERIA FOR RETURN TO PLAY

While the decision on when an athlete is ready to return to practice and competition rests primarily with the medical members of the sports medicine team, coaches can benefit from knowing the criteria used in making the decision and should play a part in the decision process. The decision is often based on a combination of the following factors.

- Adverse effects of the injury on the tissues involved and time frame for healing
- Effects of the injury on strength, endurance, flexibility, agility, and proprioception
- Effect of prolonged inactivity on cardiovascular fitness
- Effect of the injury and/or inactivity on sport-specific skills
- Psychological response to the injury

FOCAL POINT

Preparticipation Physical Evaluation

A preparticipation physical evaluation (PPE) is typically required for competitive athletes at all levels. The NCAA recommends that an athlete undergo a PPE upon entrance into the intercollegiate athletic program with an updated history obtained annually. A further PPE would only occur if warranted by the updated history or an athlete's medical condition (1). The PPE can be done in the physician's office or in a group setting where the athletes rotate through various stations with different health care providers doing assessments in their areas of expertise. The goals of the PPE include:

- Identifying medical and orthopedic problems that may place the athlete at risk for injury or illness
- Identifying problems that could affect the athlete's ability to perform
- Helping to maintain the health and safety of the athlete
- Educating athletes (and their parents) about sports injuries and other health related issues
- Meeting legal and insurance requirements
- Establishing a database and medical record for each athlete

The PPE should be conducted several weeks prior to the start of the season. This allows time for follow-up for any abnormal findings and also allows time for rehabilitation of any identified injures. Cardiovascular abnormalities that may result in sudden death of an athlete are not always detected in the PPE (2). Several organizations are addressing this and trying to develop a more standardized evaluation.

Results of the PPE are often kept in the athletic training room and are considered medical records. As such, they are subject to state and federal laws that govern patient confidentiality. Athletes can give written permission to authorize release of the information and should specify what information and to whom it can be released.

(continues)

Preparticipation Physical Evaluation *(continued)*

While the PPE provides important information about the athlete's general health and ability to participate in a sport, it does not provide specific information on the athlete's fitness. Therefore, in addition to the PPE coaches and athletic trainers should conduct preseason screenings to determine strength, cardiovascular fitness, flexibility, and sport-specific performance to provide a baseline with which comparisons can be made to determine the athlete's readiness to resume competitive sports following an injury.

1. National Collegiate Athletic Association. *Sports Medicine Handbook 2007–2008.* Available online at: http://www.ncaa.org/library/sports_sciences/sports_med_handbook/2007-08/2007-08_sports_medicine_handbook.pdf. Accessed November 29, 2007.
2. Hulkower S, Fagan B, Watts J, et al. Do preparticipation clinical exams reduce morbidity and mortality for athletes? *J Fam Pract* 2005;54:628–632.

While general guidelines have been established (21) comparing the athlete's postrehabilitation status to documented abilities prior to the injury provides the best guidance. The athlete's preseason testing on strength, cardiovascular fitness, flexibility, and sport-specific performance provides a baseline with which comparisons can be made to determine the athlete's readiness to resume competitive sports. Having sport specific preseason physical and performance requirements for which athletes are tested provides important objective data to make the necessary comparisons following rehabilitation of an injury. The return to play criteria can be made clear to the athletes at the start of the season when the testing is done.

Functional performance tests simulate, under controlled conditions, forces encountered in sports activities. They may be the best measurement tool to determine lower limb function when sophisticated laboratory equipment is not available or feasible. While not truly sport-specific, the hop tests have been proposed as the best measurement tool for lower limb function (22). They are preferred because they allow the use of the uninjured limb as a control against which return to play and competition decisions may be determined. Functional performance testing can provide objective measures of progress and measure the athlete's ability to tolerate forces.

Timing of return to play following muscle strains can be one of the more challenging decisions. There are currently no consensus guidelines for safe return to sport following a muscle strain (23). A history of a muscle injury is a risk factor for future injury (6). With a muscle strain the actual healing of the tissue is much slower than the observed function would indicate. With muscle strains return to play may not coincide with apparent recovery (24).

Rehabilitation does not stop when the athlete returns to play. Rehabilitation should not be considered complete until the athlete has successfully completed a full season following the injury (25).

SUMMARY

- Knowledge of common athletic injuries and principles of management can help the coach better understand the limitations imposed during the rehabilitation process as well as what the athlete may still be able to do during the recovery process.
- Traumatic and overuse injuries to the musculoskeletal system are common in athletics. Structures frequently injured include bones, joints, ligaments, cartilage, muscles, tendons, and bursae.
- Acute injuries are the result of sudden trauma and chronic injuries develop over time.
- The PRICE principle is used in the management of acute injuries: protection, rest, ice, compression, and elevation.
- There are three phases to the healing process of tissue: inflammatory, proliferative, and maturation. The healing rate depends on the type of tissue as well as the type and severity of injury.

- Therapeutic modalities are used to control pain and promote healing. Superficial cold and heat modalities are commonly used as well as ultrasound and electrical stimulation.
- The primary of goal of rehabilitation is to return the athlete to participation as quickly and safely as possible at the same or higher level of competition as before the injury. Restoring normal function, neuromuscular re-education and sports-specific functional progression are important elements of the rehabilitation process.
- Adherence to return to play criteria can help ensure that the athlete is ready to resume practice and competition. The coach is the most knowledgeable member of the sports medicine team in terms of knowing the physical demands of the sport. Documenting preseason sport-specific skills can provide an important baseline for post injury comparison.

References

1. Frontera WR. Epidemiology of sports injuries: implications for rehabilitation. In: Frontera WR. *Rehabilitation of Sports Injuries: Scientific Basis.* Malden, MA: Blackwell Publishing, 2005.
2. Maffulli N, Khan KM, Puddu G. Overuse tendon conditions: time to change a confusing terminology. *Arthroscopy* 1998;14: 840–843.
3. Wilder RP, Sethi S. Overuse injuries: tendinopathies, stress fractures, compartment syndrome and shin splints. *Clin Sports Med* 2004;23:55–81.
4. Wilson JJ, Best TM. Common overuse tendon problems: a review and recommendations for treatment. *Am Fam Physician* 2005; 72:811–818.
5. Crosier J, Forthomme B, Namurois M, et al. Hamstring muscle strain recurrence and strength performance disorders. *Am J Sports Med* 2002;30:199–203.
6. Croisier J. Factors associated with recurrent hamstring injuries. *Sports Med* 2004;34:681–695.
7. Järvinen TA, Järvinen TL, Kääriäinen M, et al. Muscle injuries: optimising recovery. *Best Pract Res Clin Rheumatol* 2007;21: 317–331.
8. Martinez-Hernandez A, Amenta PS. Basic concepts in wound healing. In: Leadbetter WB, Buckwalter JA, Gordon SL. *Sports-Induced Inflammation: Clinical and Basic Science Concepts.* Park Ridge, IL: American Academy of Orthopaedic Surgeons, 1990.
9. Scott A, Khan KM, Cook JL, et al. What is "inflammation?" Are we ready to move beyond Celsus? *Br J Sports Med* 2004;38:248–249.
10. Salter RB. *Textbook of Disorders and Injuries of the Musculoskeletal System,* 3rd ed. Baltimore: Williams & Wilkins, 1999: 417–497.
11. American Academy of Orthopaedic Surgeons. *Athletic Training and Sports Medicine,* 2nd ed. Rosemont, IL: American Academy of Orthopaedic Surgeons, 1991.
12. Kellaway P. The William Olser medal essay: the part played by electric fish in the early history of bioelectricity and electrotherapy. *Bull Hist Med* 1946;20:112–137.
13. Cameron MH. *Physical Agents in Rehabilitation: From Research to Practice.* St. Louis, MO: Saunders, 2003.
14. Nadler SF, Prybicien M, Malanga GA, et al. Complications from therapeutic modalities: results of a national survey of athletic trainers. *Arch Phys Med Rehabil* 2003;84:849–853.
15. Macauley DC. Ice therapy: how good is the evidence? *Int J Sports Med* 2001;22:379–384.
16. Wassinger CA, Myers JB, Gatti JM, et al. Proprioception and throwing accuracy in the dominant shoulder after cryotherapy. *J Athl Train* 2007;42:84-89.
17. Järvinen TA, Järvinen TL, Kääriäinen M, et al. Muscle injuries: biology and treatment. *Am J Sports Med* 2005;33:745–764.
18. Knapik JJ, Mawdsley RH, Ramos MU. Angular specificity and test mode specificity of isometric and isokinetic strength training. *J Orthop Sports Phys Ther* 1983;5:58–65.
19. Griffin LY. Neuromuscular training and injury prevention in sports. *Clin Orthop Relat Res* 2003;409:53–60.
20. Kegerreis S. The construction and implementation of functional progressions as a component of athletic rehabilitation. *J Orthop Sports Phys Ther* 1983;5:14–19.
21. Team physician and return-to-play issues: a consensus statement. *Med Sci Sports Exerc* 2002;34:1212–1214.
22. Clark NC. Functional performance testing following knee ligament injury. *Phys Ther Sport* 2001;2:91–105.
23. Orchard J, Best TM, Verrall GM. Return to play following muscle strains. *Clin J Sport Med* 2005;15:436–441.
24. Orchard J, Best TM. The management of muscle strain injuries: an early return versus the risk of recurrence. *Clin J Sport Med* 2002;12:3–5.
25. Brukner P, Khan K. *Clinical Sports Medicine,* 3rd ed. North Ryde, New South Wales: McGraw-Hill Australia, 2007:195.

Common Upper Limb Injuries

Upon reading this chapter, the coach should be able to:

1. Identify the basic anatomical structures and movements of the upper limb.
2. Associate particular anatomical structures with common athletic injuries of the shoulder, elbow, wrist and hand and describe the nature of those injuries.
3. Describe return to play criteria for common upper limb injuries.
4. Discuss some ways that the coach can help in the rehabilitation process and in the prevention of further injury.

Joni was just beginning her first season as a Division I gymnast. She was thrilled to have been recruited on full scholarship not only because of the athletic opportunity but because she was the first person in her family to have the chance for a college education. She was practicing her uneven bar routine and on the flyaway dismount she fell, landing on her outstretched right hand. Her coach and several teammates came running over to see if she was hurt. She had already sat up by the time they were at her side. She reassured her coach and teammates that she was okay. She said that there was some pain in her right wrist, but everything else seemed all right. Just to be certain the coach called the athletic training room and asked for an athletic trainer to come to the gym.

The examination revealed point tenderness in the anatomical snuff box with some swelling in the wrist. Joni was treated with ice, compression, and elevation of the wrist and was later seen by the team physician who ordered radiographs. While the radiographs were negative for a fracture, to Joni's relief, the physician was not convinced that a fracture of the scaphoid bone was not present and he immobilized her wrist in a cast. He said the radiographs would need to be repeated in 2 weeks. Why would the physician suspect a fracture of the scaphoid bone if the radiographs were negative? Where is the anatomical snuff box and what is the significance of point tenderness in that region?

Despite proper training and appropriate measures to prevent injuries, some will still happen. Athletic trainers and sports medicine physicians are educated in the examination and management of the various injuries that occur in athletics. Their textbooks and literature cover both common and rare injuries. The focus in this and the following two chapters will be the more commonly occurring injuries with the intent of providing the coach with a basic understanding of the nature of these injuries and return to play criteria. Evaluating the injury will not be included because it is beyond the scope of the coach. The treatments described throughout these chapters are to be administered by qualified medical personnel. Treatment of athletic injuries is also beyond the scope of the coach. Keep in mind that the timeframes provided for return to play are only approximations and can vary for each of your athletes. The principles of rehabilitation discussed in Chapter 12 apply to all of these injuries.

Sports activities can place high demands on the structures of the upper limb. When throwing, for example, the shoulder joint can reach angular velocities of more than 6,000 degrees per second (1). Upper extremity joints are not normally exposed to weight-bearing loads, but in gymnastics forces as much as two times body weight have been measured at the wrist during pommel horse exercises (2). Repeated stress to previously normal tissue can result in overuse injuries. Approximately 45% to 60% of all injuries treated in sports medicine clinics can be classified as overuse injuries (3). Injuries can also be the result of trauma.

For optimal function in the upper limb, there needs to be coordination of movement from the shoulder through the hand. The elbow needs a stable shoulder, and hand movement needs to be coordinated with movement of the elbow and shoulder. This interconnection of the joints is termed the kinetic chain. While each region will be addressed separately, keep in mind that there needs to be a coordination of movement for the athlete to perform at maximum capacity.

THE SHOULDER COMPLEX

The shoulder is an extremely complicated region. There is a high degree of mobility at the expense of stability. Overhead activities make it susceptible to a number of overuse and chronic injuries. Acute shoulder injuries are more common in contact sports such as football and wrestling. Chronic injuries are more commonly seen in volleyball, swimming, baseball, and softball (4).

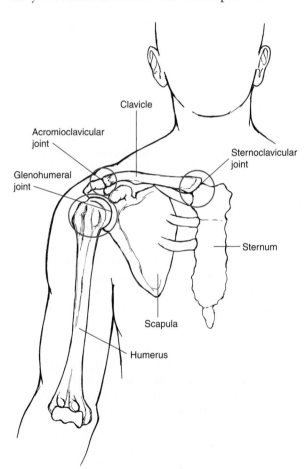

Shoulder Anatomy

The shoulder complex consists of several bones forming four distinct joints (Fig. 13.1). The clavicle serves as a strut for the shoulder to hold the arm away from the body to allow for a greater range of unencumbered movement. At one end the clavicle articulates with the sternum, forming the sternoclavicular joint, and at the other end it articulates with the scapula, forming the acromioclavicular (AC) joint. The scapula rests on the rib cage forming the scapulothoracic joint. The glenohumeral (shoulder) joint is the articulation of the humerus with the shallow glenoid fossa of the scapula. The joint is supported by a joint capsule and ligaments and receives further stabilization from the rotator cuff muscles. The bony configuration of this joint lacks stability and favors mobility.

The ball and socket configuration of the shoulder joint allows for movement in all planes of motion. In order to achieve full elevation of the arm, the scapula and humerus must function together. This is known as scapulohumeral rhythm. For every 3 degrees of elevation of the arm, 2 degrees occurs by movement at the glenohumeral joint and 1 degree by scapulothoracic upward rotation. To reach full flexion or abduction of 180 degrees, 120 degrees occurs at the glenohumeral joint and 60 degrees at the scapulothoracic joint

■ **FIGURE 13.1** Anterior view of the shoulder complex. The shoulder complex includes the clavicle, scapula, and humerus. The clavicle articulates with the sternum forming the sternoclavicular joint and with the scapula forming the acromioclavicular joint. The glenohumeral joint is the articulation of the humerus with the scapula. The scapulothoracic joint is where the scapula rests on the posterior ribs (the ribs are cut away in this figure to expose the scapula). (Modified from Oatis CA. *Kinesiology—The Mechanics and Pathomechanics of Human Movement.* Baltimore: Lippincott Williams & Wilkins, 2004.)

(Fig. 13.2). The rotator cuff muscles and the muscles that stabilize the scapula are essential for optimal function of the shoulder joint. Scapular stabilization and rotator cuff strength are important components of injury prevention.

The muscles that move the shoulder joint and scapula are illustrated in Figure 13.3. The motions of the shoulder joint can be found in Figure 13.4 and the prime movers for the shoulder joint and scapula can be found in Table 13.1.

Common Shoulder Injuries

All of the anatomical structures of the shoulder complex are susceptible to athletic injuries. Some of those that occur frequently are described below.

CLAVICLE FRACTURE

Clavicle fractures are common in sport and result from a fall on an outstretched arm or point of the shoulder or from a direct blow to the bone (5,6). There is usually a cracking sensation at the time of injury with immediate pain over the fracture site and rapid swelling. Most fractures occur in the middle third of the bone (7). The fracture is treated with immobilization in a sling or figure-eight bandage for 4 to 6 weeks (8).

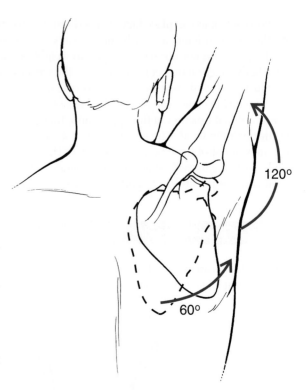

■ **FIGURE 13.2** Scapulohumeral rhythm: To reach 180 degrees of shoulder flexion or abduction, 60 degrees of motion occurs with the upward rotation of the scapula and 120 degrees occurs at the glenohumeral joint. (Modified from Hamill J, Knutzen KM. *Biomechanical Basis of Human Movement*, 2nd ed. Baltimore: Lippincott Williams & Wilkins, 2003.)

ACROMIOCLAVICULAR SPRAIN

A sprain to the acromioclavicular (AC) joint is usually the result of a fall onto the point of the shoulder or a direct blow. Traction on the arm or a fall on the outstretched hand or elbow can also lead to injury (9). The grade of the strain is dependent on the amount of damage to the supporting ligaments and is described below. These injuries have been further classified into six types and are illustrated in Figure 13.5. Grades 1 to 3 correspond to Types I to III.

- Grade 1—There is point tenderness and pain with movement, but no disruption of the AC joint.
- Grade 2—There is a tear or rupture of the AC ligament with partial displacement of the lateral end of the clavicle; there is pain, point tenderness and decreased range of motion of the shoulder.
- Grade 3—There is rupture of both ligaments that support this joint, the AC, and coracoclavicular ligaments. The pain may be greater than with a grade 2 sprain and there is more limitation of motion.

Types IV, V, and VI are subgroups of Type III and are less common. In addition to the complete rupture of both supporting ligaments there is also damage to adjacent structures and they more likely require operative management.

Treatment for a grade 1 sprain includes the use of ice and oral analgesics, rest, and a sling to provide immobilization for comfort. The sling is worn until the athlete is able to tolerate carrying the arm freely, which is typically a few days. The athlete can usually return to play in 1 to 3 weeks when nearly painless full range of motion has returned. Grade 2 injuries are treated similarly with the period of immobilization being greater, sometimes 1 to 2 weeks, and the time to return to play being increased to 4 to 6 weeks. When nearly painless full range of motion and strength have been restored, the athlete is ready to resume play (10).

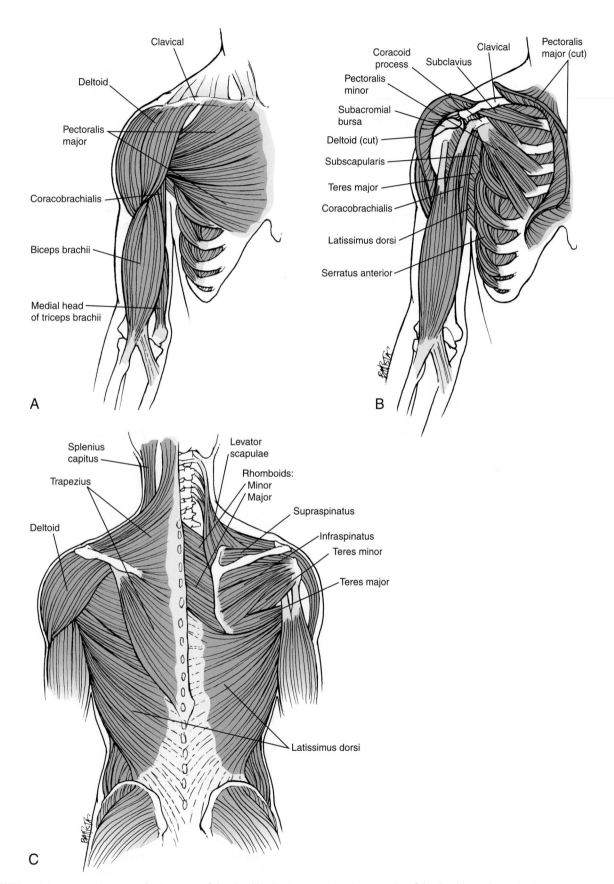

■ **FIGURE 13.3 A.** Anterior view: superficial muscles of the shoulder. **B.** Anterior view: deep muscles of the shoulder and scapula. **C.** Posterior view: superficial and deep muscles of the shoulder and scapula. (Modified from Anderson MK, Hall SJ. *Sports Injury Management*. Baltimore: Williams & Wilkins, 1995.)

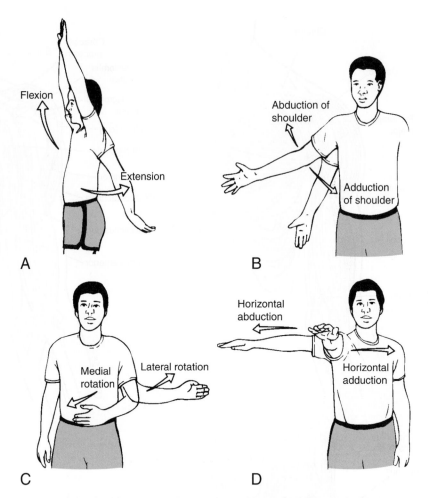

■ **FIGURE 13.4** Movements of the shoulder joint. **A.** Flexion and extension. **B.** Abduction and adduction. **C.** Medial and lateral rotation. **D.** Horizontal abduction and adduction. (Modified from Anderson MK, Hall SJ. *Sports Injury Management.* Baltimore: Williams & Wilkins, 1995.)

With a grade 3 sprain there is significant AC joint instability. Historically, these injuries were treated surgically. Because outcomes with surgery were no better than when treated nonsurgically, surgery is mostly used now when conservative treatment fails (11). A sling is worn for 2 to 3 weeks followed by gentle range of motion and strengthening exercises. Return to play criteria are the same as with grade 2 sprains and typically at least 4 to 6 weeks are needed for recovery (10).

SHOULDER DISLOCATIONS

Shoulder dislocations are very common among athletes with the majority being anterior dislocations (12). They typically occur when the arm is forced into excessive abduction and external rotation causing the humeral head to be displaced from its resting position in the glenoid fossa of the scapula (Fig. 13.6). Shoulder dislocations can also occur with a blow to the posterior shoulder or a fall on the outstretched arm. There is a sudden onset of shoulder pain and at the time of injury the athlete may experience the sensation of the shoulder 'popping out.' A dislocated shoulder requires immediate medical attention. The displacement of the humerus can cause damage to the nerves and vessels that cross the shoulder. Ice can be applied to the shoulder and the athlete should be monitored and treated for shock, if necessary, while awaiting medical care.

TABLE 13.1 Prime Movers of the Shoulder Joint	
Shoulder Movement	**Prime Movers**
Flexion	Pectoralis Major (clavicular head) Deltoid (anterior portion) Assisted by: Coracobrachialis and biceps brachii
Extension	Deltoid (posterior portion) Latissimus dorsi Teres major
Abduction	Deltoid (middle fibers) Supraspinatus
Adduction	Pectoralis major Latissimus dorsi
Horizontal Abduction	Deltoid (posterior fibers)
Horizontal Adduction	Pectoralis major
Medial Rotation	Subscapularis Pectoralis major Latissimus dorsi Teres major Deltoid (anterior portion)
Lateral Rotation	Infraspinatus Teres minor Deltoid (posterior portion)
Scapular Movement	
Abduction and upward rotation	Serratus anterior
Adduction and downward rotation	Rhomboid major and minor
Adduction	Trapezius (middle fibers) Rhomboid major
Elevation	Trapezius (superior fibers) Levator scapulae
Depression and adduction	Trapezius (inferior fibers)

Hislop HJ, Montgomery J. *Daniels and Worthingham's Muscle Testing: Techniques of Manual Examination.* St. Louis: Saunders, 2007.
Moore KL, Dalley AF. *Clinically Oriented Anatomy,* 5th ed. Philadelphia: Lippincott Williams & Wilkins, 2006.

After the shoulder is reduced (returned to its normal joint position), the arm is placed in a sling and ice is often used for the first few days to minimize swelling and pain. Analgesics may also be prescribed. When the athlete can tolerate carrying the arm, the sling can be removed. The sling is typically worn for about 3 weeks. Pendulum and isometric exercises can begin and when the pain has subsided a strengthening program is initiated. The athlete may need 6 weeks of recovery before returning to play. The athlete should have at least 90% range of motion and strength of the uninvolved side and be able to perform sport-specific tasks prior to returning to play (10).

In young athletes shoulder dislocations have a high rate of recurrence and can lead to chronic shoulder instability (13). Sometimes surgical repair is advised to limit the instability and prevent chronic dislocations. Following surgery there is a greater recovery time. The arm is usually immobilized for about 3 weeks, but passive external rotation of the arm is not begun until 6 weeks postsurgery and from there the exercise program is slowly progressed. Return to play may take 4 to 6 months (12).

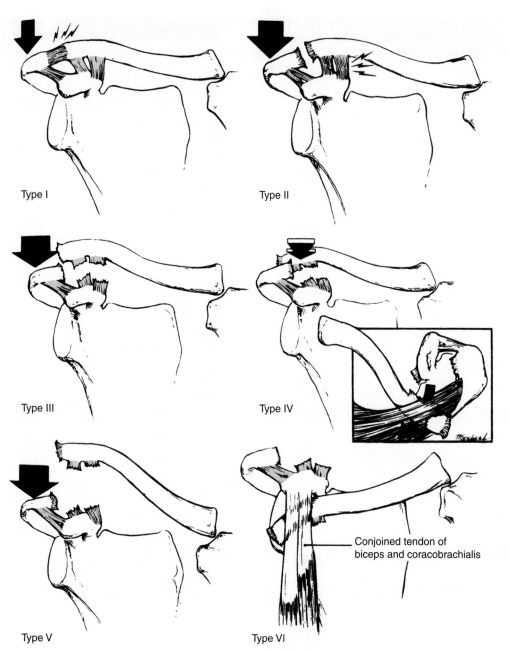

Type I

Type II

Type III

Type IV

Type V

Type VI

Conjoined tendon of
biceps and coracobrachialis

■ **FIGURE 13.5** Classification of acromioclavicular joint sprains. Type I: mild force to the point of the shoulder does not disrupt either the acromioclavicular or coracoclavicular ligaments. Type II: A greater force disrupts the acromioclavicular ligament but not the coracoclavicular ligament. Type III: A severe force disrupts both the acromioclavicular and coracoclavicular ligaments. Type IV: In addition to both ligaments being disrupted, the distal end of the clavicle is displaced posteriorly through or into the trapezius muscle. Type V: In addition to the rupture of both ligaments, the deltoid and trapezius muscle attachments are disrupted creating a major separation of the clavicle and acromion. Type VI: In addition to the disruption of both ligaments there is an inferior dislocation of the distal end of the clavicle. (Modified from Anderson MK, Hall SJ. *Sports Injury Management.* Baltimore: Williams & Wilkins, 1995.)

GLENOID LABRUM INJURIES

The glenoid labrum is a ring of fibrous tissue that is attached to the outer edge of the glenoid fossa and serves to add depth to the shallow socket and provide more stability to the glenohumeral joint. Injuries to the glenoid labrum are classified as superior labrum anterior to posterior (commonly referred to as SLAP lesions) or nonSLAP lesions. SLAP lesions are also classified as Type I to IV (14). The classification depends on the specific nature of the lesion which can vary from fraying with a degenerative appearance in Type I to a full-thickness tear of the labrum that extends into the biceps tendon in Type IV.

The glenoid labrum is typically injured by excessive or repeated traction and compression (13). Traction occurs when carrying or dropping and catching heavy objects and when lifting or stabilizing overhead objects. Athletes who engage in overhead activities such as pitchers, swimmers, and tennis players are at risk for traction injuries. Compression to the labrum can occur with a fall on an outstretched arm. The labrum can also tear in association with other injuries, such as dislocations.

Unless the injury is very minor, arthroscopic surgical repair is recommended (15). The rehabilitation program will vary depending on the specific type of lesion and repair. The overall emphasis of the rehabilitation program is on restoring and improving the dynamic stability of the glenohumeral joint and at the same time not putting any undo stresses on the healing tissue. The athlete can resume aerobic activity using the lower extremities as soon as exercise is possible without pain to the healing upper extremity. The time frame to return to play following repair of a SLAP lesion is not frequently discussed in the literature, but appears to be 9 to 12 months when done with other capsular procedures (16).

ROTATOR CUFF INJURIES

The four muscles that form the rotator cuff are the supraspinatus, infraspinatus, teres minor, and subscapularis. The mobility of the shoulder places great stress on the rotator cuff muscles. Injury to the rotator cuff is a common cause of shoulder pain in athletes, especially throwing athletes. Most rotator cuff injuries are treated conservatively for 6 weeks to 6 months before operative treatment is considered (17).

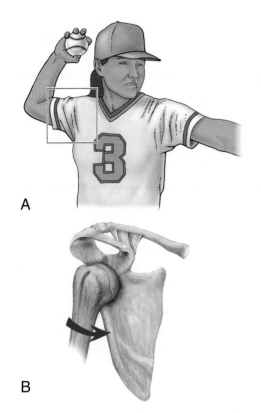

A

B

■ **FIGURE 13.6 A.** The right arm illustrates a position of abduction and external rotation. Anterior dislocations typically occur when the arm is excessively forced into this position. **B.** Anterior dislocation showing displacement of the humeral head. (A from Moore KL, Dalley AF II. *Clinically Oriented Anatomy*, 4th ed. Baltimore, Lippincott Williams & Wilkins, 1999; B, Asset provided by Anatomical Chart Co.)

Shoulder Impingement Shoulder impingement occurs when the tendons of the rotator cuff muscles, particularly the supraspinatus, are compressed due to decreased space under the coracoacromial arch (Fig. 13.7). This is most commonly seen in overhead repetitive activities. Other exacerbating factors in-

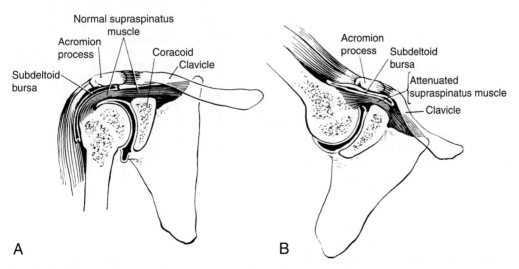

A   **B**

■ **FIGURE 13.7** Impingement of the supraspinatus tendon (anterior view). **A.** Normal position. **B.** Impingement of the tendon beneath the coracoacromial arch with abduction of the arm. (From Anderson MK, Hall SJ. *Sports Injury Management*. Baltimore: Williams & Wilkins, 1995.)

clude laxity and inflammation as well as postural malalignments. Treatment includes rest, nonsteroidal anti-inflammatory drugs (NSAIDS), and strengthening of the rotator cuff and scapular muscles. The activity that caused the problem may need to be modified and normal biomechanics should be restored to help prevent reinjury. Prior to returning to activity the athlete should be pain-free, have full range of motion and strength, and be able to confidently perform at a competitive level (18).

In addition, several modifications may be necessary during weight training exercises. Some of the common exercises, such as the bench press, shoulder press, and latissimus dorsi pulldown, may need to be modified to avoid further impingement (19). For the bench press a narrower grip should be used to avoid excessive torque on the shoulder joint. Behind the neck shoulder presses should be avoided because of stress to the glenohumeral joint structures. The posterior deltoid muscle can be targeted with other exercises such as deltoid raises, seated rows, or dumbbell rows. The latissimus dorsi behind the neck pulldown should be avoided and can be replaced with a front pulldown with the torso reclined 30 degrees (19).

Rotator Cuff Strains/Tears Minor injuries to the rotator cuff muscles are common in athletes and often involve the supraspinatus muscle. Tears often occur, alone or in combination, from repetitive microtrauma, overuse tendonitis, disuse and anatomic factors (20). Minor strains respond quickly to rest from the aggravating activity and the use of ice and other therapeutic modalities. The aggravating activity usually involves dynamic arm rotation with high velocity. Untreated strains can predispose the athlete to further rotator cuff tendon injuries. While complete and partial tears of the rotator cuff tendon are commonly seen in older athletes, they do not often occur in college or high school aged athletes unless there is a predisposition from untreated strains or a long history of shoulder impingement or instability (13).

THE ELBOW

The shoulder joint serves the purpose of positioning the arm to facilitate the action of the hand. The elbow allows for shortening and lengthening of the limb for a wider range of positioning of the hand. The elbow is prone to chronic injuries in sports such as tennis, baseball and softball. Acute injuries are more likely to happen in wrestling and gymnastics (4).

Elbow Anatomy

The elbow complex is composed of three bones, the humerus, ulna, and radius, and these bones form three separate joints that share a common joint capsule (Fig. 13.8). The humeroulnar joint is the articulation between the humerus and ulna, the humeroradial joint is between the humerus and the radius, and the proximal radioulnar joint is the articulation at the elbow between the radius and ulna. Flexion and extension of the elbow occur at the humeroulnar and humeroradial joints working together. Pronation and supination occur at the proximal radioulnar joint at the elbow along with the distal radioulnar joint at the wrist.

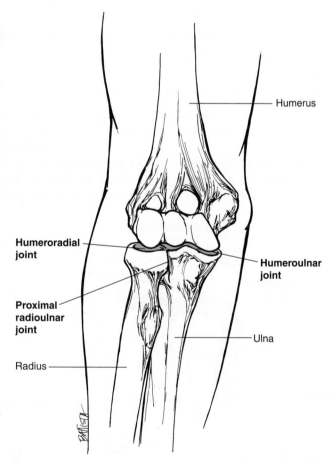

■ **FIGURE 13.8** Anterior view of elbow joint articulations. (Modified from Oatis CA. Kinesiology—*The Mechanics and Pathomechanics of Human Movement*. Baltimore: Lippincott Williams & Wilkins, 2004.)

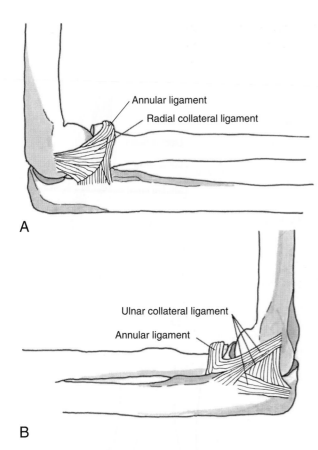

A

B

■ **FIGURE 13.9** Elbow ligaments. **A.** Lateral aspect. **B.** Medial aspect. (From Hertling D, Kessler RM. *Management of Common Musculoskeletal Disorders: Physical Therapy Principles and Methods.* Baltimore: Lippincott Williams & Wilkins, 1990).

The elbow joint is supported medially and laterally by the collateral ligaments. The ulnar collateral ligament is on the medial side of the joint connecting the humerus and ulna and the radial collateral ligament is on the lateral side connecting the humerus and radius. The anular ligament forms a sling around the head of the radius to keep it in place and allow for rotation (Fig. 13.9).

The muscles that move the elbow joint are illustrated in Figure 13.10. The motions of the elbow joint and prime movers for those motions can be found in Figure 13.11 and Table 13.2.

Common Elbow Injuries

Dislocations, muscular injuries at the proximal attachments, and ligament injuries are among the common athletic injuries seen at the elbow.

ELBOW DISLOCATIONS

Elbow dislocations are less common than shoulder dislocations and usually occur from a fall on an outstretched hand (21). Posterior dislocations are the most common and a visible deformity is apparent with the upper end of the ulna in a more posterior alignment than normal with the humerus (Fig. 13.12). Dislocations can also result in damage to the ligaments, nerves, and blood vessels that cross the elbow joint. With an elbow dislocation the athlete will experience severe pain and not be able to bend or straighten the elbow.

The injured limb should be immobilized with a splint and the athlete immediately referred to a physician for reduction of the dislocation. In the absence of medical personnel, the coach can check for a pulse at the wrist. If the pulse is absent, there is damage to a blood vessel and the athlete needs immediate emergency care. Fortunately, injuries to the blood vessels are relatively rare (12). Following reduction of an uncomplicated elbow dislocation the limb is placed in a sling or splint for approximately 1 to 3 weeks, depending on the severity. Return to play is permitted once the soft tissues have healed and the athlete has regained smooth, pain-free range of motion of the elbow and strength is equivalent to the noninjured side. Typically this occurs within 5 to 7 weeks and for the most severe cases within 8 to 10 weeks (21). Operative management of a dislocation is recommended only for baseball pitchers and when the joint remains unstable (12).

LATERAL EPICONDYLITIS (TENNIS ELBOW)

Lateral epicondylitis, often called tennis elbow, commonly refers to both acute and chronic injuries at the lateral aspect of the elbow where the wrist extensor muscles attach to the distal humerus (Fig. 13.13). Lateral epicondylitis occurs in over 50% of athletes using overhead arm motions (22). The athlete will have pain at the lateral elbow which can extend towards the hand and the pain is increased with overhead arm motion and activities that require resisted wrist extension.

Lateral epicondylitis is treated similarly to most soft tissue injuries. Pain and inflammation are controlled with rest, ice, and NSAIDS. Therapeutic modalities and deep friction massage are used to promote healing. As pain permits, strengthening exercises are done along with stretching of the wrist extensor muscles. During rehabilitation and return to play the predisposing factors should be addressed. The coach can play a vital role

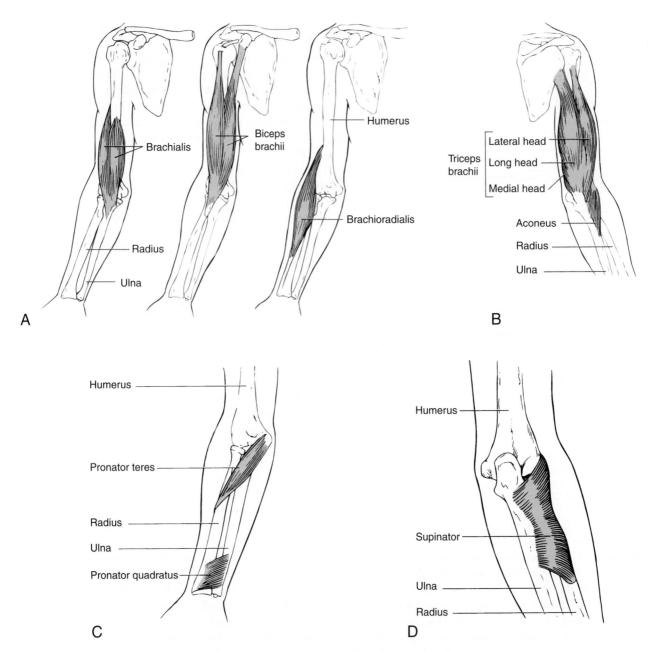

■ **FIGURE 13.10** Muscles that move the elbow joint. **A.** Flexors. **B.** Extensors. **C.** Pronators. **D.** Supinator muscle (note that the biceps brachii also supinates the forearm). (Modified from Anderson MK, Hall SJ. *Sports Injury Management*. Baltimore: Williams & Wilkins, 1995.)

FOCAL POINT

What's in a Name?

Many names are used interchangeably and incorrectly in the literature to describe epicondylar injury. While traditionally known as tennis elbow, elbow pain related to overuse of the wrist extensor muscles is more common

(continues)

What's in a Name? *(continued)*

in nontennis players than in tennis players (1). It has also been referred to as lateral epicondylitis, but that term reflects an inflammatory state and often it is more degenerative in nature. Hume et al (2) suggested the use of epicondylitis for acute injuries that result in inflammation and epicondylosis or epicondylopathy for injuries that develop over time and result in structural changes in the tendon.

1. Brukner P, Khan K. *Clinical Sports Medicine*, 3rd ed. North Ryde, New South Wales: McGraw-Hill, 2007.
2. Hume PA, Reid D, Edwards T. Epicondylar injury in sport: epidemiology, type, mechanisms, assessment, management and prevention. *Sports Med* 2006;36:151–170.

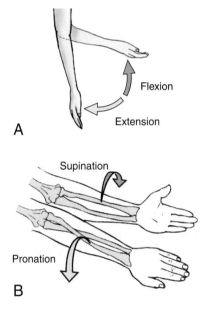

■ **FIGURE 13.11** Motions of the elbow joint. **A.** Flexion and extension. **B.** Pronation and supination.

here. Technique faults, such as a faulty backhand technique in tennis, may have predisposed the athlete to injury. In racquet sports excessively large or small grips should be avoided. Modification of playing techniques helps prevent recurrence by reducing overload forces. Counterforce bracing can also help reduce the forces on the extensor tendons (13,23). The brace can be worn during rehabilitation and return to play. The brace is applied firmly and worn over the muscles in the forearm about 2 to 4 inches below the elbow (Fig. 13.14). The brace is worn over the muscle bellies because the theory is that the brace produces a counterforce that prevents the forearm muscles from expanding fully and thus reduces the force at their tendinous insertion.

While most athletes respond to conservative treatment, occasionally surgery is required to remove degenerative tissue in the extensor tendons. Surgery is often done only after 12 months of failed conservative treatment (13). The arthroscopic technique is less traumatic than the traditional open procedure and allows for a quicker return to sports activity (24). Even though the name of this injury indicates an inflammatory process, the primary problem is usually degenerative in nature. Therefore, the use of corticosteroid injections is controversial and usually not required (13).

TABLE 13.2	Prime Movers of the Elbow and Radioulnar Joints
Elbow Movement	**Prime Movers**
Flexion	Brachialis Biceps brachii Brachioradialis
Extension	Triceps brachii Assisted by: Anconeus
Pronation	Pronator quadratus Pronator teres
Supination	Biceps brachii Supinator

Hislop HJ, Montgomery J. *Daniels and Worthingham's Muscle Testing: Techniques of Manual Examination*. St. Louis: Saunders, 2007.
Moore KL, Dalley AF. *Clinically Oriented Anatomy*, 5th ed. Philadelphia: Lippincott Williams & Wilkins, 2006.

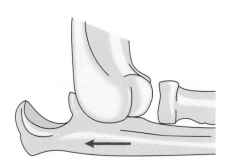

■ **FIGURE 13.12** Posterior dislocation of the elbow. Note that the articular surface of the ulna has moved posteriorly and is not in contact with the distal humerus. (From Bickley LS, Szilagyi P. *Bates' Guide to Physical Examination and History Taking*, 8th ed. Philadelphia: Lippincott Williams & Wilkins, 2003).

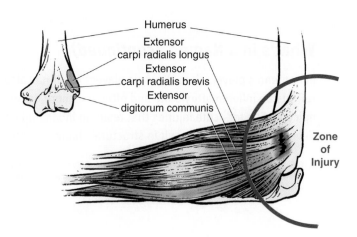

■ **FIGURE 13.13** Tennis elbow. Lateral aspect of the elbow showing the area of injury of the wrist and hand extensor muscles at their proximal attachment. (From Koval KJ, Zuckerman JD. *Atlas of Orthopedic Surgery: A Multimedical Reference*. Philadelphia: Lippincott Williams & Wilkins, 2004.)

Following treatment, return to play should occur gradually over a period of 3 to 6 weeks, depending on the severity of the injury (13). A tennis player, for example, would begin backhand strokes without a ball and then progress to hitting shorter distances and gradually hitting full length shots.

MEDIAL EPICONDYLITIS (GOLFER'S ELBOW)

Medial epicondylitis, commonly known as golfer's elbow, occurs less frequently than lateral epicondylitis (22). The athlete experiences pain and tenderness on the medial aspect of the elbow where the tendons of the wrist flexor and forearm pronator muscles attach to the medial epicondyle of the humerus. Wrist flexion and pronation result in medial elbow pain. Golfers and tennis players often develop medial epicondylitis because of the repetitive stress placed on the soft tissues of the medial elbow. Medial epicondylitis is more often seen in tennis players who use a lot of top spin because of the forced pronation with that motion (22). Conservative treatment for medial epicondylitis is similar to that of lateral epicondylitis.

ULNAR COLLATERAL LIGAMENT INJURIES

During overhead throwing the ulnar collateral ligament (UCL) at the elbow (Fig. 13.9) undergoes tremendous stress. During pitching the ligament approaches the ultimate failure load (25). Sports activities that involve overhead throwing, such as tennis serving, baseball pitching, football passing, and javelin throwing, further increase the susceptibility for UCL injury because of the repetitive stresses.

UCL injuries cause pain and tenderness to the medial aspect of the elbow and some joint swelling may also be present. The injury can be a strain or partial tear of the ligament and can occur over time or with a single incident of sudden pain while throwing. The injury is treated conservatively or operatively, depending on severity. Ice and NSAIDS are used to control pain and inflammation. A brace can be used to prevent further strain to the ligament. During the acute phase of rehabilitation the goals are to restore normal range of motion and maintain or improve muscular strength. At 4 to 6 weeks postinjury the athlete can gradually increase activity. At 6 to 7 weeks postinjury the athlete may be able to begin an advanced strengthening program (26). The athlete is ready to return to competition when asymptomatic with the increased activity.

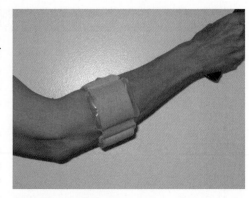

■ **FIGURE 13.14** Counterforce brace used to help alleviate tennis elbow symptoms. Note that the brace is worn over the muscle bellies distal to the elbow joint.

Little League Elbow

Over 25 years ago the term *Little Leaguer's elbow* was coined to describe a medial epicondyle fracture at the growth plate caused by pitching in the adolescent athlete. Now Little League elbow is used as a catch-all term for several injury patterns at the elbow.

Prevention is the best treatment for Little League elbow and one of the best ways to ensure that young athletes can grow up to play at the high school and college level. Youth league coaches and parents need to be educated about proper warm-up, conditioning and off-season training. Breaking pitches should not be thrown until at least the age of 13 (1). These throws place undue stress on the still developing anatomical structures, particularly with poor throwing mechanics.

In an effort to help decrease injuries, Little League International implemented new rule changes effective for the 2007 season. Pitch counts will be imposed by age group and rest days will be defined based on the number of pitches in a game (2).

League Age	Pitches allowed per day
17–18	105
13–16	95
11–12	85
10 and under	75

This is an important step in helping to reduce injuries. However, there are no rules for frequency and intensity of practice pitches which must be monitored by parents and coaches. Players should also be discouraged from joining multiple leagues to increase their playing time.

Little League elbow should be treated with rest from pitching for at least 4 to 6 weeks and during that time the athlete can engage in general conditioning activities (3). Modalities and nonsteroidal anti-inflammatory drugs can be used to decrease pain and inflammation and sometimes a brace is used. Following the rest period a slow, progressive throwing program can begin within pain-free limits. The average time to return to competitive pitching is 12 weeks (3).

1. Olsen SJ, Flesig GS, Dun S, et al. Risk factors for shoulder and elbow injuries in adolescent baseball pitchers. *Am J Sports Med* 2006;34:905–912.
2. Little League Online. *Regulation and Rule Changes for 2007*. Available online at http://www.littleleague.org/media/pitch_count_08-25-06.asp. Accessed January 2, 2007.
3. Benjamin HJ, Briner WW. Little League elbow. *Clin J Sport Med* 2005;15:37–40.

When symptoms persist or when the injury is severe, surgical intervention may be needed. The rehabilitation program will vary depending on the surgical technique. The elbow is usually placed in a posterior splint for the first week to protect the healing structures. For the next 4 or 5 weeks a functional brace is used and rehabilitation includes a progressive range of motion and strengthening program leading to return to play activities. An interval throwing program can begin at about 4 months and the athlete may return to competitive throwing around 9 months following surgery (27).

THE WRIST AND HAND

The wrist and hand are commonly injured in sports (28). The injuries range from fractures which more commonly occur in contact sports or falls on to the outstretched hand to overuse injuries often seen in racquet sports, gymnastics, and golf. Most injuries seem to occur during competition as opposed to practice and each sport has its own injury pattern (28). Sports with higher risk of hand injury include football, gymnastics, wrestling and basketball (29). Finger trauma is common in ball handling sports.

Coaches and athletes often minimize the importance of proper evaluation and treatment of what appears to be only a minor injury. Since injuries to the wrist and hand may not interfere with sports participation that primarily relies on the lower extremities, these injuries are often overlooked. Untreated, hand and wrist injuries can result in future disabling deformities. Hand and wrist injuries need to be evaluated, treated, and protected from further injury during the healing process.

Strength and conditioning programs often do not include exercises for the hands. Squeezing a rubber ball or spring device can help strengthen the fingers. Small dumbbells can be used to strengthen the wrist flexors and extensors. Another protective measure is learning the correct way to fall, especially in collision sports or those in which falling is routine. Athletes should learn to roll as they hit the ground so the force is transmitted to the larger and better protected joints to avoid impact to the hand or wrist (30).

Wrist and Hand Anatomy

While the arm has one bone and the forearm has two bones, each wrist and hand has 26 bones along with multiple ligaments and muscles. The intricate structure of this region allows for precise, skilled movement, but also makes it complex.

The proximal row of wrist bones articulate with the radius and ulna of the forearm and the distal row articulates with the five metacarpal bones. Each metacarpal bone articulates distally with the corresponding proximal phalanx forming the metacarpophalangeal (MCP) joints. Each finger has three phalanges (proximal, middle, and distal) and the thumb has two (proximal and distal). See Figure 13.15.

A complex series of ligaments attach all adjacent bones in the wrist and hand. Both extrinsic (originating outside the hand) and intrinsic (contained within the hand) muscles are responsible for the movement of the wrist and hand. In general, the muscles on the palmar surface cause flexion and those on the dorsal (posterior) surface cause extension. The intrinsic muscles also abduct and adduct the digits and allow the thumb to oppose each of the fingers. The muscles that move the wrist and finger joints are illustrated in Figure 13.16. The motions of the wrist and fingers and prime movers for those motions can be found in Figure 13.17 and Table 13.3.

Common Wrist and Hand Injuries

Numerous injuries occur in the wrist and hand. Entire books are devoted to these injuries and

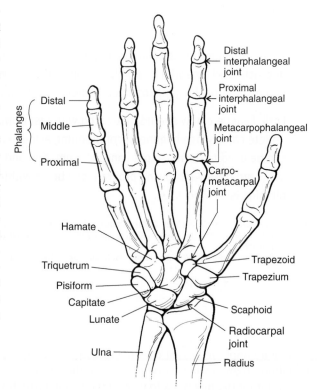

■ **FIGURE 13.15** Anterior view of the bones and joints of the right wrist and hand. (From Hamill J, Knutzen KM. *Biomechanical Basis of Human Movement*, 2nd ed. Baltimore: Lippincott Williams & Wilkins, 2003.)

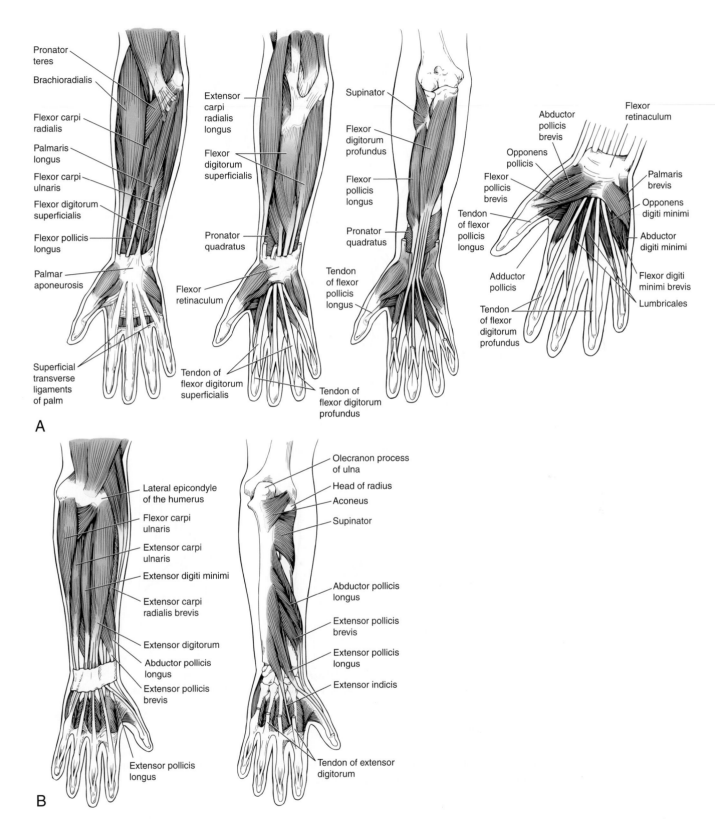

■ **FIGURE 13.16** Muscles of the wrist and hand. **A.** Superficial and deep anterior muscles. **B.** Superficial and deep posterior muscles. (From Anderson MK, Hall SJ. *Sports Injury Management*. Baltimore: Williams & Wilkins, 1995.)

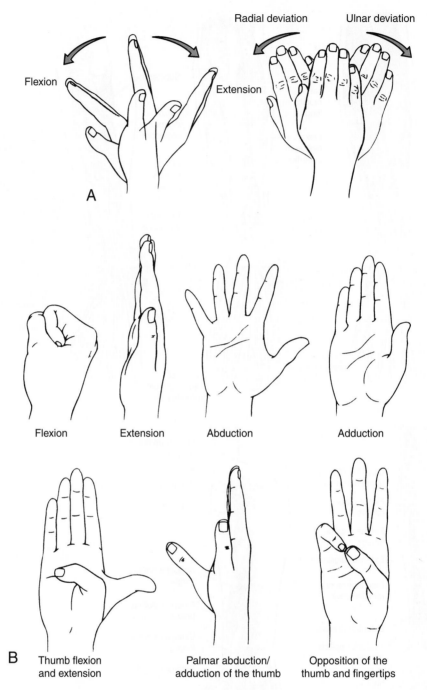

■ **FIGURE 13.17 A.** Motions of the wrist. **B.** Motions of the hand. (From Anderson MK, Hall SJ. *Sports Injury Management*. Baltimore: Williams & Wilkins, 1995.)

physicians as well as physical and occupational therapists specialize in treating hand injuries. This section will cover some of the more commonly seen injuries in sports.

SCAPHOID FRACTURES

A scaphoid fracture is the most common and most problematic fracture of the wrist in athletes (31). A fall onto the outstretched hand is a common mechanism of injury. This fracture can be difficult to diagnose because it may not be apparent on initial radiographs. Radiographs can be repeated in 2 weeks when the fracture line may be more apparent. Magnetic resonance imaging can also be used at the time of injury to better detect the fracture. Sometimes these fractures fail to unite despite treatment, but if untreated,

TABLE 13.3 Prime Movers of the Wrist and Finger Joints

Wrist Movement	Prime Movers
Flexion	Flexor carpi radialis Flexor carpi ulnaris
Extension	Extensor carpi radialis longus Extensor carpi radialis brevis Extensor carpi ulnaris
Abduction	Abductor pollicis longus Flexor carpi radialis Extensor carpi radialis longus Extensor carpi radialis brevis
Adduction	Extensor carpi ulnaris Flexor carpi ulnaris
Finger Movement	
Flexion—Metacarpophalangeal joints	Lumbricals Dorsal interossei Palmar interossei
Extension—Metacarpophalangeal joints	Extensor digitorum Extensor indicis Extensor digiti minimi
Flexion—Proximal interphalangeal joints	Flexor digitorum superficialis
Flexion—Distal interphalangeal joints	Flexor digitorum profundus
Extension—Interphalangeal joints	Extensor digitorum, lumbricals and interossei via the extensor digital expansion
Finger abduction	Dorsal interossei Abductor digiti minimi
Finger adduction	Palmar interossei
Flexion—Metacarpophalangeal joint of thumb	Flexor pollicis brevis
Flexion—Interphalangeal joint of thumb	Flexor pollicis longus
Extension—Metacarpophalangeal joint of thumb	Extensor pollicis brevis
Extension—Interphalangeal joints of thumb	Extensor pollicis longus
Thumb abduction	Abductor pollicis longus Abductor pollicis brevis
Thumb adduction	Adductor pollicis
Opposition	Opponens pollicis Opponens digiti minimi

Hislop HJ, Montgomery J. *Daniels and Worthingham's Muscle Testing: Techniques of Manual Examination*. St. Louis: Saunders, 2007.
Moore KL, Dalley AF. *Clinically Oriented Anatomy*, 5th ed. Philadelphia: Lippincott Williams & Wilkins, 2006

nonunion of the fragments is likely (32). If there is uncertainty, the wrist should be immobilized in a cast for 2 weeks and then reassessed.

With a scaphoid fracture the athlete will have tenderness in the anatomical snuff box (Fig. 13.18) with decreased range of motion of the wrist, swelling, and pain with wrist extension. Treatment typically includes cast immobilization for 2 to 4 months. The cast should be evaluated every 2 weeks or so to be certain it is still immobilizing the wrist. Displaced and unstable fractures may require surgery. Return to play decisions are based on the type of fracture and nature of the sport. Athletes involved in noncontact sports and being managed with cast immobilization can return immediately. In contact sports return to play with cast immobilization may need to be delayed for 6 weeks to allow for initial healing of the fracture (10).

INJURY TO THE ULNAR COLLATERAL LIGAMENT OF THE THUMB

This injury is commonly called a game-keeper's thumb or skier's thumb (Fig. 13.19) and is caused by a forced abduction and hyperextension of the thumb. As with other ligament injuries the severity can range from a minor sprain to a complete rupture. With this injury there will be swelling and tenderness along the ulnar collateral ligament on the medial aspect of the metacarpophalangeal joint of the thumb. Minor injuries can be treated with a thumb spica splint (Fig. 13.20) until pain and tenderness resolve. Partial tears are typically treated with a thumb spica cast for 4 to 6 weeks. Complete ruptures can be repaired surgically but may also resolve with cast immobilization of at least 6 weeks (10). Following surgery the thumb is immobilized in a spica cast for 4 to 6 weeks followed by protective splinting during sports activities for another 3 months (13).

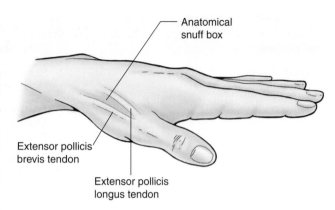

■ **FIGURE 13.18** Anatomical snuff box. The scaphoid bone is located in the area between the tendons and there is tenderness to palpation when the bone is fractured. (From Moore K, Dalley A. *Clinically Oriented Anatomy*, 4th ed. Baltimore: Lippincott Williams & Wilkins, 1999.)

Return to play is allowed once the thumb is comfortable and protected in a cast (10). If thumb immobilization is not possible in the sport, then return to play is delayed until healing is complete and the joint is stable. Once the cast is removed, a range of motion and strengthening program is initiated. Athletes returning to contact sports should use a thermoplastic thumb spica splint during play until their rehabilitation is complete (10).

METACARPAL FRACTURES

Metacarpal fractures can occur at the head, neck or shaft of the bones and usually result from a direct blow. A fracture of the neck of the 5th metacarpal (small finger) is known as a boxer's fracture. Most of these fractures are stable and can be treated conservatively. Unstable fractures may require surgery. These fractures are usually treated with immobilization for about 3 weeks followed by an additional 3 weeks with a removable thermoplastic splint. Following either surgical or conservative treatment, athletes are held out of contact sports for 2 to 3 weeks to allow for initial healing. Return to play can then occur with a playing cast (10).

PROXIMAL INTERPHALANGEAL JOINT INJURIES

The proximal interphalangeal (PIP) joint is the most often injured joint in sports (33). Injuries to this joint include sprains of the collateral ligaments, dislocations, fracture dislocations, and injury to the palmar (also known as volar) plate. The palmar plate is a thick, fibrous ligament on the palmar surface of the joint. The athlete typically reports a "jammed" finger. Often these injuries are assumed to be a simple sprain and are treated on the sideline by buddy taping the injured finger to the adjacent finger (Fig. 13.21). The problem with this approach is missing a more serious injury. Untreated, 2 to 3 months later the athlete will have a painful, stiff and deformed finger that has been called "The Coach's Finger" (34). By having all injuries of this joint appropriately evaluated, you can help prevent the consequences of undertreating these injuries.

Sprains can be treated with buddy taping or splinting and range of motion exercises. Athletes can return to play immediately in sports where playing with a splint is possi-

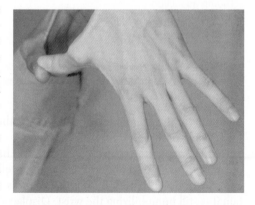

■ **FIGURE 13.19** Gamekeeper's or skier's thumb. This injury is a result of a sprain or rupture of the ulnar collateral ligament of the thumb. (From Anderson MK, Hall SJ. *Sports Injury Management*. Baltimore: Williams & Wilkins, 1995.)

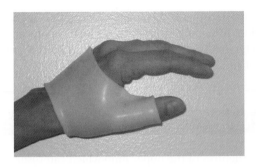

■ **FIGURE 13.20** Thumb spica splint to protect a healing ulnar collateral ligament of the thumb.

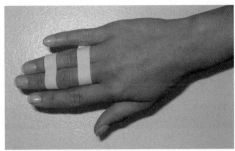

■ **FIGURE 13.21** Buddy taping of fingers to support the proximal interphalangeal joint.

ble. When full range of motion is needed, return to play is in about 20 to 21 days. If there is laxity in the joint, splinting may be needed for 2 to 3 weeks and return to full play may require 4 to 6 weeks (33).

Stable dislocations are immobilized for 2 to 3 days and return to play may be allowed after that with immobilization or buddy taping. Stable fracture dislocations are immobilized for 3 weeks and return to play with protective immobilization can then occur as tolerated by the athlete (10). Unstable fracture dislocations may keep the athlete from play for 6 to 8 weeks (33).

MALLET FINGER

Mallet finger, also known as baseball finger, is the rupture of the distal extensor tendon (Fig. 13.22). It occurs when the distal interphalangeal (DIP) joint is actively extended and the distal phalanx is forced into flexion (35). These injuries are common in ball catching sports. There can be a simple tendon rupture at the bony attachment or a piece of bone can fracture with the tendon attached. With this injury the athlete cannot fully extend the distal phalanx of the finger at the DIP joint. The middle finger is most commonly involved, but this injury can occur to any of the fingers. With a rupture or small avulsion fragment the injury is treated with a split to immobilize the DIP joint. The splint is worn for at least 6 to 8 weeks. Once full active DIP extension is regained, the splint can be gradually withdrawn. Sports participation is possible with this injury as long as the DIP joint is firmly immobilized in extension and the joint is protected from further injury (35). The treating physician should provide consent for participation.

JERSEY FINGER

A jersey finger is the avulsion of the flexor digitorum profundus from its attachment on the distal phalanx (Fig. 13.23). It received its name from a common mechanism of injury. When tackling and pulling on someone's jersey, the finger is forced into extension while the DIP is being actively flexed. The ring finger is most commonly involved, but this injury can occur with any finger (35). With this injury the athlete

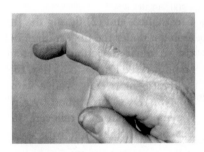

■ **FIGURE 13.22** Mallet finger. The distal extensor tendon is ruptured and the athlete is not able to extend the distal phalanx (From Anderson MK, Hall SJ. *Sports Injury Management*. Baltimore: Williams & Wilkins, 1995.)

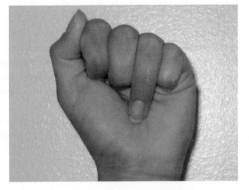

■ **FIGURE 13.23** Jersey finger. With an avulsion of the flexor digitorum profundus from its attachment on the distal phalanx, the athlete will not be able to actively flex the distal interphalangeal joint.

cannot flex the distal phalanx while the PIP is held in extension. Unlike mallet finger, this injury usually requires surgery to reattach the tendon to its insertion. After surgery, return to contact sports and sports requiring the use of the injured hand may take 4 to 6 months (10). Return to play can be earlier for athletes whose sports will not place the injured finger at risk for further injury.

SUMMARY

- Sports activities can place high demands on the structures of the upper limb which can result in both overuse and acute injuries.
- The shoulder complex has four articulations and its structure favors mobility over stability.
- Common injuries to the shoulder complex include clavicular fractures, acromioclavicular joint sprains, shoulder dislocations, glenoid labrum tears, and rotator cuff injuries.
- At the elbow, joint flexion and extension occur at the humeroulnar and humeroradial joints and pronation and supination occur at the radioulnar joint.
- Posterior dislocations, lateral epicondylitis (tennis elbow), medial epicondylitis (golfer's elbow), and injuries to the ulnar collateral ligament are among the athletic injuries that commonly occur at the elbow joint.
- The hand is complex with many bones, ligaments, and muscles to allow for precise, skilled movements.
- Hand injuries are common in sports and are often minimized and overlooked. This can lead to disabling deformity. Hand and wrist injuries, even seemingly minor ones, need to be evaluated, treated, and protected from further injury during the healing process.
- Fractures can occur in the wrist bones, metacarpals, and phalanges. The scaphoid is the most often fractured bone in the wrist. Metacarpal fractures occur at the head, neck, or shaft of the bone. Ligament injuries can occur to the ulnar collateral ligament of the thumb (gamekeeper's thumb or skier's thumb) as well as at the proximal and distal interphalangeal joints. A mallet finger occurs when there is a rupture of the distal extensor tendon. A jersey finger is the avulsion of the flexor digitorum profundus. These are some of the many injuries that occur in the wrist and hands.
- Coaches can play a vital role in the prevention and rehabilitation of common injuries by focusing on proper technique and ensuring that injured athletes adhere to return to play criteria.

References

1. Fleisig GS, Kingsley DS, Loftice JW, et al. Kinetic comparison among the fastball, curveball, change-up, and slider in collegiate baseball pitchers. *Am J Sports Med* 2006;34:423–430.
2. Markolf KL, Shapiro MS, Mandelbaum BR, et al. Wrist loading patterns during pommel horse exercises. *J Biomech* 1990; 23: 1001–1011.
3. Frontera WR. Epidemiology of sports injuries: implications for rehabilitation. In: Frontera WR. *Rehabilitation of Sports Injuries: Scientific Basis*. Malden, MA: Blackwell Publishing, 2003.
4. Flegel MJ. *Sport First Aid: A Coach's Guide to Preventing and Responding to Injuries*, 3rd ed. Champaign, IL: Human Kinetics, 2004.
5. Post M. Current concepts in the treatment of fractures of the clavicle. *Clin Orthop* 1989;245;89–101.
6. Gómez JE. Upper extremity injuries in youth sports. *Pediatr Clin N Am* 2002;49:593–626.
7. Postacchini F, Gumina S, De Santis P, et al. Epidemiology of clavicle fractures. *J Shoulder Elbow Surg* 2002;11:452–456.
8. Denard PJ, Koval KJ, Cantu RV, et al. Management of midshaft clavicle fractures in adults. *Am J Orthop* 2005;34:527–536.
9. Garretson RB, Williams GR. Clinical evaluation of injuries to the acromioclavicular and sternoclavicular joints. *Clin Sports Med* 2003;22:239–254.
10. Kovacic J, Bergfeld J. Return to play issues in upper extremity injuries. *Clin J Sport Med* 2005;15:448–452.
11. Bradley JP, Elkousy H. Decision making: operative versus nonoperative treatment of acromioclavicular joint injuries. *Clin Sports Med* 2003;22:277–290.
12. Burra G, Andrews JR. Acute shoulder and elbow dislocations in the athlete. *Orthop Clin N Am* 2002;33:479–495.
13. Brukner P, Khan K. *Clinical Sports Medicine*, 3rd ed. North Ryde, New South Wales: McGraw-Hill, 2007.
14. Snyder SJ, Karzel RP, Del Pizzo W, et al. Slap lesions of the shoulder. *Arthroscopy* 1990;6:274–279.
15. Wilk KE, Reinold MM, Dugas JR, et al. Current concepts in the recognition and treatment of superior labral (SLAP) lesions. *J Orthop Sports Phys Ther* 2005;35:273–291.
16. Park HB, Lin SK, Yokota A, et al. Return to play for rotator cuff injuries and superior labrum anterior posterior (SLAP) lesions. *Clin Sports Med* 2004;23:321–334.

17. Bytomski JR, Black D. Conservative treatment of rotator cuff injuries. *J Surg Orthop Adv* 2006;15:126–131.

18. Myers JB. Conservative management of shoulder impingement syndrome in the athletic population. *J Sport Rehabil* 1999;8:230–253.

19. Fees M, Decker T, Snyder-Mackler L, et al. Upper extremity weight-training modifications for the injured athlete. *Am J Sports Med* 1998;26:732–742.

20. Wilk KE, Harrelson GL, Arrigo C. Shoulder rehabilitation. In: Andrews JR, Harrelson GL, Wilk KE. *Physical Rehabilitation of the Injured Athlete*, 3rd ed. Philadelphia: Saunders, 2004.

21. Rettig AC. Traumatic elbow injuries in the athlete. *Orthop Clin N Am* 2002;33:509–522.

22. Field LD, Savoie FH. Common elbow injuries in sport. *Sports Med* 1998;26:193–205.

23. Hume PA, Reid D, Edwards T. Epicondylar injury in sport: epidemiology, type, mechanisms, assessment, management and prevention. *Sports Med* 2006;36:151–170.

24. Dlabach JA, Baker CL. Lateral and medial epicondylitis in the overhead athlete. *Op Tech Ortho* 2001;11:46–54.

25. Fleisig GS, Andrews JR, Dillman CJ, et al. Kinetics of baseball pitching with implications about injury mechanisms. *Am J Sports Med* 1995;23:233–239.

26. Wilk KE, Arrigo CA. Rehabilitation of elbow injuries. In: Andrews JR, Harrelson GL, Wilk KE. *Physical Rehabilitation of the Injured Athlete,* 3rd ed. Philadelphia: Saunders, 2004.

27. Wilk KE, Reinold MM, Andrews JR. Rehabilitation of the thrower's elbow. *Clin Sports Med* 2004;23:765–801.

28. Rettig AC. Epidemiology of hand and wrist injuries in sports. *Clin Sports Med* 1998;17:401–406.

29. Posner MA. Hand injuries. In: *The Upper Extremity in Sports Medicine*, 2nd ed. St. Louis, MO: Mosby, 1995.

30. Press JM, Wiesner SL. Prevention: conditioning and orthotics. *Hand Clinics* 1990;6:383–392.

31. Retig AC. Athletic injuries of the wrist and hand. Part 1: traumatic injuries of the wrist. *Am J Sports Med* 2003;31:1038–1048.

32. Barton N. Sports injuries of the hand and wrist. *Br J Sports Med* 1997;31:191–196.

33. Rettig AC. Athletic injuries of the wrist and hand. Part II: overuse injuries of the wrist and traumatic injuries to the hand. *Am J Sports Med* 2004;32:262–273.

34. McCue FC, Andrews JR, Hakala M, et al. The coach's finger. *J Sport Med* 1974;2:270–275.

35. Hong E. Hand injuries in sports medicine. *Prim Care Clin Office Pract* 2005;32:91–103

Common Lower Limb Injuries

Upon reading this chapter, the coach should be able to:

1. Identify the basic skeletal and muscular structure of the hip, thigh, knee, leg, ankle, and foot.
2. Describe the etiology of common injuries to the hip, thigh, knee, leg, ankle, and foot.
3. Recognize many of the common lower limb injuries.
4. Describe basic techniques of lower limb injury prevention.
5. Participate in functional rehabilitation techniques for lower limb injuries.
6. Discuss return to play criteria and typical rehabilitation requirements for injured athletes.

Antonio was the best player on his high school soccer team. The years he had spent playing with his friends in Puerto Rico had paid off. After he moved with his parents to Florida at age 12, he immediately became part of his school's soccer program. His school had made the playoffs in his final year. Early in the second half, as he went to kick a ball just off the ground, an opposing player kicked him directly in the front of his thigh. Antonio went down immediately. The pain was severe and when he tried to get up, his leg was not working properly. Unfortunately, the school's athletic trainer had been assigned to the football team that day. The coach helped Antonio off the field and checked out his leg. Redness and swelling had already appeared. The coach knew his soccer well but little about sports medicine. Antonio's coach needed him back in the game and encouraged him to walk around for a while. "Try to loosen it up," he said. Antonio limped around for awhile but had trouble jogging. The coach decided that massage might loosen up the leg and got one of the other players to massage Antonio's thigh. This went on for a while but Antonio never did get back into the game. His team won and was scheduled to play in the finals the next day.

Antonio's parents drove him home after the game. Later that evening the athletic trainer called and told Antonio not to massage the thigh but to put ice on it. Antonio wakened the next day to a leg that was very stiff. He could feel a lump on the front of his leg. He went outside and tried to loosen up but to no avail. He showed up for the game and the athletic trainer told him he could not play and treated him with ice and compression. The soccer season ended that day but Antonio's injury did not. Within a few weeks the knot in his thigh got harder and upon a visit to his physician was told that he had a calcium deposit in his thigh. Myositis ossificans was the diagnosis and his physician told him he might need surgery. Myositis ossificans can be caused by a direct blow resulting in an intramuscular hematoma. The athlete normally recalls a particular trauma that initiates the symptoms. The hematoma is complicated by bone formation within the muscle. The bone formation may be attached to the femur but can also have no connection.

The preceding is a perfect example of why coaches need basic sports medicine training. In fact, Antonio's coach did the exact opposite of the recommended treatment. Ice and compression would have decreased the bleeding in Antonio's thigh. Massage and exercise increased blood flow to the thigh and resulted in a considerable hematoma. When in doubt, conservative treatment is the answer. One can rarely go wrong with simple rest and ice.

Lower body injuries represent the majority of injuries in sport. Injuries to the hip, thigh, knee, leg, ankle, and foot are rather common. For example, Table 14.1 represents just four common NCAA sports (1). Even in the sport of football in which there are multiple upper body contacts while blocking and tackling, lower limb injuries prevail. Although many of these injuries are the result of contact, in college football, noncontact injuries represent a substantial number of injuries per year. In sports like soccer, basketball, track and field, and baseball/softball, noncontact injuries are very common. Athletes need strong symmetrically developed hips, knees, and ankles that are well coordinated for running, jumping, turning, and stopping. Overuse injuries have become much more widespread and coaches need to schedule recovery into all workout schedules. Extensive resistance training of the upper body with secondary preparation of the lower body is a serious training error. The primary measure coaches can utilize to prevent such injuries is the proper conditioning of the lower body.

THE HIP COMPLEX

The hip joint is a ball and socket joint similar to the shoulder. Motion is allowed in the basic planes of motion plus oblique planes. The head of the femur is quite pronounced and fits into a fairly deep socket on the hip. This structure combined with the fact that the pelvic girdle is not nearly as mobile as the shoulder girdle, restricts the movement of the femur. This combination of structure as well as the heavy musculature surrounding the hip makes the hip joint extremely stable.

Hip Anatomy

At birth the ilium, ischium, and pubis are fairly distinct but eventually fuse together into one structure. The pelvic girdle is composed of these three bones on each side of the hip and the sacrum at the sacroiliac joint. A convenient method of reviewing the muscles of the hip is to observe their relationship to the hip joint. Those muscles that are anterior to the joint generally flex the hip while those muscles that are posterior extend the hip. The muscles on the medial side adduct while the abductors are located on the lateral side of the hip. In addition, because of each muscle's unique spatial relationship and line of pull, many hip muscles perform multiple movements. For example, the gluteus maximus is a powerful extensor of the hip but can also outwardly rotate the femur. Table 14.2 details those muscles that are primarily involved in the basic movements of the hip. Figure 14.1 identifies the principal muscles about the hip.

Common Hip and Thigh Injuries

Muscle strains and contusions are the predominant injuries to the hip and thigh. Fractures of the femur are rare in most sports but do occur occasionally in downhill skiing and football. Although athletic injuries about the hip occur less frequently than other injuries to the extremities, hip and thigh injuries can have

TABLE 14.1 Percent of Injuries by Sport in NCAA Practice and Competition		
Sport	**Practice**	**Competition**
Football	56.9	51.1
Men's Basketball	62.3	59.4
Women's Basketball	66.9	53.6
Men's Soccer	51.1	54.8
Women's Soccer	70.0	60.0
Softball	41.5	38.3

TABLE 14.2	Hip Joint Muscles and Their Actions	
Movement	**Prime Movers**	**Location**
Flexion	Iliopsoas Rectus Femoris Pectineus Sartorius	Anterior
Extension	Gluteus Maximus Semitendinosus Semimembranosus Biceps Femoris	Posterior
Adduction	Adductor Magnus, Longus, Brevis Gracilis Pecineus	Medial
Abduction	Gluteus Medius Tensor Fascia Latae	Lateral
Outward Rotation	Gluteus Maximus Six Outward Rotators (Piriformis, Obturator internus, Obturator externus, Quadratus femoris, Gemellus superior, Gemellus inferior)	Posterior
Inward Rotation	Gluteus Minimus Tensor Fascia Latae	Anterior-Lateral

Hislop HJ, Montgomery J. *Daniels and Worthingham's Muscle Testing: Techniques of Manual Examination*. St. Louis, MO: Saunders, 2007.

a profound impact on performance in those sports requiring running and jumping. Additionally, extensive rehabilitation time is involved with many of these injuries (2).

MUSCLE STRAINS

Muscle strains at the hip usually occur to those muscles causing hip flexion or adduction (groin strains) (2). Groin injuries are labeled such because most of these muscles originate on the pubis and pain is felt in the groin area. Adductor strains are slightly more common than hip flexion strains and these tend to be more prevalent in sports that require oblique movements of the femur. For instance, adductor strains for soccer players are rather common, amounting to 10% to 15% of all injuries in men and women's collegiate soccer (1). Ice hockey players and breaststroke swimmers are also particularly susceptible. Muscle strains to the hip account for only 1.7% of football injuries, 2.3% of basketball injuries, and 3.0% of softball injuries (1).

Adductor strains are graded similar to other injuries. A strain is graded as first-degree if pain is minimal along with a loss of strength and minimal restriction of motion. Second-degree strains result in tissue damage that seriously compromises the function of the muscle but does not result in total loss of strength or function. Third-degree is a complete disruption of the muscle with accompanying loss of function (3). Fortunately, first-degree strains tend to be the most frequent. Unfortunately, groin strains tend to require extensive rehabilitation and time to heal. Since these injuries tend to recur, it is best to allow complete recovery before athletes return to play. Coaches can be involved in this rehabilitation process by supervising strength training (see Focal Point: Can Groin Strains be Prevented?) and having the athlete participate in lower speed drills that functionally prepare the athlete to return to play. The adductor muscles are recruited more when an athlete changes directions, so drills that require the athlete to change direction are particularly effective. Make sure the athlete is properly warmed up and without pain prior to performing such drills.

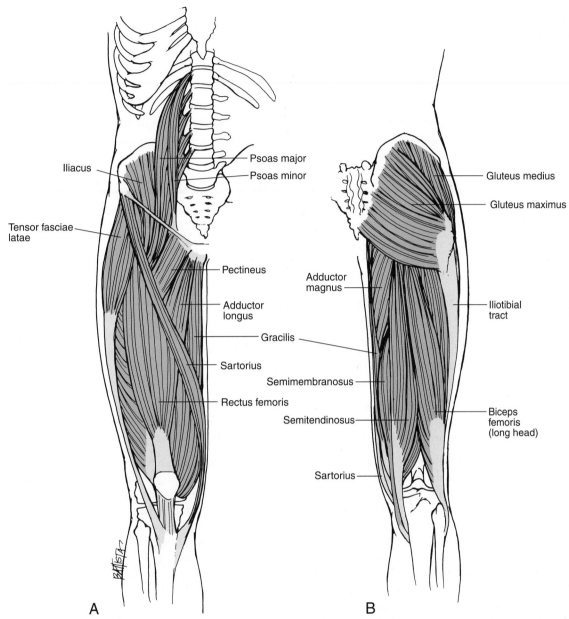

A   B

■ **FIGURE 14.1** Muscles of the hip. **A.** Anterior view of hip shows hip flexors and hip adductors. **B.** Posterior view illustrates the gluteus maximus and medius plus hamstrings. (Modified from Oatis CA. *Kinesiology—The Mechanics and Pathomechanics of Human Movement*. Baltimore: Lippincott Williams & Wilkins, 2004.)

FOCAL POINT

Can Groin Strains be Prevented?

Due to the nature of skating, adductor muscle strains are a common problem in ice hockey. In a series of studies at Lenox Hill Hospital in New York, researchers measured the strength of the adductor muscle group in ice hockey players. Prior to the season adduction and abduction strength was measured along with adductor

(continues)

Can Groin Strains be Prevented? *(continued)*

flexibility. Researchers found that a player was 17 times more likely to sustain an adductor injury if the strength in the hip adductors was 80% or less of the abductor strength. Uninjured players tended to have more equal abduction/adduction strength. Flexibility was unrelated to injury. Researchers then took 38 "at risk" players identified by muscle strength imbalance and administered a 6 week program of exercises designed to increase the functional strength of the adductor muscles. Athletes involved in the intervention program received significantly less adductor injuries as a result.

Tyler TF, Nicholas SJ, Campbell RJ, et al. The association of hip strength and flexibility with the incidence of adductor muscle strains in professional ice hockey players. *Am J Sport Med* 2001;29(2):124–128.

Tyler, TF, Nicholas SJ, Campbell RJ, et al. The effectiveness of a preseason exercise program to prevent adductor muscle strains in professional ice hockey players. *Am J Sport Med* 2002;30:680–683.

Groin injuries are fairly prevalent in breaststroke swimmers but these groin injuries are probably different than for soccer and ice hockey athletes (4). Groin injuries to swimmers are the result of microtraumas due to repetitive adduction against the water. In one study, researchers surveyed almost 300 competitive swimmers and found that 42.7% who compete in breaststroke have been unable to participate in breaststroke training at some point in the year due to hip adduction injury. Grote et al suggested two preventative measures:

1. Make sure all athletes have a proper, supervised warm-up
2. Education of the athletes. For example, they found that many athletes tend to "swim through the pain" and this just causes further injury. The more athletes trained the more they were injured (4).

From our point of view, these injuries are clear examples of overuse and are best treated by prevention.

Hip flexor strains usually occur to the iliopsoas muscle and are more prevalent in sports that require rapid, particularly forward, acceleration. Hip flexor strains also involve extensive time out of competition and practice. Since most sports require quick forward acceleration coaches should be aware of prevention techniques for hip flexor injuries. First, athletes must be warmed up properly prior to high speed activities. Second, fatigue is another factor leading to increased susceptibility to muscle strain. As athletes begin to tire, they become more susceptible. A gradual increase in training intensity eventually leading to high-speed running which also includes full-speed starts and stops, should be one goal of training. Activities that will specifically enhance the hip flexors include hill and/or stair running. For uphill running to be effective in injury prevention, the speed of the run should replicate what is expected in competition. That is, hill running should be short and intense so that the fast twitch muscles utilized in sprinting are trained. In addition, the athletes should not be overly fatigued when performing this type training.

FOCAL POINT

High Hamstring Strains in Distance Runners

As discussed in Chapter 2 and in this chapter, hamstring strains normally occur during the eccentric phase of contraction during high speed running. This type of muscle strain is usually quite abrupt, with the athlete in

(continues)

High Hamstring Strains in Distance Runners *(continued)*

severe and immediate pain. These injuries occur during high speed running and are often indicated by a quick deceleration where the athlete quickly begins to hobble and occasionally falls. Another type of hamstring strain can occur but is more related to overuse, developing gradually after long and repetitive distance running. The athlete often feels pain in the buttock and occasionally develops back pain. In fact, athletes (and physicians) may actually suspect back pain rather than a hamstring injury. However, the athlete often experiences considerable pain at the base of the pelvic girdle (ischial tuberosity) where the hamstrings originate. Physicians at Stanford University recently reported on a case of a middle-distance runner with such a problem. The authors discuss the difficulty in diagnosing such an injury and also suggest that treatment is difficult. They treated the athlete with a corticosteroid injection followed by extensive rehabilitation including eccentric exercises and core strengthening of the pelvic girdle. The athlete returned to running without symptoms.

Fredericson M, Moore W, Guillet M, et al. High hamstring tendinopathy in runners. *Phys Sportsmed* 2005;33(5):[np]

Hamstring injuries are among the most common injuries in sport and present serious problems to athletes. One study reported that hamstring strains were the third most frequent orthopaedic injury after ankle and knee injuries (5). Hamstring injuries also tend to recur and the highest risk of recurrence is in the first few weeks upon returning to play. Orchard and Best studied several hundred Australian footballers to determine the frequency of recurrence following hamstring injury (6). The reinjury rate was 12.6% during the first week and 8.1% during the second week. The cumulative risk for the entire season was 30.6%, clearly indicating the ongoing problem of a hamstring strain.

All three hamstring muscles are bi-articular, involving major movements at the hip and knee. Of the three hamstrings, the biceps femoris is slightly more complicated since it has two heads. Conversely, of the four quadriceps muscles, only the rectus femoris is bi-articular. Since running involves repeated hip flexion/extension and knee flexion/extension, the coordination of the bi-articular hamstrings is very complex. It is no surprise that hamstring injuries tend to occur during high speed activities. A muscular analysis of the hamstrings during high speed running reveals a very intricate series of concentric and eccentric muscle contractions intertwined with relaxation. Hamstring injuries tend to occur during that phase of the running cycle when the hamstrings are contracting eccentrically to decrease the velocity of the rapidly extending leg (7).

Because of the possibly devastating effects of hamstring strains on subsequent performance, we strongly suggest that coaches put considerable effort into the prevention of hamstring injuries. Since hamstrings are frequently injured in the eccentric phase of contraction, we suggest that the exercise demonstrated in Figure 2.2 be part of athlete's pre- and inseason training. Askling et al found that athletes who performed eccentric strength training significantly reduced the incidence of hamstring injuries (7). Coaches must take care to include hamstring resistance exercises when designing strength training programs for their athletes. Running backwards is another good training activity for the hamstrings.

Returning to play following a hamstring injury depends on how serious the injury is. In the study by Sherry and Best, athletes returned to competition in 3 to 5 weeks (8). We recommend that athletes recovering from hamstring injuries supplement traditional rehabilitation with trunk stabilization and agility exercises followed by icing (see From the Athletic Training Room: A Comparison of Two Hamstring Rehabilitation Programs). Watch the athlete carefully during the early stages of return. If the athlete starts to feel twinges or pulls then he/she is not ready to return and it is best to continue rehabilitation. An early return to competition following hamstring strain may actually result in an eventual reduction in playing time.

FROM THE ATHLETIC TRAINING ROOM

A Comparison of Two Hamstring Rehabilitation Programs

Researchers at the University of Wisconsin recently compared two methods of rehabilitation following hamstring injury. The standard hamstring rehabilitation program (ST) has consisted of static stretching, progressive hamstring resistance exercise, and icing. They compared this standard technique with a program (AS) consisting of progressive agility and trunk stabilization exercises and icing. The average time to return to sports for athletes in the ST group was 37.4 days while the time for athletes in the AS group was 22.2 days. Furthermore, about half of the athletes in the ST group were reinjured during the first 2 weeks after return to play while none of the athletes in the AS group suffered a recurrence during the first 2 weeks after return. One year after return to sport 70% of the athletes in the ST group had suffered a recurrent injury while only 7.7% of the athletes in the ST group suffered a reinjury. Coaches are often not involved in the rehabilitation process, but can easily be included when the treatment begins to include sport specific activities like agility exercises.

Sherry MA, Best TM. A comparison of 2 rehabilitation programs in the treatment of acute hamstring strains. *J Orthop Sports Phys Ther* 2004;34:116–125.

CONTUSIONS

Blows to the front of the thigh are fairly common in sport, especially in contact sports such as football, soccer, lacrosse, and ice hockey. Thigh pads are the obvious way to prevent these injuries and are mandatory in some sports. Coaches should not allow athletes to participate in practice without thigh pads. For instance, NCAA football data indicates that 3.4% of thigh contusions occur during games, but 2.0% also occur in practice (1). Athletes need to be protected in games and practice. Blows to the quadriceps are the most common contusions and range from slight to severe. Normally, there is immediate swelling and reduction in movement. The effect of a blow to the quadriceps is swift, and the athlete needs to be treated quickly rather than waiting for the practice or game to end. Early treatment reduces recovery time.

Before the athlete returns to play they should be functionally prepared to undergo all activities without pain. In addition, coaches should expect the athlete to wear some sort of protection and to insist that they keep the protection on until complete recovery. In one study, researchers at West Point found that the average disability time was 13 days for mild, 19 days for moderate, and 21 days for severe contusions. They also found that 9% developed myositis ossificans and that a delay in treatment was one of the related factors (9).

FROM THE ATHLETIC TRAINING ROOM

Acute Compartment Syndrome of the Thigh

Compartment syndrome is normally associated with increased compartmental pressure in the leg. However, other compartments exist in the human and can also suffer compartment syndrome. A recent article in the *Physician and Sportsmedicine* describes the case of a healthy 17-year-old soccer goalkeeper who sustained a direct blow to his left thigh during a collision with another player. He experienced immediate pain but kept playing. Following the game he continued to get worse despite good treatment. He couldn't walk the next morning and went to the emergency room. Pain continued to increase as pressure worsened; he began to lose sensation in his thigh and a diagnosis of acute compartment syndrome was made.

(continues)

Acute Compartment Syndrome of the Thigh *(continued)*

About 22 hours post injury the athlete underwent surgery to three compartments of his thigh. Fasciotomy (cutting the fascia surrounding the muscle) was performed. The incisions were loosely secured to accommodate further swelling and the patient had an immediate decrease in pain. Sensation began to return. Three days later the athlete was returned to surgery to close the incisions. Six months postsurgery he returned to play at his preinjury state.

Acute compartment syndrome can be quite dangerous and requires prompt attention. Even with proper on field treatment (ice and rest but **not elevation** is the norm), the condition can progress and may lead to irreversible damage, renal failure, and possibly death. A simple blow to the leg can be devastating.

Golden D, Flik K, Turner D, Bach B, Sawyer J. Acute compartment syndrome of the thigh in a high school soccer player. *Phys Sportsmed* 2005;33(12):19–24.

THE KNEE JOINT

Often called the largest and most complex joint in the body, the integrity of the knee joint is of great interest to athletes and coaches. Finnish researchers have indicated that injuries to the knee joint are the most frequent athletic injury that requires surgery (10). Repeated injuries to the knee are also related to a higher incidence of osteoarthritis in later life. The primary motions of the knee joint are flexion and extension, but some rotation of the tibia is possible when the knee is in the flexed position.

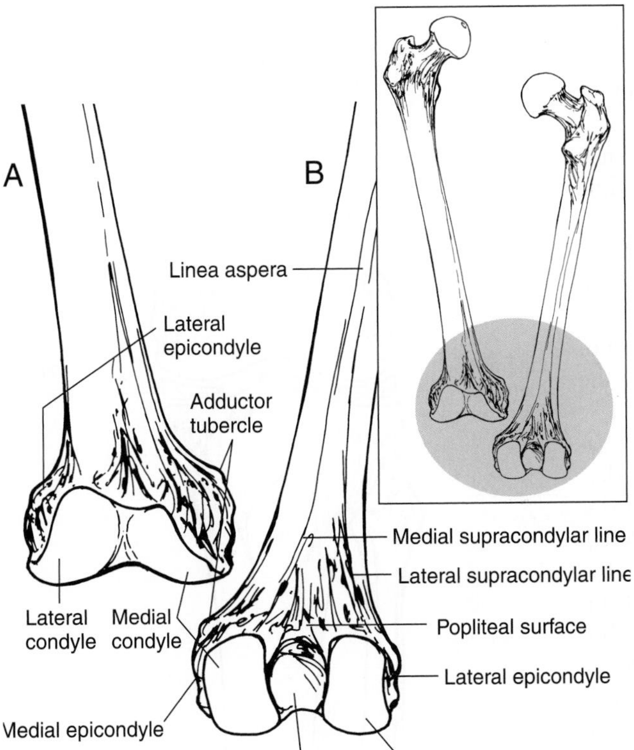

Knee Joint Anatomy

The knee joint is composed of the femur, tibia, and patella. Anatomists indicate that the knee joint is actually composed of three joints: two tibio-femoral joints and the joint between the patella (kneecap) and the femur. The two concave surfaces of the femoral condyles (Fig. 14.2) make contact with the convex surfaces of the tibial plateau (Fig. 14.3). The knee has two important articular discs located on the tibial plateau that are very central toward maintaining stability. They deepen the articular surface and serve as a main shock absorber by increasing the surface area in addition to providing cushioning. In total, the menisci cover about 50% of the articular surface. Figure 14.4 indicates that the medial meniscus is larger than the lateral meniscus. Figure 14.5 illustrates that the menisci are wedge shaped (thicker on the periph-

■ FIGURE 14.2 Bones of the posterior thigh. **A.** Anterior view of femur indicates the medial and lateral condyles. **B.** Posterior view of femur reveals condyles plus intercondylar fossa. (Modified from Oatis CA. *Kinesiology—The Mechanics and Pathomechanics of Human Movement.* Baltimore: Lippincott Williams & Wilkins, 2004.)

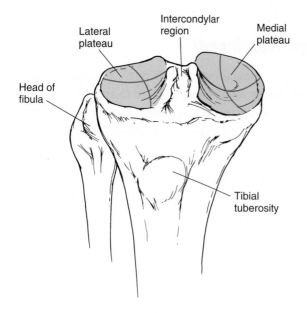

FIGURE 14.3 The tibial plateau: anterior view of tibia indicating the medial and lateral plateaus of the tibia. (Modified from Oatis CA. *Kinesiology—The Mechanics and Pathomechanics of Human Movement*. Baltimore: Lippincott Williams & Wilkins, 2004.)

FIGURE 14.4 Knee menisci: superior view of medial and lateral menisci. (Modified from Oatis CA. *Kinesiology—The Mechanics and Pathomechanics of Human Movement*. Baltimore: Lippincott Williams & Wilkins, 2004.)

ery) helping to create a more stable joint. Removal of the meniscus (meniscectomy) increases the friction within the knee and decreases the contact area (therefore increasing force per area) of the femur on the tibia (11).

The patella is an important bone of the knee since it acts to protect the front of the femur while also improving the angle at which the quadriceps tendon connects to the tibia. The patella can be dislocated. In fact, most cases of suspected knee dislocation are actually dislocations of the patella. An important aspect of the patella is its ability to properly track on the femur. Improper tracking of the patella is one issue of concern.

The knee joint is supported by four main ligaments: the tibial (medial—MCL) and fibular (lateral—LCL) collateral ligaments and the anterior and posterior cruciates (ACL and PCL). Additionally, the popliteal ligaments reinforce the knee posteriorly. The tibial collateral ligament stabilizes the medial side of the knee while the fibular collateral stabilizes the lateral side. As shown in Figure 14.6, the tibial collateral is larger than the fibular collateral. Another important aspect is that the medial meniscus attaches to the medial collateral ligament. The cruciates (Fig. 14.7) provide anterior-posterior stability and are located on the inside of the knee. If either of the cruciates is severely strained or ruptured, the tibia will tend to slide forward or backward (drawer sign) with respect to the femur. If the tibia tends to move for-

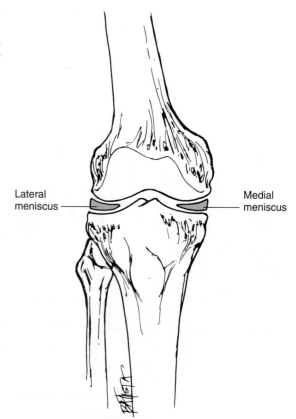

FIGURE 14.5 Anterior view of menisci: menisci are wedge shaped and create a more stable surface. (Modified from Oatis CA. *Kinesiology—The Mechanics and Pathomechanics of Human Movement*. Baltimore: Lippincott Williams & Wilkins, 2004.)

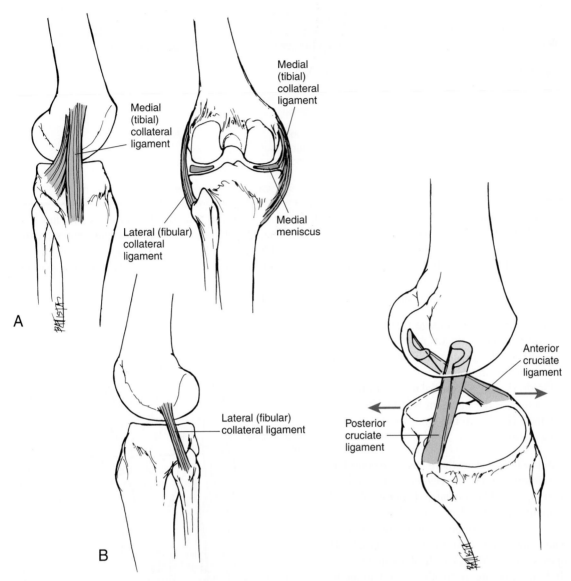

■ **FIGURE 14.6** Collateral ligaments of the knee. **A.** The MCL is large and attaches to the medial meniscus as well as the tibia and femur. **B.** The LCL is smaller and attaches to the fibula and femur. (Modified from Oatis CA. *Kinesiology—The Mechanics and Pathomechanics of Human Movement*. Baltimore: Lippincott Williams & Wilkins, 2004.)

■ **FIGURE 14.7** The cruciate ligaments of the knee. (Modified from Oatis CA. *Kinesiology—The Mechanics and Pathomechanics of Human Movement*. Baltimore: Lippincott Williams & Wilkins, 2004.)

ward then the anterior cruciate (ACL) is compromised, while the posterior cruciate (PCL) is injured if the tibia can slide backward on the femur.

The primary muscles of the knee (Table 14.3) are four quadriceps muscles (Fig. 14.8) on the anterior side (knee extension) and the three hamstring muscles (knee flexion) on the posterior side. The quadriceps are uni-articular, except for the rectus femoris, while the hamstrings are all bi-articular. Because of the mass of the quadriceps and their mechanical advantage at the knee, knee extension is more powerful than knee flexion. All four quadriceps muscles attach to the tibia via the patella tendon, while each hamstring has an independent insertion below the knee. As shown in Figure 14.9 the semimembranosus and semitendinosus each insert on the medial side of the knee and the biceps femoris inserts on the lateral side.

COMMON KNEE INJURIES

Injuries to the knee are rather common in most sports, representing about 14.19% of collegiate football injuries, 14% of men's soccer injuries, and around 20% for women's soccer (1). Injuries to the knee also

TABLE 14.3   Knee Joint Muscles and Their Actions

Movement	Prime Movers	Location
Extension	Rectus Femoris Vastus Lateralis Vastus Intermedius Vastus Medialis (VMO)	Anterior
Flexion	Biceps Femoris Semimembranosus Semitendinosus	Posterior

Hislop HJ, Montgomery J. *Daniels and Worthingham's Muscle Testing: Techniques of Manual Examination*. St. Louis, MO: Saunders; 2007.

tend to represent more severe injuries, involving more surgery and time off. For instance, studies have found that 29% of severe soccer injuries were to the knee (12). Due to the nature of joint stresses while turning and stopping, as well as the tendency to receive blows to the outside of the leg, injuries to the tibial collateral ligament (MCL) and the menisci are the most common knee injuries. Anterior cruciate ligament (ACL) injuries are also common.

Knee sprains are quite common and these are graded into three levels:

- Grade I: there is damage (tearing) to the ligament but little or no change in the length of the ligament. That is, the ligament is not stretched.
- Grade II: There is partial tearing of the ligament plus the ligament is stretched.
- Grade III: There is a complete tear of the ligament.

In the last 20 years there has been considerable progress in the management of knee ligament injuries. The medial and lateral collateral ligaments appear to have a very healthy ability for healing and surgical intervention is normally unnecessary (13). In fact, even Grade III injuries to the MCL can heal spontaneously. MCL injuries are normally treated immediately with early rehabilitation. Peterson and Renstrom have suggested that return to play is normally accomplished in 3 to 8 weeks. They also suggest that Grade I MCL injuries may only take 1 to 2 weeks to recover and a little longer for Grade II injuries (14).

Unlike the collateral ligaments, cruciate ligaments do not self-heal and often require surgical reconstruction. The ACL is injured far more frequently than the posterior cruciate and can be the result of direct trauma, but more likely the result of some form of rapid deceleration. The athlete often has a sudden pain and will hear a "pop" upon injury. The knee may give way and many people are fooled since it is not unusual for the athlete to walk off the field or court after sustaining an ACL injury. Surgery is usually postponed for a few weeks until the athlete

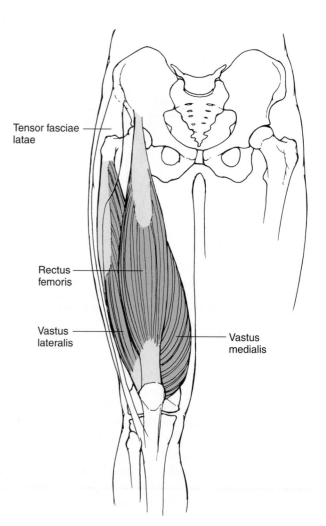

Tensor fasciae latae

Rectus femoris

Vastus lateralis

Vastus medialis

■ **FIGURE 14.8** The quadricep muscles of the knee. The vastus intermedius is not shown as it lies under the rectus femoris. (Modified from Oatis CA. *Kinesiology—The Mechanics and Pathomechanics of Human Movement*. Baltimore: Lippincott Williams & Wilkins, 2004.)

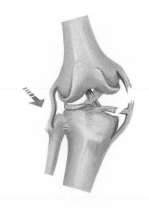

■ FIGURE 14.9 The unhappy triad: a knee injury involving a torn MCL, torn medial meniscus, and ruptured ACL. (Asset provided by Anatomical Chart Co.)

has regained range of motion and strength. Fortunately, surgical treatments have advanced considerably over the past 20 years and most people (80% to 90%) can return to their pre-injured state following surgery. Time of recovery is quite varied but normally lasting at least 6 months (14). In one extensive follow-up study of athletes who had received ACL reconstruction surgery 81% had returned to play within 12 months. Of these, 89% claimed to function at a level equal to pre-injury (or higher) (15).

Simultaneous injuries to the MCL and ACL are not that uncommon. In addition, the medial meniscus—because it is attached to the MCL—can be injured as well. This condition, often labeled "The Unhappy Triad," is illustrated in Figure 14.9. Following such an injury the routine is often to treat the MCL first, followed later by surgery to repair the ACL and meniscus, if necessary.

The best prevention of knee injuries is a program of strengthening and proprioceptive training. Since so many injuries to the knee occur during the deceleration phase of stopping, landing, and turning, athletes need to practice these activities often and at high speed. Although some athletes may possess some intrinsic factors that make them more susceptible, all athletes can gain from a program that improves the ability of muscles surrounding the knee to work better.

Meniscus injuries are also common problems of the knee. It has been reported that about 10%–15% of all orthopaedic surgeries are to repair meniscus lesions. Some years ago surgeons routinely removed the entire meniscus upon tearing. Fortunately, surgical techniques have improved. The common practice is to protect as much of the meniscus as possible to help stabilize the knee and reduce the susceptibility to arthritis. Typical arthroscopic knee meniscus surgery involves removal of the affected tissue. Occasionally a torn meniscus results in a locked knee in which the torn section lodges in the joint preventing normal motion. These injuries usually require surgery soon after the injury. Recovery from meniscus surgery depends on the degree of damage. Prior to returning to competition and practice, the athlete should have almost full range of motion, strength, and agility. This often takes about 2 to 6 weeks, but can be as long as 12 to 16 weeks if the athlete suffers a large posterior tear (14).

Patellofemoral pain syndrome (pain around the patella) is fairly common in athletes and often caused by overuse. Athletes occasionally have patella knee pain as a result of direct trauma. However, one of the primary causes of patellofemoral pain is tracking of the patella on the femur. Females, because of their wider hips and increased "Q" angle (Chapter 3), tend to have more patella tracking problems than males. Individuals with hypermobile joints tend to have more patella tracking problems (16). As with most soft tissue problems, patella problems are graded by the degree of pathology involved. Patella tracking problems are often treated by attempts to strengthen the knee extensors on the medial side of the knee (vastus medialis), various types of braces, and NSAIDs. Athletes with these problems should be discouraged from performing exercises that require extensive knee flexion since this tends to exacerbate the problem. Exercises such as deep squats or knee bends and squat jumps should be avoided. Peterson and Renstrom have suggested that patellofemoral pain is one of the most difficult problems to manage in sports (14). There is often a long period of rehabilitation and occasionally the problem heals itself. Athletes must be prepared to change their training habits and avoid up- and downhill running.

Iliotibial band syndrome (ITBS) is occasionally called "Runner's Knee" since it seems to occur more frequently in runners. The tensor fascia latae muscle (Fig. 14.8) is interesting since it does not have a bony attachment but inserts into the iliotibial band. The iliotibial band inserts into the lateral portion of the tibial condyle. When the knee is in extension the iliotibial band is anterior to the lateral epicondyle of the femur. However, at about 30 degrees flexion, the band passes over this epicondyle causing some friction. This condition is pronounced when athletes do an extensive amount of downhill running or when running on an uneven surface, such as the side of a cambered road. ITBS is fairly easy for athletic trainers to diagnose since the pain is localized to the lateral side of the knee. Coaches can help with this problem by making sure athletes run on even surfaces and frequently switch directions when running around indoor tracks. Improving the flexibility of the iliotibial band is also important. Figure 14.10 illustrates one exercise for stretching the iliotibial band.

LEG, ANKLE, AND FOOT

A quick observation of the human skeleton reveals an analogy between the leg, ankle, and foot and the forearm, wrist, and hand. The number of bones and joints is similar but the stress on the lower body is much greater. As a result, the frequency of injuries to the lower body is much greater. Running and jumping predominate in many sports, and proper conditioning and footwear are essential in the prevention of injury.

Leg Anatomy

The tibia and fibula compose the bones of the leg, but the tibia bears the predominate weight (Fig. 14.11). The foot is composed of 26 bones grouped as the seven tarsal bones, five metatarsals, and 14 phalanges. The ankle joint is the articulation of the tibia and fibula with the most superior bone in the foot, the talus. The tibia and fibula form a saddle over the talus, helping to stabilize the ankle. The bones of the foot are arranged to create longitudinal and transverse arches. The arches have strong ligament support and serve as shock absorbers during weight bearing. The bottom of the foot is composed of a plantar fascia which runs longitudinally from the heel (calcaneous) to the first of the phalanges.

The movements of the foot (Fig. 14.12) include dorsi- and plantar flexion which occur at the ankle joint. Inversion (foot turns in) and eversion (foot turns out) occur in the joint below the talus (sub-talar joint). Foot supination and pronation are combination movements of the foot. Pronation is the combination of eversion, foot abduction, and dorsiflexion, while supination is the combination of inversion, foot adduction, and plantarflexion. There is also slight external rotation of the tibia during supination and slight internal rotation of the tibia during pronation. During running, the heel strikes the ground with the foot in the supinated position and leaves the ground in the pronated position. This action when running from supination to pronation is one primary source of injury to the foot and leg.

The muscles of the leg possess an interesting and somewhat problematic characteristic; they are enclosed in four, rather inflexible, compartments restricted by connective tissue (Fig. 14.13). The muscles in the anterior compartment are the tibialis anterior, extensor hallucis longus, extensor digitorum longus, and fibularis (peroneus) tertius. These muscles primarily cause dorsiflexion at the ankle as well as toe extension. Also encased in the anterior compartment are the blood vessels and nerves that supply the anterior leg muscles and foot. There are two posterior compartments: the deep and superficial. The deep one is composed of the tibialis posterior as well as the flexor hallucis longus and the flexor dig-

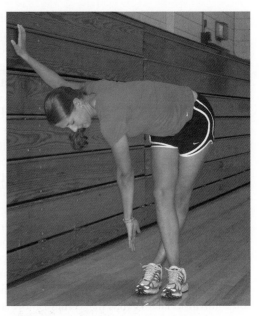

■ **FIGURE 14.10** Iliotibial band stretch. Stretch the left ITB by placing the left foot behind the right and then stretching toward the floor on the right side.

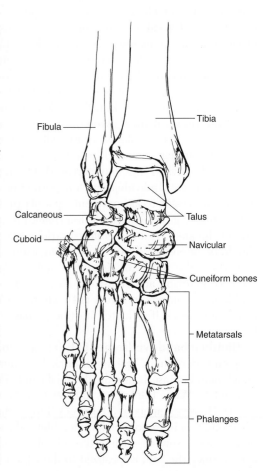

■ **FIGURE 14.11** Anatomy of the foot and ankle. (Modified from Oatis CA. *Kinesiology—The Mechanics and Pathomechanics of Human Movement*. Baltimore: Lippincott Williams & Wilkins, 2004.)

itorum longus. Nerves and blood supply are also incased in this compartment. The soleus (a broad deep calf muscle) and the gastrocnemius (the bi-articular superficial calf muscle) compose the posterior superficial compartment. On the lateral side of the leg the fibularis (peroneus) longus, fibularis (peroneus) brevis, and fibular (peroneal) nerve are located in the lateral compartment. With the exception of the gastrocnemius and the soleus, all of the muscles of the leg perform multiple functions at the foot (Table 14.4). These two muscles of the calf (sometimes called the triceps surae) attach to the Achilles tendon which inserts onto the calcaneous (heel). These two muscles are capable of exerting tremendous tension on the Achilles tendon.

INJURIES TO THE LEG AND FOOT

Injuries to this area of the body occur frequently and range from mild heel blisters to broken tibias. Since most ground reaction forces are transmitted through the foot, ankle, and leg, proper footwear, protection, and conditioning are imperative for injury prevention. As a result of high repetition training, overuse injuries—such as stress fractures—have become commonplace.

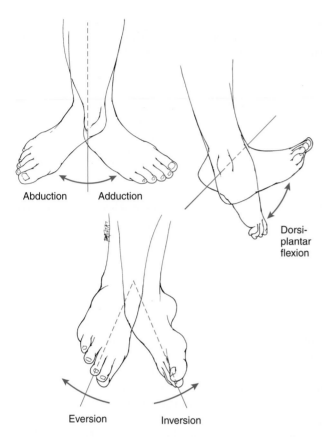

■ **FIGURE 14.12** Movements of the foot. (Modified from Oatis CA. *Kinesiology—The Mechanics and Pathomechanics of Human Movement*. Baltimore: Lippincott Williams & Wilkins, 2004.)

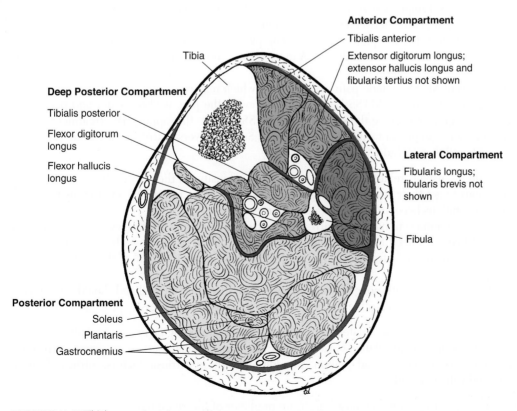

■ **FIGURE 14.13** Tibial compartments.

TABLE 14.4   Leg Muscles and Their Actions

Movement	Prime Movers	Compartment
Dorsiflexion	Tibialis Anterior Extensor Hallucis Longus Extensor Digitorum Longus	Anterior
Plantar Flexion	Tibialis Posterior Flexor Hallucis Longus Gastrocnemius Soleus	Deep Posterior Deep Posterior Superficial Posterior Superficial Posterior
Inversion	Tibialis Anterior Tibialis Posterior	Anterior Deep Posterior
Eversion	Fibularis Tertius Fibularis Longus Fibularis Brevis	Anterior Lateral Lateral

Hislop HJ, Montgomery J. *Daniels and Worthingham's Muscle Testing: Techniques of Manual Examination.* St. Louis, MO: Saunders, 2007.

Tibial stress injuries (often called "shin splints") are among the most common leg injuries. Shin splints has been a general term for pain to the tibia. However, as suggested, "The term 'shin splints' describes a symptom of exercise-induced shin pain; it is not a diagnosis" (17). Medial tibial stress syndrome (MTSS) has been advocated as one term to replace shin splints (17). Regardless of the nomenclature, exercise induced pain to the tibia represents 10% to 20% of all injuries in runners and approximately 60% of overuse injuries of the leg (18–20). Pecina and Bojanic prefer to call these tibial syndromes "runner's leg," because of their frequency in runners (21).

Most of these tibial stress injuries are the result of a maladaptive remodeling process. The normal response of increased stress to the bones as a result of running and jumping is an increase in the metabolic activity of the bone involved. Bones encounter mechanical stress and remodel in a well-defined sequence resulting in bones better able to withstand stress. Maladaptation occurs when the bones do not remodel quickly enough for the subsequent stresses applied. The athlete has either been stressed too much with training or not given enough time between training sessions for proper adaptation to occur. The bone then becomes inflamed (periostitis), complete with pain. The pain is most often felt on the medial tibia and therefore the term medial tibial stress syndrome. A more serious form of maladaptation is the occurrence of stress fractures.

Typical symptoms of MTSS include pain early in a run which may resolve as the run continues. Pain returns following the workout. As MTSS becomes more severe the pain is also greater and persistent. Coaches should attempt to recognize the symptoms of MTSS early so that appropriate treatment can be started. Early treatment can prevent subsequent problems. Several adverse extrinsic factors are related to the onset of MTSS and they include:

- Training methods—usually related to abrupt increases in intensity. At the start of the season coaches are often anxious to get their athletes in shape, but a sharp increase in activity is not easily tolerated by athletes. Adaptations become negative rather than positive.
- Surfaces—training on uneven, banked, or irregular surfaces such as grass. Changes in surface are also problematic and coaches need to reduce the intensity and volume of training when athletes change surfaces. In one study of stress fractures, switching surfaces was common to all of the injured athletes (22).
- Footwear—worn out shoes with poor shock absorption. The shoe must fit well and should not be used except for training. In some cases, athletes need orthotics to help control excessive pronation/supination.

Of the preceding extrinsic factors related to tibial stress injuries, training errors are probably the most frequent as well as the most controllable. Coaches must plan for a gradual increase in exercise stress accompanied by recovery to allow for adaptation. In addition to these extrinsic factors, intrinsic factors, unique to each individual, include:

- Previous injury—prior injury is the most significant predictor of future injury.

- Muscle strength and flexibility—fatigue increases bone stress so athletes in poor condition may fatigue earlier and be more susceptible to damage. Likewise, athletes need good dorsi-flexion strength as well as plantar flexion. Some athletes with lower dorsi-flexion range of motion are more prone to injury (23,24).
- Low bone density—low bone density is more often related to female athletes, especially those who have menstrual irregularities. Low bone density is often related to the "female triad," characterized by the combination of disordered eating, amenorrhea, and osteoporosis (25,26).

Stress fractures can happen to almost any bone but tend to occur more often in the tibia. The metatarsal bones and the calcaneus (heel) are also susceptible, especially in runners and jumpers. Tibial stress fractures often resemble MTSS though the pain tends to be more localized. Stress fractures are more serious and long lasting. As the condition progresses the pain intensifies and persists throughout the day and night. Physicians will normally use radiographs to diagnose stress fractures, but these only test positive after a few weeks. Although the causes of stress fractures are similar to those mentioned above for MTSS, it has been estimated that training errors account for 22% to 75% of stress fractures (21).

The time needed to return to play is related to the severity of the problem. Athletes with fairly mild MTSS may only need a few days of rest. However, the athlete and coach need to monitor discomfort and work closely with the athletic trainer. A good rule is to resume training at about 50% of pre-injury levels and to gradually increase intensity if the athlete tends to be pain free. Athletes with stress fractures often need about 6 weeks before they can return to activity (27).

Lower extremity compartment syndromes are occasionally confused with shin splints but these conditions are more severe, and fortunately, less frequent. The lower leg muscles lie in compartments and the pressure inside these compartments can occasionally increase, resulting in significant discomfort and swelling. A typical scenario for this injury is that the exercise may lead to increased volume. If the fascia surrounding the muscle is noncompliant, the pressure in the compartment increases resulting in decreased blood flow to the muscle, impaired muscle function, and weakness. Another scenario is that when an athlete overtrains their muscles, there is muscle damage and fluid leakage, causing increased compartmental pressure.

Although compartment syndromes can occur in many different areas, they tend to happen more frequently in the anterior and posterior portions of the lower leg. These syndromes can be acute or chronic. Acute compartment syndrome is often caused by a direct blow, resulting in trauma and bleeding within the compartment. This tends to happen more often in the anterior compartment. Sometimes these conditions are very serious (both blood flow and nerve conduction are impeded) and can require emergency surgery (fasciotomy) to relieve pressure. Chronic compartment syndrome is more frequent and often related to overuse, especially in endurance runners (21). For instance, in one study of 100 cases of compartment syndrome, 70% were runners (28).

The initial treatment of compartment syndrome is usually conservative and involves icing after exercise and strain reduction. Unfortunately, this is difficult to accomplish in active athletes. Athletes can continue to cross-train if the problem is not exacerbated. Unfortunately, conservative treatment is not that successful and the athlete frequently undergoes surgery. If the affected compartment is one of the more superficial ones (anterior or lateral) then the prognosis is good and rehabilitation lasts about 7 months. However, if the deep posterior compartment is affected the prognosis is more varied and rehabilitation may take as long as 16 months (29).

Achilles tendon disorders are more widespread in sports requiring extensive running and jumping. The Achilles tendon is the tendon for the two powerful plantar flexors (gastrocnemius and soleus) on the posterior lower leg and inserts onto the back of the foot at the calcaneus. The Achilles tendon is the strongest tendon in the body as tremendous tension can be exerted during plantar flexion. Walking, running, and jumping all require repetitive tension on the Achilles tendon and injury to this important tendon can seriously disrupt performance. Achilles disorders (tendinopathies) include, but are not limited to, tendonitis (acute inflammation), tendinosis (chronic degeneration normally caused by overuse), tenosynovitis (inflammation of the surrounding sheath), and rupture. With the exception of tendon rupture, determining the exact disorder and cause is quite difficult and the subject of considerable debate. A recent review indicated that the exact cause of Achilles tendon disorders is largely unknown (30).

Inflammation of the Achilles tendon and/or the sheath around it is often an acute problem and the result of an abrupt increase in physical activity. These inflammations are frequently related to the beginning of a season or a change in activity. Insertional tendonitis is another form of inflammation and occurs at the insertion of the tendon at the heel. Achilles inflammations are treated in the typical method to relieve inflammation. Athletes should cross-train during periods of treatment. Prognosis is generally good as athletes with acute inflammation can return to play in about 1 to 2 weeks. Injury recurrence is fairly low if the athlete does not repeat the same activity that resulted in the original inflammation.

Chronic tendon problems are normally the result of overuse (tendinosis) and present more troubles. In some respects, tendinosis is analogous to the stress fractures discussed earlier. That is, tendinosis has been described as a failure of the cell matrix to adapt to the trauma (stress) placed upon the tendon. Although stress fractures are related to bone formation, tendinosis is related to a loss of collagen. There is little evidence of inflammation although chronic tendon problems are routinely and mistakenly called tendonitis. Training errors, such as a sudden increase in mileage, excessive uphill running (which places severe stress on the Achilles tendon), and extensive use of interval training are common causes of tendinosis. Individuals with flat or hyperpronated feet tend to have more problems (31).

Since training errors are a common cause of tendinosis, treatment should involve some moderation of training, primarily a reduction in activity. Fortunately, most cases can be treated without surgery and respond well to conservative treatment. If cessation of training is required, the athlete can continue training by stationary cycling and water jogging. If pain is reduced, then the athlete can progress to machines that place a bit more stress on the Achilles, like stair-climbing, cross-country ski machines, or elliptical machines. Mild cases of tendinosis simply require a reduction in mileage. One recommendation is to cut back to 25% of the usual mileage and then increase about 10% a week depending on symptoms (31). Further treatment of tendinosis should involve attention to alignment problems and the strengthening of tendon and muscle. The use of orthotic foot inserts has proven to be quite effective for relieving painful Achilles symptoms (31).

Recently, researchers in Scandinavia have had excellent success utilizing eccentric training to improve the Achilles tendon. In one study, elite soccer players were treated with high-resistance eccentric training for 12 weeks. The eccentric training apparently improved collagen synthesis in the injured tendon (but not in the uninjured tendon) and all players successfully returned to play at the end of the treatment (32). A second study, utilizing eccentric calf muscle training, indicated that 89% of athletes with mid-portion Achilles tendon problems (the common tendinosis problem) were back to pre-injury activity at the end of training. Interestingly, individuals with Achilles pain at the insertion (possibly an inflammation problem) were not helped (33). Figure 14.14 demonstrates an easy eccentric exercise specific to the Achilles tendon.

We recommend a multi-focused treatment for overuse injuries to the Achilles tendon including:

- modification of training
- attention to alignment
- eccentric training

One of the most common causes of pain on the bottom of the heel is **plantar fasciitis** (34). Distance runners are particularly affected (35). The bottom of the foot contains a fairly broad fascia that originates under the calcaneus (heel) on the medial side and extends out over the bottom of the foot to the toes. The plantar fascia (Fig. 14.15) forms the longitudinal arch of the foot and provides arch support as well as shock absorption. Plantar fasciitis involves local inflammation and pain is often confined to the heel on the medial side. Commonly, the first few steps in the morning are particularly painful and individuals with this condition will tend to walk on their toes upon wakening. Walking barefoot on hard surfaces is particularly painful.

The causes of plantar fasciitis are still unclear although studies have suggested several factors that tend to be related. For example, individuals with limited dorsiflexion seem to be more at risk, as well as individuals who are heavier (36). In runners, plantar fasciitis is often thought to be associated with repeated microtraumas caused by excessive running, hard surfaces, or poor shoes (37). Athletes with worn out or defective training shoes are also susceptible. In one interesting study researchers identified an athlete with a classic case of plantar fasciitis (38). After observation of the athlete's shoes, the authors noticed that a heel counter had been improperly glued into the shoe. The athlete was taught how to examine shoes, treated, and released without further problems. The authors concluded that proper assessment of athletic shoe construction may prevent such injuries.

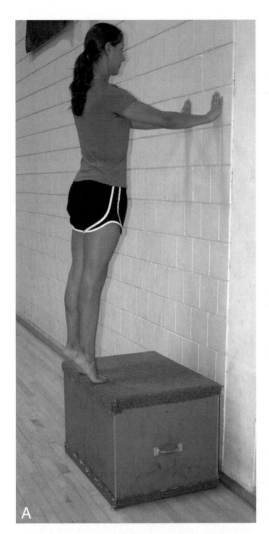
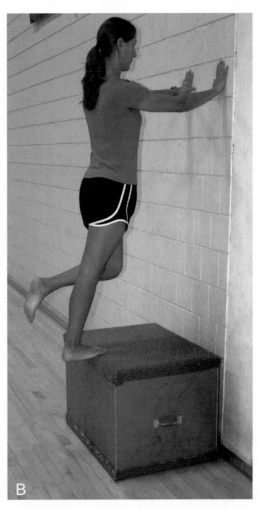

■ **FIGURE 14.14** Eccentric exercise for Achilles. **A.** Stand with toes on edge and plantar flex both ankles. **B.** Then lower slowly on one foot to provide eccentric contractions of posterior leg muscles.

Conservative treatment is the norm for plantar fasciitis although a few cases eventually require surgery. Interestingly, most cases simply resolve themselves after about a year regardless of treatment (39). Treatments for plantar fasciitis include rest, heat, NSAIDs, stretching the Achilles tendon and plantar fascia, heel cups, orthotics, night splints to passively dorsiflex the foot, ice, and taping. In one study of over 400 patients with plantar fasciitis the best treatment reported was a short leg walking cast. Apparently rest and the position of the walking cast promoted fairly rapid heeling. The minimal period to wear the cast was 3 weeks. Heat and plastic heel cups were judged to be less effective (40). Unfortunately, the causes as well as the treatment are still a subject of debate.

Certainly, some modification of training should be implemented to prevent further problems. Athletes should be educated to make a careful observation of their footwear and not to wear their running shoes except for training. Athletes should not overlook early symptoms of plantar fasciitis since early treatment is best. A chronic injury of this nature often takes up to 6 months to recover (14).

Turf toe is an injury that has increased in frequency with the advent of artificial surfaces. This injury normally occurs when the athlete comes to a sudden stop during which the player's shoe stops suddenly (due the increased friction of the artificial surface) but the foot in the shoe continues moving forward and the toes extend quickly. As a result, the ligaments under the big toe are stretched. There is often swelling and considerable pain at the base of the big toe. This condition can be quite excruciating and seriously impedes the player since rapid movements require the athlete to push off the big toe.

The athletic trainer will normally ice the toe and apply some sort of compression. The athlete is often removed from weight bearing on the injured foot for several days after which the athlete can return to walking. A slow return to play is required for recovery which often takes 2 to 4 weeks. Athletes are often encouraged to wear a firm shoe upon return to play since highly flexible shoes do not adequately protect excessive toe extension.

ANKLE SPRAINS

Ankle sprains are undoubtedly the most common sports injury accounting for approximately 17% of soccer injuries and 25% of basketball injuries (1). Athletes in all sports that require quick stops, starts, and turns are susceptible. Most ankle sprains are unrelated to contact and approximately 80% occur to the lateral side of the ankle (41). Improper footwear can result in a more susceptible athlete, particularly shoes that are too narrow. If an athlete's foot tends to bulge out the sides of a shoe, it is too narrow and less stable. It appears that the field shoe with the lowest incidence of ankle sprains (the same shoe recommended to reduce knee sprains) is the soccer-style shoe. This shoe has fairly wide cleats (about 14) and has a polyurethane sole (42). Obviously, a smooth playing surface helps reduce ankle injuries.

Strengthening the muscles around the ankle using proprioceptive techniques (such as balance disks—see Chapter 2) helps an athlete prevent ankle sprains. Athletes differ in their proprioceptive abilities. You can evaluate this by having the athletes balance on one foot with their eyes closed. Athletes who have trouble maintaining their balance have poor proprioception (43). Fortunately, proprioception can be improved by balance drills, jumping drills (practice landing on one foot without losing balance), and strengthening of the surrounding musculature. Prevention of ankle sprains by taping and/or bracing is especially recommended for susceptible individuals and athletes who have been previously injured. However, tape tends to decrease in support as the game or practice continues, but braces can be tightened. Coaches need to educate athletes who wear braces and low-top shoes to re-tighten their ankle braces as practices and games continue (41).

The typical sprained ankle occurs as a result of simultaneous plantar flexion and inversion. Because of its position on the front of the foot, the anterior talofibular ligament (Fig 14.16) is the most commonly torn ligament (about 2/3 of all ankle injuries). If the injury is more severe, the ligament that attaches the calcaneus to the fibula (calcaneofibular) is also injured. One of the primary reasons athletic trainers often palpate the ankle after injury is to determine which ligaments have been injured. Medial ankle sprains occur when the foot is everted and usually externally rotated, tearing the deltoid ligament. Occasionally plantar flexion and inversion may also be accompanied by rotation and an injury to the syndesmosis (the anterior and posterior tibiofibular ligament along with the interosseous membrane) occurs. This is the "high ankle sprain" mentioned occasionally in the media. A fracture of the fibula often accompanies this injury.

Treatment for ankle sprains includes ice and a compression bandage (sometimes a cast). Athletes are encouraged

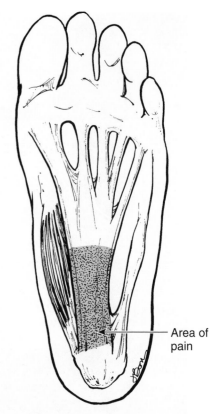

■ **FIGURE 14.15** Plantar fasciitis. Note the area of pain with plantar fasciitis. (Reprinted with permission from Baker CL. *The Hughston Clinic Sports Medicine Book*. Baltimore: Williams & Wilkins, 1995:604.)

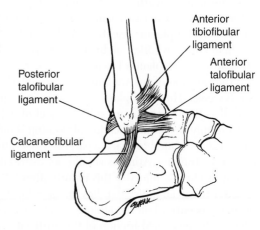

■ **FIGURE 14.16** Lateral ankle ligaments. (From Bucholz and Heckman JD. *Rockwood & Green's Fractures in Adults*, 5th ed. Baltimore: Lippincott Williams & Wilkins, 2001.)

to start functional rehabilitation fairly early. Occasionally, one or two crutches are utilized to help athletes resume their gait. The time required to return to play is related to the degree of tearing and the number of ligaments involved. A typical suggestion is that Grade I injuries require about 1 to 2 weeks, Grade II about 2 to 3 weeks, and up to 8 weeks for a Grade III injury. Normally, the ankle will be either taped or braced upon return to play. A program of proprioceptive and strength training is advised.

SUMMARY

- Injuries to the lower body are the most frequent sports injuries and are best prevented by proper protection and conditioning.
- Since injuries tend to recur, the best treatment is prevention.
- Groin muscle strains are fairly common in ice hockey and soccer and can be reduced by developing hip adduction strength.
- Hamstring injuries normally occur during high-speed running and can be reduced by an eccentric muscle strengthening program.
- Overuse hamstring injuries also occur to distance runners resulting in considerable pain in the lower buttocks.
- Knee injuries are the most serious of the lower limb injuries and require the most surgeries.
- Knee injuries can be reduced by strengthening and proprioceptive exercises.
- Collateral ligaments tend to heal themselves while the cruciates do not.
- Surgery to the cruciates tends to be quite successful and most athletes can play at pre-injury levels 12 months postsurgery.
- Shin splints is a common phrase for a host of lower leg problems, but commonly associated with medial tibial stress, an overuse injury.
- Abrupt changes in training should be avoided since such training often results in injury. When athletes change training surfaces they should reduce the volume and intensity of training.
- Compartment syndromes, whether in the lower leg or thigh, can be extremely serious and require immediate treatment.
- Many Achilles tendon problems are not inflammations but overuse injuries. Good rehabilitation results have been found utilizing eccentric strength training of the calf muscles.
- Most ankle sprains occur to the lateral side of the ankle. Bracing and proprioceptive training should be part of the rehabilitation.
- The most common injury to the bottom of the foot is plantar fasciitis and is an inflammation of the fascia under the foot. A walking cast for 3 weeks has been shown to be effective treatment.

References

1. NCAA Injury Surveillance System. Available online at http://www1.ncaa.org/membership/ed_outreach/health-safety/iss/index. html. Accessed March 3, 2008.
2. Anderson K, Strickland S, Warren R. Hip and groin injuries in athletes. *Am J Sports Med* 2001;29(4):521–533.
3. Tyler TF, Nicholas SJ, Campbell RJ, et al. The association of hip strength and flexibility with the incidence of adductor muscle strains in professional ice hockey players. *Am J Sports Med* 2001;29(2):124–128.
4. Grote K, Lincoln TL, Gamble JG. Hip adductor injury in competitive swimmers. *Am J Sports Med* 2004;32(1):104–108.
5. Canale ST, Cantler ED, Sisk TD, et al. A chronicle of injuries of an American intercollegiate football team. *Am J Sports Med* 1981;9:384–389.
6. Orchard JW, Best TM. The management of muscle strain injuries: an early return versus the risk of recurrence. *Clin J Sports Med* 2002;12:3–5.
7. Askling C, Karlsson J, Thorstensson A. Hamstring injury occurrence in elite soccer players after preseason strength training with eccentric overload. *Scand J Med Sci Sports* 2003;13(4):244–250.
8. Sherry MA, Best TM. A comparison of 2 rehabilitation programs in the treatment of acute hamstring strains. *J Orthop Sports Phys Ther* 2004;34(3):116–125.
9. Ryan JB, Wheeler JH, Hopkinson WJ, et al. Quadriceps contusions. West Point update. *Am J Sports Med* 1991;19(3):299–304.
10. Sandelin J. Acute sports injuries requiring hospital care. *Br J Sports Med* 1986;20:99–102.
11. Sutton FS, Thompson CH, Lipke J, et al. The effect of patellectomy on knee functions. *J Bone Joint Surg* 1976;58:537–540.

12. Chomiak J, Junge A, Peterson L, et al. Severe injuries in football players: influencing factors. *Am J Sports Med* 2000;28:S58–S68.

13. Woo SL, Vogrin TM, Abramowitch SD. Healing and repair of ligament injuries in the knee. *J Am Acad Orthop Surg* 2000;8: 364–372.

14. Peterson L, Renstrom P. *Sports Injuries: Their Prevention and Treatment*, 3rd ed. London: Martin Dunitz, 2001.

15. Smith FW, Rosenlund EQ, Aune AK, et al. Subjective functional assessments and the return to competitive sport after anterior cruciate ligament reconstruction. *Br J Sports Med* 2004;38(3):279–284.

16. al-Rawi Z, Nessan AH. Joint hypermobility in patients with chondromalacia patellae. *Rheumatology* 1997;36:1324–1327.

17. Couture CJ. Tibial stress injuries: decisive diagnosis and treatment of 'shin splints.' *Phys Sportsmed* 2002;30(6):29–36.

18. Blue JM, Matthews LS. Leg injuries. *Clin J Sport Med* 1997;16(3):467–478.

19. Batt ME. Shin splints: a review of terminology. *Clin J Sport Med* 1995;5(1):53–57.

20. Bates P. Shin splints: a literature review. *Br J Sport Med* 1985;(19(3):132–137.

21. Pecina MM, Bojanic I. *Overuse Injuries of the Musculoskeletal System*, 2nd ed. New York: CRC Press, 2004.

22. Kang L, Belcher D, Hulstyn M. Stress fractures of the femoral shaft in women's college lacrosse: a report of seven cases and a review of the literature. *Br J Sport Med* 2005;39:902–906.

23. Messier SP, Pittala KA. Etiologic factors associated with selected running injuries. *Med Sci Sports Exerc* 1988;20(5):501–505.

24. Krivickas LS. Anatomical factors associated with overuse sports injuries. *Sports Med* 1997;24(2):132–146.

25. Teitz C, Hu S, Arendt E. The female athlete: evaluation and treatment of sports-related problems. *J Am Acad Orthop Surg* 1997;5:87–96.

26. Voss L, Fadale P, Hulstyn M. Exercise-induced loss of bone density of athletes. *J Am Acad Orthop Surg* 1998;6:349–357.

27. Beck BR. Tibial stress injuries: an etiological review for the purposes of guiding management. *Sports Med* 1998;26(4):265–279.

28. Detmer DE. Chronic shin splints: classification and management of medial tibial stress syndrome. *Sports Med* 1986;3(6): 436–446.

29. Wallensten R. Results of fasciotomy in patients with medial tibial syndrome or chronic anterior-compartment syndrome. *J Bone Joint Surg* 1983;65:1252–1255.

30. Wilder RP, Sethi S. Overuse injuries: tendinopathies, stress fractures, compartment syndrome, and shin splints. *Clin Sports Med* 2004;23(1):55–81.

31. Schepsis AA, Jones H, Haas, AL. Achilles tendon disorders in athletes. *Am J Sport Med* 2002;30(2):287–305.

32. Langberg H, Ellingsgaard H, Madsen T, et al. Eccentric rehabilitation exercise increases peritendinous type I collagen synthesis in humans with Achilles tendinosis. *Scand J Med Sci Sports* 2007;17(1):61–66.

33. Fahlstrom M, Jonsson P, Lorentzon R, et al. Chronic Achilles tendon pain treated with eccentric calf-muscle training. *Knee Surg Sports Traumatol Arthrosc* 2003;11(5):327–333.

34. Singh D, Angel J, Bentley G, et al. Fortnightly review. Plantar fasciitis. *BMJ* 1997;315:172–175.

35. Kibler WB, Goldberg C, Chandler TJ. Functional biomechanical deficits in running athletes with plantar fasciitis. *Am J Sport Med* 1991;19:66–71.

36. Riddle DL, Pulisic M, Pidcoe P, et al. Risk factors for plantar fasciitis: a matched case-control study. *J Bone Joint Surg* 2003;85-A(5):872–877.

37. Rome K. Anthropometric and biomechanical risk factors in the development of plantar heel pain—a review of the literature. *Phys Ther Rev* 1997;2:123–134.

38. Wilk BR, Fisher KL, Gutierrez W. Defective running shoes as a contributing factor in plantar fasciitis in a triathlete. *J Orthop Sports Phys Ther* 2000;30(1):21–28.

39. Buchbinder R. Plantar fasciitis. *N Engl J Med* 2004;350(21):2159–2166.

40. Gill LH, Kiebzak GM. Outcome of nonsurgical treatment for plantar fasciitis. *Foot Ankle Int* 1996;17:527–532.

41. Rovere GD, Clarke TJ, Yates CS, et al. Retrospective comparison of taping and ankle stabilizers in preventing ankle injuries. *Am J Sports Med* 1988;16(3):228–233.

42. Roy SP. Evaluation and treatment of the stable ankle sprain. *Phys Sportsmed* 1977;5:60–63.

43. Irvin R, Iversen D, Roy S. *Sports Medicine*, 2nd ed. Boston: Allyn & Bacon, 1998.

Head and Spine Injuries

Upon reading this chapter, the coach should be able to:

1. Identify the basic anatomical structures of the head and spine and movements of the spinal column.
2. Discuss recognition and management of concussion and the role of the coach.
3. Recognize the seriousness of intracranial hemorrhage.
4. Explain the prevention and management of acute spinal cord injuries.
5. Describe stingers and criteria for return to play.
6. Discuss common causes and management of low back pain in the athlete.
7. Describe training techniques that may promote back health and help avoid injury to the low back.

Dave was in his senior year of high school. He was a stand-out player on the football team and was look-ing forward to playing college ball the following year. He was tackled on the last play of the first half of an important game and struck his head on the ground. He was not feeling well during halftime and had a headache, but he did not tell his coach. He did not want to risk being kept from playing during the second half. Four minutes into the third quarter he received a helmet-to-helmet hit that knocked him backwards. He walked off the field complaining of a severe headache. Moments later he collapsed and lapsed into a coma with rapidly dilating pupils. He was rushed to the hospital where a computed tomography brain scan indicated diffuse swelling of the brain and a small subdural hematoma. A surgical attempt to decrease the elevated intracranial pressure and remove the hematoma was not successful. He was pronounced brain dead 3 days later. Was this tragedy preventable?

While the head and spine are subject to a variety of injuries, this chapter will focus on a few injuries that coaches may commonly see in their athletes as well as those with serious consequences. Ways to help pro-tect the low back from injury are also discussed.

HEAD ANATOMY

The skull is the skeleton of the head and the most complex bony structure in the body (Fig. 15.1). It is formed by 22 bones, 21 of which are firmly bound together. The mandible articulates with the temporal bone at the temporomandibular joint (commonly referred to as TMJ) to allow movement of the jaw for eating and speaking. Eight of the 22 bones are paired so there is a total of 14 named bones in the skull.

FROM THE ATHLETIC TRAINING ROOM

Nasal Fractures

In college sports, the nasal bone is the most commonly fractured facial bone. Epistaxis (nosebleed) usually occurs with the fracture. Bony fragments can obstruct the nasal airway. The blow that caused the fracture could also result in a concussion. Therefore, the athlete with a nasal fracture should always be checked for signs of concussion.

The fractured nose will be swollen and deformity is usually present, especially if the force was lateral. Treatment includes controlling bleeding, applying ice, and referring the athlete to the physician for further examination and reduction of the fracture. Within a few days the athlete with an uncomplicated fracture can safely return to play with a nose guard or gauze splinting.

The skull forms the bony protection of the brain. The meninges are three layers of membranes on the outer surface of the brain that further protect it and are comprised of the dura mater, arachnoid mater and pia mater. Cerebrospinal fluid occupies the space between the arachnoid mater and pia mater and helps to dissipate shocking forces on the brain (Fig. 15.2).

ATHLETIC HEAD INJURIES

Closed head injuries are common in sports. An estimated 300,000 mild to moderate traumatic sports-related brain injuries occur each year in the United States (1). The types of sports-related brain injuries treated in emergency departments include concussion, postconcussion syndrome, second impact syndrome, and intracranial hemorrhage (2).

FROM THE ATHLETIC TRAINING ROOM

Scalp Lacerations Bleed Profusely!

The scalp is the outer covering of much of the skull and is highly vascularized. Because of all the blood vessels, lacerations can result in profuse bleeding, even when the wound is minor or superficial. The coach should not be overly alarmed by this bleeding, but steps must be taken to control the bleeding (see Chapter 16). If the bleeding cannot be stopped, the emergency medical services system should be activated as uncontrolled bleeding of the scalp can become life threatening. The athlete needs to be monitored and treated for shock as needed. The wound must also be treated appropriately to prevent a scalp infection which could spread to the underlying bone or the cranial cavity.

The athletic trainer will clean and evaluate the wound and decide if the athlete needs further medical care or if the athlete can return to play. A gaping wound in which the edges do not touch may require sutures and the athlete should be referred to a physician. An athlete should also be referred to a physician if the wound cannot be completely cleaned or if a foreign body is embedded in the wound. If the wound is on the face, disfiguration is a concern. If the bleeding is stopped, the wound is cleaned, the edges are touching, and there is no concern about disfiguration, the athlete can return to play with the wound appropriately bandaged.

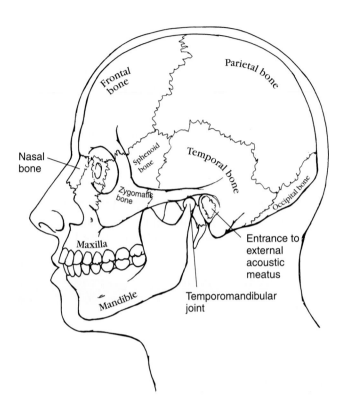

■ FIGURE 15.1 Lateral view of the skull. (Modified from Oatis CA. *Kinesiology—The Mechanics and Pathomechanics of Human movement.* Baltimore: Lippincott Williams & Wilkins, 2004.)

Both acceleration-deceleration (linear) and rotational (angular) mechanisms can occur when a force is applied to the brain. Usually one mechanism predominates depending on the nature of the impact. Acceleration-deceleration forces tend to be more common in contact sports. The boxing hook punch and similar mechanisms impart rotary forces (3).

Concussion

Concussion is the most common sports related head injury and can occur in any sport, not just collision and contact sports (2). A concussion is a brain injury and is sometimes called mild traumatic brain injury (MTBI). Concussion has been defined as a complex pathophysiological process that affects the brain and is induced by traumatic biomechanical forces (4). A concussion results in a functional disturbance and is not associated with a structural injury. A bump, blow, or jolt to the head can cause a concussion. The injury is caused by direct contact (bump or blow) to the head or contact elsewhere with the force being transmitted to the head (jolt).

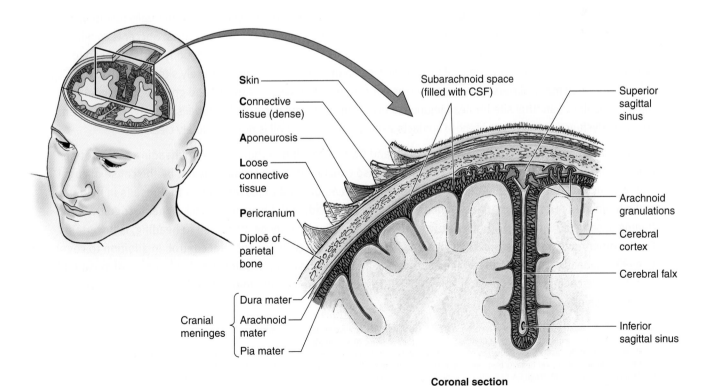

Coronal section

■ FIGURE 15.2 Layers of the scalp and the meninges. Note the subarachnoid space filled with cerebrospinal fluid. (Reprinted from Moore KL, Dalley AF. *Clinically Oriented Anatomy*, 4th ed. Baltimore: Lippincott Williams & Wilkins, 1999.)

Concussion is a serious injury and can occur without the loss of consciousness. Amnesia, not loss of consciousness, appears to be a better predictor of outcome following a sports-related concussion (5). Being able to recognize a concussion when it first occurs, along with proper management, can help prevent further injury and even death. Coaches can play an important role in both the recognition and management. Of the estimated 300,000 sports-related brain injuries that occur each year, most are concussions (1). However, the number may be greater as some concussions go unrecognized and some are not reported because the athlete does not want to be held from play. The risk of sustaining a concussion is almost six times greater for athletes with a history of concussion compared to those who have not had a prior concussion (6).

SIGNS AND SYMPTOMS

If an athlete experiences a bump, blow, or jolt to the head, the coaching staff should be on the alert for certain signs of injury or symptoms reported by the athlete. Sometimes the athlete does not experience the symptoms until days or weeks later. Common signs and symptoms are listed in Table 15.1. Although

FOCAL POINT

Soccer: Heading for Injury?

Soccer is one of the most popular team sports and unique in that it is the only field sport in which the unprotected head is used to control and advance the ball. Controversy exits regarding the safety of heading the ball.

The force of the impact is based on the equation: $F = ma$ where F is the force of impact, m is the mass of the ball and a is the acceleration of the ball. Prior to the 1970s, the ball was leather and absorbed water from the wet ground, considerably increasing the mass of the ball. The balls currently in use are synthetic and are resistant to water absorption.

Some of the conflicting findings can be attributed to studying athletes who played with leather balls resulting in an increased force of impact. Other problems are related to methodological errors in the studies. Soccer is considered a contact sport. Concussions are common and mostly occur from head to head (or other body parts) or head to ground impact (1). Contact with the goal posts is less common. The penalty area is a likely site on the field for head injury when many players compete for a cross or corner kick or when a forward and goalkeeper collide. Near the midfield line is another site for head injuries to occur when players compete for airballs. Distinguishing when cognitive dysfunction is a result of these contacts versus heading the ball is not completely clear.

In their critical review of the literature, Kirkendall and Garrett concluded that purposeful heading could not be blamed for reported cognitive deficits (1). Putukian also concluded that heading may not be the cause of cognitive dysfunction, but the act of heading leads to head to head or head to player contact that results in mild traumatic brain injury (2). Other studies found the frequency of heading did have an impact on neurocognitive functioning in some athletes (3,4). However, whether the deficits could only be attributed to heading, is uncertain. On the other hand, in a different study heading had no impact on tests for postural control. In addition to cognitive effects, heading may negatively impact the neck and cervical spine. Heading may lead to a predisposition to degenerative changes in the cervical spine (5). Further studies are needed to determine the long term effects of frequent use of heading in soccer.

1. Kirkendall DT, Garrett WE. Heading in soccer: integral skill or grounds for cognitive dysfunction? *J Athl Train* 2001;36:328–333.
2. Putukian M. Heading in soccer: Is it safe? *Current Sports Medicine Reports* 2004;3:9–14.
3. Webbe FM, Ochs SR. Recency and frequency of soccer heading interact to decrease neurocognitive performance. *Appl Neuropsychol* 2003;10:31–41.
4. Witol AD, Webbe FM. Soccer heading frequency predicts neuropsychological deficit. *Arch Clin Neuropsychol* 2003;18:397–417.
5. Mehnert MJ, Agesen T, Malanga GA. "Heading" and neck injuries in soccer: a review of biomechanics and potential long-term effects. *Pain Physician* 2005;8:391–397.

TABLE 15.1   Signs and Symptoms of Concussion

Signs Observed by Coaching Staff	Symptoms Reported by Athlete
Appears dazed or stunned	Headache
Confused about assignment	Nausea or vomiting
Forgets plays	Dizziness or difficulty with balance
Unsure of game, score or opponent	Double or fuzzy vision
Moves clumsily	Hearing problems or ringing
Answers questions slowly	Sensitivity to light or noise
Loses consciousness	Feeling sluggish, drowsy or low energy
Exhibits behavior or personality change	Feeling foggy or groggy
Forgets events prior to impact (retrograde)	Concentration or memory problems
Forgets events after impact (anterograde)	Confusion
	More emotional than usual

Information compiled from: Lovell MR, Collins MW, Iverson GL, et al. Grade 1 or "ding" concussions in high school athletes. *Am J Sports Med* 2004;32:47–54 and McCrory P, Johnston K, Meeuwisse W, et al. Summary and agreement statement of the 2nd International Conference on Concussion in Sport, Prague 2004. *Clin J Sport Med* 2005;15:48–55.

headache is the most commonly reported symptom, a concussion may occur without a headache. Often, a postconcussion headache becomes worse with physical exertion (7). The athlete should be kept from play until cleared by the athletic trainer and/or physician.

PREVENTION

Coaches can play an important role in helping to prevent concussions and properly managing them when they do occur. Safety must always come first. Coaches can teach safe playing techniques and make sure that athletes wear proper protective equipment that is well maintained and fits properly. Coaches can help ensure that players follow rules that have been established to decrease head injuries. They can also establish a climate of no tolerance for violence in sports.

While helmet use can decrease the incidence of skull fracture and major head trauma, it does not prevent, and may even increase, the incidence of concussion, especially if it does not fit properly (8). Mouthguards create a separation between the mandible and temporal bone. They may provide some cushioning effect from impact and lessen the energy transmission from the jaw and facial area to the cranial vault (9). Whether mouthguards actually provide any protection against concussion is not clear. However, they should be used to decrease the risk of dental and facial injury (10,11).

Athletes should be discouraged from playing injured. After a bump, blow, or jolt to the head, athletes should not be allowed to continue to play even if they say they are fine. Even a seemingly minor blow should be evaluated by a health care professional.

Coaches can foster a climate where the well-being of each player is of utmost importance. Athletes should be encouraged to report head injures that occurred in other sports or activities. Players can be taught the signs and symptoms and be reminded to tell the coaching staff if they suspect a teammate may have signs of a concussion. Teammates may be the first to observe the signs.

Strength training has been advocated for the prevention of cervical spine injuries (12). There is currently no clear evidence that strengthening the neck muscles can help reduce concussions (13). However, since neck muscle strengthening may reduce the impact forces to the brain and provide other benefits to the athlete, such conditioning may be considered.

CLASSIFICATION

For clinical purposes, concussion is usually categorized into three types or grades: mild (I), moderate (II), or severe (III). Many classification schemes have been proposed with three of them being used most commonly (Table 15.2) (14–16). A problem with these scales is that loss of consciousness is associated with more severe injuries and that may not be the case. At the 1st International Symposium on Concussion in Sport, abandoning these scales was recommended in favor of using combined measures of recovery to determine injury prognosis and individually guide return to play decisions (13).

At the 2nd International Conference on Concussion in Sport, a new classification system was proposed (4). For management purposes, concussion may be categorized as either simple or complex.

Simple Concussion

- Progressively resolves without complication over 7 to 10 days
- Other than limiting playing or training while symptomatic, no other intervention is needed during the recovery period and the athlete typically resumes sport activity without further problems
- The athlete rests until all symptoms resolve and then engages in a graded program of exertion before returning to sport
- These athletes can be managed by primary care physicians or certified athletic trainers working under medical supervision
- Most common type of concussion

Complex Concussion

- Athletes suffer persistent symptoms, including persistent symptom recurrence with exertion
- Specific sequelae occur such as concussive convulsions, prolonged loss of consciousness (>1 minute), or prolonged cognitive impairment
- Includes athletes who suffer multiple concussion over time or when repeated concussions occur with progressively less impact force
- Formal neuropsychological testing should be considered
- These athletes should be managed by a multidisciplinary team with expertise in concussive injury

MANAGEMENT AND RETURN TO PLAY

Sports where there is a high risk of head injury or concussion should include baseline neurological screening as part of the preparticipation examination. Having that information available is invaluable when making postinjury assessments and return to play decisions. If there is access to computerized neuropsychological testing (Table 15.3), it can provide even more precise data because the multiple forms used within the testing reduces practice effects. The baseline data provide the best benchmark for measuring postinjury recovery for the individual athlete. Recent research that used ImPACT, a computerized test battery, found that cognitive performance deficits following concussion in high school and college athletes persisted for 7 to 14 days in some cases (17). This indicates that cognitive recovery may take longer than previously believed and athletes may be returning to play prematurely.

TABLE 15.2	Concussion Grading Scales		
	Mild—I	**Moderate—II**	**Severe—III**
Cantu (1)	No loss of consciousness; post-traumatic amnesia <30 min	<5 min loss of consciousness or post-traumatic amnesia >30 min, but <24 hours	≥5 min loss of consciousness or ≥24 hours of posttraumatic amnesia
Colorado Medical Society (2)	No loss of consciousness; confusion without amnesia	No loss of consciousness; confusion with amnesia	Loss of consciousness
American Academy of Neurology (3)	No loss of consciousness; transient confusion; symptoms or mental status abnormalities resolve in <15 min.	No loss of consciousness; transient confusion; symptoms or mental status abnormalities last >15 min	Loss of consciousness

1. Cantu RC. Guidelines for return to contact sports after a cerebral concussion. *Phys Sportsmed* 1986;14(10):75–83.
2. Sports Medicine Committee, Colorado Medical Society. *Guidelines for the Management of Concussion in Sports.* May 1990 (revised May 1991).
3. Quality Standards Subcommittee of the American Academy of Neurology. Practice parameter: the management of concussion in sports (summary statement). *Neurology* 1997;48:581–585.

TABLE 15.3 Computerized Neuropsychological Tests Used in Concussion Management

Neuropsychological Test	Contact Information
Automated Neuropsychological Assessment Metrics (ANAM)	National Rehabilitation Hospital Washington, DC kirby@ou.edu or schlegel@ou.edu
CogState Sport	CogState Ltd. New Haven, CT www.cogstate.com
Concussion Resolution Index	HeadMinder, Inc. New York, NY www.headminder.com
Immediate Postconcussion Assessment and Cognitive Testing (ImPACT)	ImPACT Applications, Inc. Pittsburgh, PA, online at www.impacttest.com

Acute Management The time of the initial incident needs to be recorded. If an athletic trainer or other medical personal are not present, the coach needs to do this and call for assistance. When a concussion is suspected and an athletic trainer or physician is not present, the primary role of the coach is to ensure that the athlete is immediately seen by an athletic trainer or physician (18). Coaches should only do what they are qualified to do in the case of an emergency.

A systematic on-the-field examination is done to assess for adequate airway, breathing and circulation (see Chapter 16). Once breathing and circulation are established, neurological assessment is done to determine mental status and neurological deficit. The cervical spine and skull should also be examined for associated injury. If an athlete is unconscious, a cervical spine injury must also be suspected and spinal precautions must be used in movement and transport of the athlete (see Chapter 16).

The brief on-the-field examination allows medical personnel to determine whether emergency transport is needed or if the athlete can be further evaluated on the sidelines (8). The Sport Concussion Assessment Tool (SCAT) can be used for both sideline assessment by physicians and athletic trainers and can also be used for educational purposes (Fig. 15.3) (4).

Following a concussion, an athlete should not be left alone and should be monitored regularly for deterioration during the initial few hours following the injury. The coach can help ensure that parents, teammates, or roommates are aware of the athlete's condition and have contact numbers and instructions should the condition of the athlete deteriorate. The athlete should not consume alcohol during the postconcussive period. During the first few days following the injury both physical and cognitive rest are required. Activities that require concentration may exacerbate symptoms and delay recovery (4).

Return to Play Because concussions do not result in structural changes in the brain, currently there are no imaging techniques that are widely available to help determine recovery. Over the next several years this will hopefully change. Rather than relying on published guidelines, the focus has shifted to an individualized approach for making return to play decisions (7). Return to play decisions should be made based on neurocognitive testing and ideally the results are compared to baseline testing. These tests include evaluation of mental processing speed and accuracy, reaction time, and postural stability. When there is a rapid reduction of symptoms, most athletes are able to return to play within 5 to 10 days after the initial concussion (19). While a team approach (physician, athletic trainer, coach, and athlete) is best for determining readiness for return to play, the ultimate decision rests with the physician. When there are multiple concussions during a season or career, the physician makes the decision to disqualify the athlete for the remainder of the season or career on an individual basis taking into account multiple factors.

Following a concussion, return to play follows a stepwise process (4):

1. Complete rest. Proceed to step 2 once asymptomatic.
2. Light aerobic exercise (e.g., walking or stationary cycling); no resistance training.
3. Sport specific exercise (e.g., running in soccer, skating in hockey); at steps 3 and 4 resistance training is added progressively.

4. Noncontact training drills.
5. Full contact training after cleared by physician.
6. Game play.

With this stepwise progression, the athlete proceeds to the next level the following day only when asymptomatic at the current level. If postconcussion symptoms occur with the activity, the athlete should drop back to the previous asymptomatic level and try to progress again the following day. Using this progression, the athlete would return to play a minimum of 5 days following the onset of being symptom-free.

POSTCONCUSSION SYNDROME

Athletes who have sustained a concussion can have symptoms that persist for days or even months. Common complaints include persistent headache, irritability, inability to concentrate, dizziness, vertigo, impaired memory and general fatigue (9). The symptoms tend to be aggravated by exercise. Precisely why the symptoms persist is not understood. There is no clear treatment and most symptoms are self-limiting. The athlete should not be allowed to return to play until all symptoms have resolved. Athletes with persistent symptoms should undergo further neurocognitive testing and imaging of the brain to rule out more serious head injuries discussed below.

Sport Concussion Assessment Tool (SCAT)

This tool represents a standardized method of evaluating people after concussion in sport. This Tool has been produced as part of the Summary and Agreement Statement of the Second International Symposium on Concussion in Sport, Prague 2004

Sports concussion is defined as a complex pathophysiological process affecting the brain, induced by traumatic biomechanical forces. Several common features that incorporate clinical, pathological and biomechanical injury constructs that may be utilized in defining the nature of a concussive head injury include:
1. Concussion may be caused either by a direct blow to the head, face, neck or elsewhere on the body with an 'impulsive' force transmitted to the head.
2. Concussion typically results in the rapid onset of short-lived impairment of neurological function that resolves spontaneously.
3. Concussion may result in neuropathological changes but the acute clinical symptoms largely reflect a functional disturbance rather than structural injury.
4. Concussion results in a graded set of clinical syndromes that may or may not involve loss of consciousness. Resolution of the clinical and cognitive symptoms typically follows a sequential course.
5. Concussion is typically associated with grossly normal structural neuroimaging studies.

Post Concussion Symptoms
Ask the athlete to score themselves based on how they feel now. It is recognized that a low score may be normal for some athletes, but clinical judgment should be exercised to determine if a change in symptoms has occurred following the suspected concussion event.

It should be recognized that the reporting of symptoms may not be entirely reliable. This may be due to the effects of a concussion or because the athlete's passionate desire to return to competition outweighs their natural inclination to give an honest response.

If possible, ask someone who knows the athlete well about changes in affect, personality, behavior, etc.

Remember, concussion should be suspected in the presence of ANY ONE or more of the following:
• Symptoms (such as headache), or
• Signs (such as loss of consciousness), or
• Memory problems
Any athlete with a suspected concussion should be monitored fro deterioration (i.e., should not be left alone) and should not drive a motor vehicle.

For more information see the "Summary and Agreement Statement of the Second International Symposium on Concussion in Sport" in the April, 2005 edition of the Clinical Journal of Sport Medicine (vol 15), British Journal of Sports Medicine (vol 39), Neurosurgery (vol 59) and the Physician and Sportsmedicine (vol 33). This tool may be copied for distribution to teams, groups and organizations.
©2005 Concussion in Sport Group

The SCAT Card
(Sport Concussion Assessment Tool)
Athlete Information

What is a concussion? A concussion is a disturbance in the function of the brain caused by a direct or indirect force to the head. It results in a variety of symptoms (like those listed below) and may, or may not, involve memory problems or loss of consciousness.

How do you feel? You should score yourself on the following symptoms, based on how you feel now.

Post Concussion Symptom Scale	None		Moderate		Severe	
Headache	0	1	2 3	4	5	6
"Pressure in head"	0	1	2 3	4	5	6
Neck Pain	0	1	2 3	4	5	6
Balance problems or dizzy	0	1	2 3	4	5	6
Nausea or vomiting	0	1	2 3	4	5	6
Vision problems	0	1	2 3	4	5	6
Hearing problems / ringing	0	1	2 3	4	5	6
"Don't feel right"	0	1	2 3	4	5	6
Feeling "dinged" or "dazed"	0	1	2 3	4	5	6
Confusion	0	1	2 3	4	5	6
Feeling slowed down	0	1	2 3	4	5	6
Feeling like "in a fog"	0	1	2 3	4	5	6
Drowsiness	0	1	2 3	4	5	6
Fatigue or low energy	0	1	2 3	4	5	6
More emotional than usual	0	1	2 3	4	5	6
Irritability	0	1	2 3	4	5	6
Difficulty concentrating	0	1	2 3	4	5	6
Difficulty remembering	0	1	2 3	4	5	6

(follow up symptoms only)

	None		Moderate		Severe	
Sadness	0	1	2 3	4	5	6
Nervous or Anxious	0	1	2 3	4	5	6
Trouble falling asleep	0	1	2 3	4	5	6
Sleeping more than usual	0	1	2 3	4	5	6
Sensitivity to light	0	1	2 3	4	5	6
Sensitivity to noise	0	1	2 3	4	5	6
Other: _____	0	1	2 3	4	5	6

What should I do?
Any athlete suspected of having a concussion should be removed from play, and then seek medical evaluatoin.

Signs to watch for:
Problems could arise over the first 24-48 hours. You should not be left alone and must go to a hospital at once if you:
• Have a headache that gets worse
• Are very drowsy or can't be awakened (woken up)
• Can't recognize people or places
• Have repeated vomiting
• Behave unusually or seem confused; are very irritable
• Have seizures (arms and legs jerk uncontrollably)
• Have weak or numb arms or legs
• Are unsteady on your feet; have slurred speech
Remember, it is better to be safe. Consult your doctor after a suspected concussion.

What can I expect?
Concussion typically results in the rapid onset of short-lived impairment that resolves spontaneously over time. You can expect that you will be told to rest until you are fully recovered (that means resting your body and your mind). Then, your doctor will likely advise that you go through a gradual increase in exercise over several days (or longer) before returning to sport.

■ **FIGURE 15.3** The Sport Concussion Assessment Tool (SCAT) is a two-sided card with information for the athlete on one side and an evaluation form for medical personnel on the other side. (Reprinted from McCrory P, Johnston K, Meeuwisse W, et al. Summary and agreement statement of the 2nd International conference on Concussion in Sport, Prague, 2004. *Clin J Sport Med* 2005;15:48–55.) *(continues)*

SECOND IMPACT SYNDROME

Second impact syndrome (SIS) is the rapid swelling of the brain when a second injury to the head is sustained before symptoms of the initial injury have resolved. The second impact can be minimal and not involve any direct contact with the head. The autoregulatory system of the blood in the brain is disrupted with the second impact leading to rapid swelling and increasing intracranial pressure. The athlete may look stunned and may not initially lose consciousness. Within 15 seconds to several minutes following the injury the athlete's condition degrades rapidly. The pupils dilate, eye movement is lost, there is loss of consciousness leading to coma, and respiratory failure ensues. The usual time frame for this to occur following the second impact is 2 to 5 minutes (20). This is a life-threatening injury that must be addressed within 5 minutes at an emergency facility.

Sport Concussion Assessment Tool (SCAT)

The SCAT Card
(Sport Concussion Assessment Tool)
Medical Evaluation

Name: _____   Date _____

Sport/Team: _____   Mouth guard? Y N

1) SIGNS
Was there loss of consciousness or unresponsiveness?   Y   N
Was there seizure or convulsive activity?   Y   N
Was there a balance problem / unsteadiness?   Y   N

2) MEMORY
Modified Maddocks questions (check correct)

At what venue are we? __; Which half is it? __; Who scored last?__

What team did we play last? __; Did we win last game? __?

3) SYMPTOM SCORE
Total number of positive symptoms (from reverse side of the card) = _____

4) COGNITIVE ASSESSMENT

5 word recall		Immediate	Delayed
	(Examples)		(after concentration tasks)
Word 1 _____	cat	____	____
Word 2 _____	pen	____	____
Word 3 _____	shoe	____	____
Word 4 _____	book	____	____
Word 5 _____	car	____	____

Months in reverse order:
Jun-May-Apr-Mar-Feb-Jan-Dec-Nov-Oct-Sep-Aug-Jul   (circle incorrect)
or
Digits backwards (check correct)
5-2-8   3-9-1   _____
6-2-9-4   4-3-7-1   _____
8-3-2-7-9   1-4-9-3-6   _____
7-3-9-1-4-2   5-1-8-4-6-8   _____

Ask delayed 5-word recall now

5) NEUROLOGIC SCREENING

	Pass	Fail
Speech	____	____
Eye Motion and Pupils	____	____
Pronator Drift	____	____
Gait Assessment	____	____

Any neurologic screening abnormality necessitates formal neurologic or hospital assessment

6) RETURN TO PLAY
Athletes should not be returned to play the same day of injury. When returning athletes to play, they should follow a stepwise symptom-limited program, with stages of progression. For example:
1. rest until asymptomatic (physical and mental rest)
2. light aerobic exercise (e.g. stationary cycle)
3. sport-specific exercise
4. non-contact training drills (start light resistance training)
5. full contact training after medical clearance
6. return to competition (game play)

There is approximately 24 hours (or longer) for each stage and the athlete should return to stage 1 if symptoms recur. Resistance training should only be added in the later stages. Medical clearance should be given before return to play.

Instructions:
This side of the card is for the use of medical doctors, physiotherapists or athletic therapists. In order to maximize the information gathered from the card, it is strongly suggested that all athletes participating in contact sports complete a baseline evaluation prior to the beginning of their competitive season. This card is a suggested guide only for sports concussion and is not meant to assess more severe forms of brain injury. **Please give a COPY of this card to the athlete for their information and to guide follow-up assessment.**

Signs:
Assess for each of these items and circle Y (yes) or N (no).

Memory: If needed, questions can be modified to make them specific to the sport (e.g. "period" versus "half")

Cognitive Assessment:
Select any 5 words (an example is given). Avoid choosing related words such as "dark" and "moon" which can be recalled by means of word association. Read each word at a rate of one word per second. The athlete should not be informed of the delayed testing of memory (to be done after the reverse months and/or digits). Choose a different set of words each time you perform a follow-up exam with the same candidate.
Ask the athlete to recite the months of the year in reverse order, starting with a random month. Do not start with December or January. Circle any months not recited in the correct sequence.
For digits backwards, if correct, go to the next string length. If incorrect, read trial 2. Stop after incorrect on both trials.

Neurologic Screening:
Trained medical personnel must administer this examination. These individuals might include medical doctors, physiotherapists or athletic therapists. Speech should be assessed for fluency and lack of slurring. Eye motion should reveal no diplopia in any of the 4 planes of movement (vertical, horizontal and both diagonal planes). The pronator drift is performed by asking the patient to hold both arms in front of them, palms up, with eyes closed. A positive test is pronating the forearm, dropping the arm, or drift away from midline. For gait assessment, ask the patient to walk away from you, turn and walk back.

Return to Play:
A structured, graded exertion protocol should be developed; individualized on the basis of sport, age and the concussion history of the athlete. Exercise or training should be commenced only after the athlete is clearly asymptomatic with physical and cognitive rest. Final decision for clearance to return to competition should ideally be made by a medical doctor.

For more information see the "Summary and Agreement Statement of the Second International Symposium on Concussion in Sport" in the April, 2005 Clinical Journal of Sport Medicine (vol 15), British Journal of Sports Medicine (vol 39), Neurosurgery (vol 59) and the Physician and Sportsmedicine (vol 33). ©2005 Concussion in Sport Group

■ **FIGURE 15.3** *(continued)* The Sport Concussion Assessment Tool (SCAT)

The mortality rate with SIS is 50% (9); therefore, prevention is essential! An athlete should never be allowed to participate until all symptoms of a previous head injury have resolved. Preferably, the athlete should be asymptomatic, both during exertion and at rest, for an entire week prior to returning to play (20). This condition usually occurs in adolescents and is uncommon in adults (21). Athletes under age 18 should therefore be managed more conservatively than the more mature athlete.

Some controversy exists about SIS. McCrory contends there is no evidence to support the existence of this syndrome and suggests the diffuse cerebral swelling occurs as a rare and catastrophic complication of a single brain impact and is more common in adolescents and children (22). Cantu (21) adamantly opposes the views of McCrory (22) and has provided further documented cases of SIS. With such serious consequences, we need to err on the side of caution. Without further evidence to support McCrory's claims, precautions and guidelines related to the prevention of SIS should be followed.

Intracranial Hemorrhage

Intracranial hemorrhage (epidural, subdural, intracerebral, and subarachnoid) is the most severe type of athletic head injury and the leading cause of death following an athletic head injury (2). Rapid and aggressive treatment is needed to prevent a fatal outcome. Unlike concussions, these injuries can be diagnosed with computed tomography (CT) scanning or magnetic resonance imaging (MRI).

EPIDURAL HEMATOMA

Epidural hematomas are more commonly seen in sports where helmets are not worn. An epidural hematoma is the result of bleeding with an accumulation of blood between the dura and skull (inside the skull, but outside the covering of the brain; Fig. 15.4A). It is the most rapidly progressing intracranial hematoma and is usually a result of a direct blow. The bleeding is often caused by a skull fracture which lacerates the middle meningeal artery or vein. Sometimes there is a lucid interval, often preceded by a loss of consciousness (20). This clinical picture makes it crucial for any athlete who sustains a blow to the

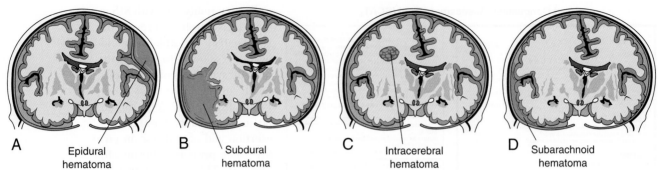

■ **FIGURE 15.4** Intracranial bleeding can lead to accumulation of blood (hematoma) in different locations within the skull depending on the nature of the impact. **A.** Epidural hematoma—between the skull and dura. **B.** Subdural hematoma—between the dura and surface of the brain. **C.** Intracerebral hematoma—within the brain. **D.** Subarachnoid hematoma—within the subarachnoid space. (Adapted from Smeltzer SC, Bare BG. *Textbook of Medical-Surgical Nursing,* 9th ed. Philadelphia: Lippincott Williams & Wilkins, 2000.)

head to be observed for an adequate time period. The lucid interval can give a false picture of the athlete's status. As the hematoma forms, neurological deterioration will ensue. If left alone, the signs of deterioration will be missed and the athlete will not receive appropriate emergency medical care. The lesion usually becomes obvious within 2 hours of the injury and if the clot is promptly removed, full recovery is possible (23). An athlete who receives a head injury must be observed closely for several hours, preferably 24 hours.

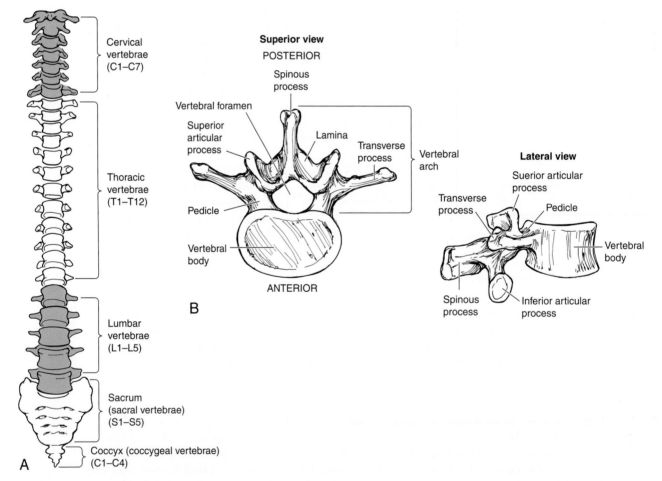

■ **FIGURE 15.5 A.** Anterior view of the spinal column showing the vertebrae of each region. **B.** Superior and lateral view of the 5th lumbar vertebra. Note the vertebral body anteriorly and the vertebral arch posteriorly. The spinal cord passes through the vertebral foramen. (Modified from Oatis CA. *Kinesiology—The Mechanics and Pathomechanics of Human Movement.* Baltimore: Lippincott Williams & Wilkins, 2004.)

SUBDURAL HEMATOMA

A subdural hematoma is located between the dura and surface of the brain and results from torn blood vessels that run in that region (Fig. 15.4B). Acceleration and deceleration forces from a blow cause the vessels to tear. Subdural hematomas are more common than epidural hematomas and are associated with severe neurologic disability and death (3). When the hematoma causes associated injury to the brain tissue, there can be irreversible brain damage even with successful removal of the hematoma (3).

There are both acute and chronic forms of subdural hematoma. The acute subdural hematoma forms within 48 to 72 hours after injury. With an acute subdural hematoma there is often loss of consciousness and neurological signs can be dependent on the area of the brain that is damaged. A chronic subdural hematoma occurs in a later time frame with a more variable presentation (3). A headache is common. Other neurological symptoms can be mild and imperceptible. If an athlete sustains a head injury and weeks later still does not seem right, a CT scan can provide a definitive diagnosis. This is important since recognition and removal can lead to full recovery (23).

INTRACEREBRAL HEMATOMA

Intracerebral hematoma involves bleeding into the substance of the brain, usually from a torn artery (Fig. 15.4C). There may be no loss of consciousness and the athlete may have a persistent headache, confusion, or retrograde (before the injury) amnesia. If the symptoms persist, further evaluation is necessary. The athlete will require close observation and possibly surgery (20). These are the least common of the intracranial hematomas, but are commonly found in boxers.

SUBARACHNOID HEMORRHAGE

Subarachnoid hemorrhage is seen in athletes less frequently than the other types. The bleeding occurs in the subarachnoid space (Fig. 15.4D). A severe headache is the primary symptom and may be accompanied by neck stiffness, vomiting, or nausea.

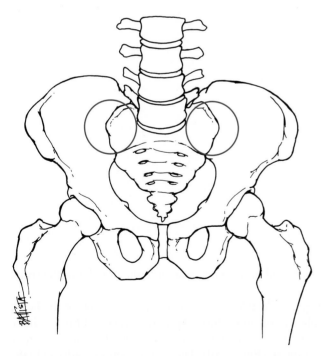

■ **FIGURE 15.6** Anterior view of the distal spinal column and bony pelvis indicating the location of the sacroiliac joints. These joints connect the lower limbs to the axial skeleton. (Modified from Oatis CA. *Kinesiology—The Mechanics and Pathomechanics of Human Movement.* Baltimore: Lippincott Williams & Wilkins, 2004.)

SPINE ANATOMY

The spine is a column of 33 bones. Most have intervening discs and some are fused together. There are 7 cervical, 12 thoracic, and 5 lumbar vertebrae. The sacrum (5 fused bones) and the coccyx (4 fused bones) form the distal portion of the spinal column (Fig. 15.5). The spine connects with the hip bones at the sacroiliac joints (Fig. 15.6). The normal spine is not a straight column, but has anterior-posterior curves (Fig. 15.7). The discs that are located between the vertebrae are composed of the outer annulus fibrosus and the inner nucleus pulposus (Fig. 15.8).

The anterior and posterior longitudinal ligaments connect the vertebral bodies, and the interspinous, supraspinous, and intertransverse ligaments connect the arches of the vertebra. The spinal cord passes through the vertebral foramen located between the vertebral bodies and arches. The column of vertebrae form a canal for the spinal cord (vertebral canal). The spinal nerves exit the vertebral

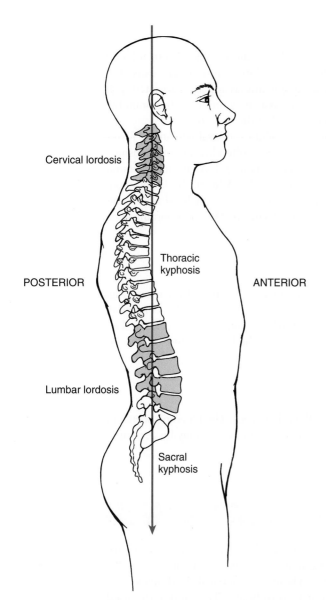

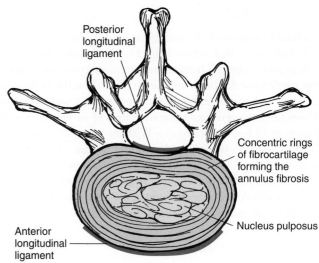

■ **FIGURE 15.8** A top view of a vertebra illustrating the nucleus pulposus in the center of the intervertebral disc surrounded by the annulus fibrosus. (Modified from Oatis CA. *Kinesiology—The Mechanics and Pathomechanics of Human Movement.* Baltimore: Lippincott Williams & Wilkins, 2004.)

■ **FIGURE 15.7** A side view of the spinal column illustrating the normal lordosis in the cervical and lumbar spine (anteriorly convex) and normal kyphosis in the thoracic spine and sacrum (posteriorly convex). (Modified from Oatis CA. *Kinesiology—The Mechanics and Pathomechanics of Human Movement.* Baltimore: Lippincott Williams & Wilkins, 2004.)

canal through the intervertebral foramina (Fig. 15.9) and provide innervation to the muscles of the trunk and limbs.

The spinal column provides a partly rigid and partly flexible axis for the body and a pivot for the head. It functions to protect the spinal cord and also plays a role in posture, supporting the weight of the body and locomotion. The motion between any two adjacent vertebrae is limited, but together the column or regions are able to flex, extend, laterally flex, and rotate (Fig. 15.10). The motion between adjacent vertebrae occurs primarily at the discs and facets joints (Fig. 15.11).

The muscles in the back are arranged in three layers. The superficial layer is comprised of the posterior muscles of the upper limb (see Chapter 13). The intermediate layer contains muscles that assist in respiration. The deep layer has the true or intrinsic muscles of the back (Fig. 15.12). These muscles extend, laterally flex and rotate the vertebral column. The abdominal muscles flex the spine.

CERVICAL SPINE INJURIES

Injuries to the cervical spine include catastrophic damage to the spinal cord as well as less serious transient injuries to the spinal nerves. The muscles and ligaments of the cervical region are also susceptible to sprains, strains and contusions.

Spinal Cord Injury

Fortunately, spinal cord injuries are not a common athletic injury, but because they are catastrophic they will be mentioned here briefly. According to the National Spinal Cord Injury Statistical Center, approximately 11,000 new cases of spinal cord injury occur each year with 8.7% of the injuries occurring during sporting activities (24). The percent that occur during organized sports versus recreational activities is not clear. Over time the percentage of injuries due to sports has decreased. This may possibly be due in part to improved equipment and rule changes.

The most common mechanism of injury is a blow to the top of the head with the neck flexed. The force results in a crushing of the vertebral bodies or a dislocation of the facet joints which can damage the spinal cord. Since spear tackling was banned from football, the incidence of serious cervical injuries has decreased dramat-

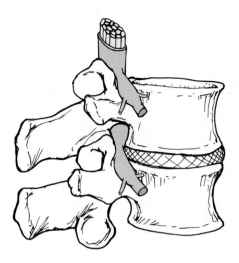

■ **FIGURE 15.9** Lateral view of a spinal segment illustrating the spinal nerve exiting the intervertebral foramen. Note the spinal cord passing through the vertebral canal. (Modified from Oatis CA. *Kinesiology—The Mechanics and Pathomechanics of Human Movement*. Baltimore: Lippincott Williams & Wilkins, 2004.)

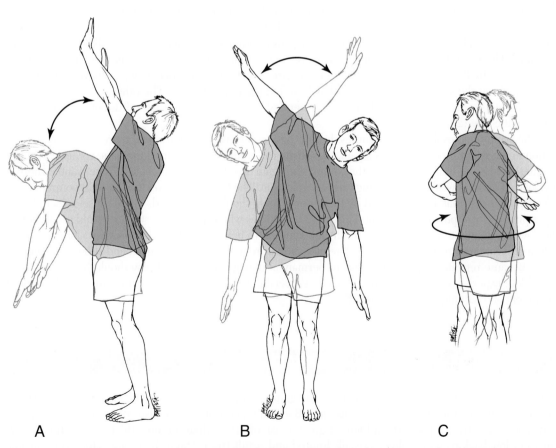

A   B   C

■ **FIGURE 15.10** While the movement between each individual vertebra is limited, working together the vertebrae are a considerable range of motion. The spine is able to flex and extend **(A)**, laterally flex **(B)**, and rotate **(C)**. (Modified from Hamill J, Knutzen KM. *Biomechanical Basis of Human Movement*, 2nd ed. Baltimore: Lippincott Williams & Wilkins, 2003).

ically. Coaches and parents must continue to be vigilant in educating athletes about the dangers of spear tackling.

An athlete who is down on the field should never be moved until spinal cord injury is ruled out. For an unconscious athlete, where volitional movement and testing are not possible, a cervical spine injury must be assumed until it can be proven otherwise. Cardiopulmonary resuscitation may be necessary and transport guidelines outlined in Chapter 16 must be followed.

These cervical spine injuries are catastrophic and can result in permanent paralysis or death. Perhaps that is why they receive more attention in the press. However, ligament sprains and muscle strains and contusions are much more common (see Chapter 12).

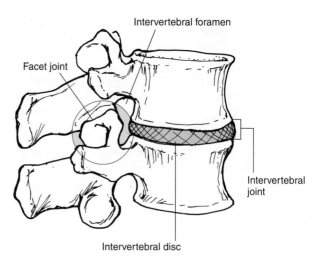

■ FIGURE 15.11 Adjacent vertebrae articulate at both the intervertebral discs anteriorly and the paired facet joints posteriorly allowing movement between each segment of the spinal column. (Modified from Oatis CA. *Kinesiology—The Mechanics and Pathomechanics of Human movement.* Baltimore: Lippincott Williams & Wilkins, 2004.)

Stingers

Stingers or burners are an injury to the brachial plexus (the large network of nerves that innervates the upper limb) or the nerve roots as they exit the cervical vertebrae. The injury causes a sudden radiating pain and numbness in the limb and associated local weakness is possible. Stingers only affect one side of the body. Usually the symptoms are transient and only last a few seconds or minutes. This injury is very common in football players and can be seen in athletes in other sports such as basketball, ice hockey, and wrestling. There are two common mechanisms of injury. One is traction on the nerves of the brachial plexus caused by the arm and neck moving in opposite directions which occurs when there is downward displacement of the shoulder while the neck is flexed to the opposite side. The other is a compression of the nerve roots when the head and neck are extended in a posterior and lateral direction towards the symptomatic side (25).

If the symptoms resolve within minutes, full strength and sensation return, and there is no limitation of motion in the neck or increase in neck pain, the athlete can return to play during the same contest (26). The athlete should be re-examined during the contest and again over the next few weeks to determine if there is any delayed onset of weakness requiring further evaluation. The C5 and C6 level are the most commonly involved, so muscles that are innervated by these nerve roots should be checked. These muscles include the supraspinatus, infraspinatus, deltoid and biceps (25). Athletes who experience a stinger should use a protective device to limit lateral neck flexion and hyperextension to help prevent another incident along with possible modification of playing technique. A rehabilitation program can include neck and shoulder strengthening. Because repeated injuries may lead to permanent damage, cessation of play should be considered if the athlete experiences three or more stingers, especially within the same season or after implementing equipment and technique adjustments (26).

LOW BACK PAIN

Low back pain is a very common problem in the general population with nearly 85% of people experiencing an episode at least once in their lifetime. Back pain and injuries are also common in athletes and some sporting activities place the athlete at greater risk of injury than the nonathlete (27). Most occurrences of low back pain in athletes are self-limited and result from strains or sprains. However, chronic or recurrent symptoms may be associated with degenerative lumbar disc disease or spondylolysis and related lesions (28). The sacroiliac joint can also be a cause of low back and buttock pain. Low back injuries

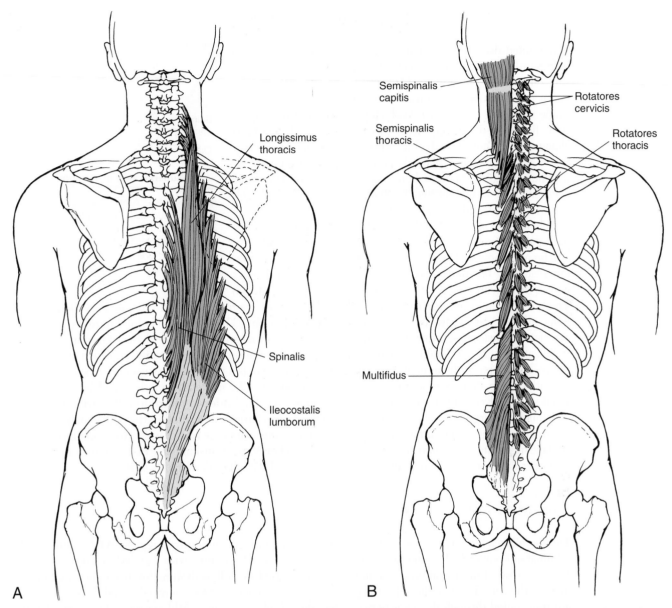

■ FIGURE 15.12 A. The erector spinae muscles are the primary extensors of the vertebral column. From lateral to medial the three columns of muscles are the iliocostalis, longissimus and spinalis. **B.** Deep to the erector spinae is the transversospinal muscle group. These muscles occupy the space between the transverse and spinous processes of the vertebrae and include the semispinalis, multifidus and rotators muscles. (Modified from Oatis CA. *Kinesiology—The Mechanics and Pathomechanics of Human Movement.* Baltimore: Lippincott Williams & Wilkins, 2004.)

infrequently occur from a single event. More commonly they are a result of excessive loading over time which eventually leads to tissue failure. Athletes who have sustained a low back injury are 3 to 6 times more likely to have another low back injury than other athletes (29). Proper conditioning may play an important role in prevention.

Lumbar Strains and Sprains

Similar to the general population, muscle strains and ligament sprains are the most common back injuries in athletes (30). Following a strain or sprain a short rest period of 1 to 2 days is recommended along with intervals of icing during the acute phase. This is followed by gentle and progressive stretching and strengthening exercises. The athlete gradually increases activity and can return to full play when pain-free and has normal range of motion, strength, and endurance (28).

Herniated Disc

A herniated disc occurs when the nucleus portion of the disc bulges or leaks out through fissures in the annulus and puts pressure on a nerve root (Fig. 15.13). Axial loading, usually with rotation is a common mechanism of injury. It rarely occurs from single incidence of excessive load. Repeated cycles of compression, flexion and torsional loading can result in degenerative changes in the annulus which can eventually result in a herniation. Genetics may also play a large role in susceptibility to disc degeneration (31). Sports where disc injuries more commonly occur include weight lifting, football, hockey, volleyball, golf, throwing sports, and racquet sports (32).

When a disc is herniated the athlete will often experience low back pain that radiates down one of the lower limbs. There can also be numbness and tingling as well as weakness in the muscles innervated by the nerve root that is impinged. In most cases, nonsurgical treatment is recommended as the first approach.

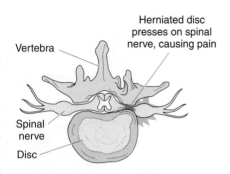

■ FIGURE 15.13 A herniated disc causes pain when the nucleus penetrates the layers of the annulus and puts pressure on the adjacent spinal nerve. (Modified from Willis MC. *Medical Terminology: The Language of Health Care.* Baltimore: Williams & Wilkins, 1996:133.)

Treatment includes limited rest and activity modifications, exercise, and anti-inflammatory medications. Some athletes are also treated with lumbar steroid injections (33). Ice can be helpful to relieve pain and associated muscle spasm. Extension exercises are a key component in the early phases of treatment. Spinal stabilization exercises should be included in the rehabilitation program prior to return to activity. Surgery can be considered if the athlete does not improve or if there is a progressive worsening of symptoms.

With conservative treatment return to play decisions must be made on an individual basis. Symptoms should be resolved and strength and range of motion regained prior to return to full activity. Return to play following surgical intervention depends on the type of surgery and whether the athlete plays noncontact or contact sports. For noncontact sports the time frame can range from 6 weeks to 3 months (33). For contact sports the timeframe can be 2 to 6 months. When a spinal fusion is necessary, return to play can be 1 year for noncontact sports and is not recommended for full contact sports (33).

Sacroiliac Joint Pain and Dysfunction

The sacroiliac joint (SIJ) can be a source of pain in the low back and buttock region. While there is only minimal movement at this joint, when it is not moving properly, asymmetries and dysfunction may result. Pain can result from irritation or inflammation of the joint as well as dysfunction from abnormal movement at the joint. Because the SIJ is the point of connection between the bony pelvis and the spine, forces are transmitted through this joint between the lower limbs and spine. Athletes who play sports that involve unilateral loading may be at increased risk (34). Kicking and throwing, skating, gymnastics, and golfing are examples of activities with unilateral loading. Trauma, such as a fall onto the buttocks, can lead to SIJ dysfunction. A marked increase in intensity, frequency, or duration of an activity can also lead to injury of the SIJ (34).

Treatment in the acute phase includes pain control with rest, anti-inflammatory medications and icing. Relative rest includes avoiding running and excessive walking as they can provoke SIJ pain. Avoiding single leg stance activities can help alleviate symptoms (34). Mobilization by the athletic trainer or physical therapist is done to correct mechanical dysfunctions. When necessary, exercises to correct strength and muscle length imbalances are included in the rehabilitation program. The coach can be involved in the rehabilitation to help analyze technique to see if faulty form may be contributing to the excessive stress being placed on the SIJ. When an athlete does not respond to conservative treatment, sometimes the joint is injected with a corticosteroid.

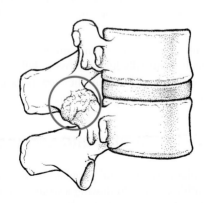

■ FIGURE 15.14 Spondylolysis showing a defect in the pars interarticularis portion of the lamina. (Adapted from Neil O. Hardy. Westpoint, CT.)

FOCAL POINT

Bench Rest: Bad for the Back?

In many team sports athletes warm-up and stretch prior to the game. Those who do not start sit on the bench until they are substituted into the game. Often times the bench is low to the ground without any back support which encourages sitting with a flexed spine. Prolonged sitting has been linked to low back pain and prolonged flexion can compromise spine stability.

In addition, more recent research has shown that when a warm-up is followed by bench rest there is increased stiffness in some motions of the lumbar spine (1). This could have implications for both low back health and performance. While further research is needed to determine the length of time needed for the increased stiffness to occur as well as testing a larger number of athletes, coaches should be aware that sitting on the bench may be detrimental to their athletes' backs. Further research is also needed to determine if there are postures or activities athletes can engage in while waiting to return to play that may prevent the stiffness in the low back.

1. Green JP, Grenier SG, McGill SM. Low-back stiffness is altered with warm-up and bench rest: implications for athletes. *Med Sci Sports Exerc* 2002;34:1076–1081.

There are no universally established return to play criteria with SIJ lesions. Generally, the athlete should be able to play at full capacity within pain tolerance.

Spondylolysis

Spondylolysis is a stress fracture in the pars interarticularis of the vertebra (the part of the lamina between the superior and inferior articular processes) and is a common cause of low back pain in adolescent athletes (Fig. 15.14). Athletes will have pain which worsens with activity, especially extension of the lumbar spine. There is usually a gradually worsening pain with no specific injurious event (35). Repetitive hyperextension, as seen in gymnastics or with football linemen, may predispose an athlete to the development of spondylolysis (36).

Treatment for spondylolysis varies, but often includes the use of a brace worn 23 hours a day (37). Rehabilitation includes trunk stabilization and pelvic flexibility exercises, and all hyperextension maneuvers of the spine are avoided. After 4 to 6 weeks the athlete can return to play wearing the brace if pain free with extension (35,37). Brace wear can be slowly reduced over the next few months if the pain does not return.

TRAINING THE BACK TO AVOID INJURY

Because of the high prevalence of back pain among athletes, using training techniques that are less likely to put the spine at risk and incorporating appropriate spinal stabilization exercises into the training regimen can be beneficial. Contraction of the abdominal and spine extensor muscles can increase the load on the intervertebral discs. The safest spinal stabilization program uses exercises that maximally engage the muscles with the minimal stress on the spine.

Many injuries to the low back are associated with the end range of motion of the spine. Therefore, maintaining a neutral spine with its normal curvature may reduce the risk of injury (38). Maintaining a neutral spine is important not only in exercises for the back, but in all activities. For example, when stretching the hamstring muscles, a neutral spine should be maintained rather than allowing the spine to flex (Fig. 15.15).

In most sports, exercises to increase the range of motion of the spine are not warranted. Spine mobility should be emphasized rather than stretching at the end of range. There is little evidence to support the notion that trunk flexibility can improve the health of the back or prevent injury.

Endurance of the muscles that support the spine should be the initial emphasis of exercise rather than strength. Decreased strength does not appear to be related to the development of low back pain, but endurance is associated with back health. Athletes should first train for endurance of the back supporting muscles and then progress to strengthening exercise (39). We do not recommend the use of weight machines for strengthening the abdominal and spine extensor muscles. Functionally, they bear little resemblance to any motions used in athletic activities and put the spine at great risk for future injury.

Training that requires a large amount of spinal motion should be avoided first thing in the morning. After a night of bed rest the disc is at its maximum size with increased stresses on the annulus. First thing in the morning is the most dangerous time to perform exercises with full forward bending (39). This is particularly problematic for rowers who like to train in the early morning hours. If early morning training cannot be avoided, rising earlier and slowly progressing the load on the spine is advised.

Following a back injury, each athlete needs an individualized exercise program based on the specific needs of the athlete, the nature of the injury, and the sport in which the athlete is engaged. There is no one size fits all exercise prescription. The same can be true for conditioning and preparing athletes for back health and competition. There is, however, a series of exercises that should form the foundation of low back exercise. Higher level exercises can build on these. The remainder of this chapter will outline these exercises. These exercises have been shown to challenge the abdominal and back extensor muscles with less compressive load to the spine than other exercises (40). For higher level exercises the reader is referred elsewhere (39,40).

Flexion-Extension Exercise

This exercise is often known as the cat or cat/camel stretch (Fig. 15.16) and should be performed first. The athlete slowly cycles through flexion and extension in a hands and knees position. This is a motion exercise and not a stretch so pushing at the end ranges should be avoided. Five to six cycles within a pain free range provide a warm-up for the spinal segments.

Curl-Up

The curl-up exercise targets the rectus abdominis muscle and is performed maintaining a neutral spine (Fig. 15.17). To help maintain the neutral spine and stabilize the pelvis the hands are placed under the lumbar region. One knee is bent and the other remains straight which also helps maintain the neutral spine. The bent and straight leg can be switched half-way through the repetitions. The curl-up is performed by lifting the head and shoulders off the supporting surface. The head should maintain alignment with the spine. Each curl is held for about 8 seconds. This helps build endurance along with multiple repetitions. Because sustained muscle contraction does not allow adequate blood flow to the muscle, holding each curl-up for longer than 8 seconds is not recommended.

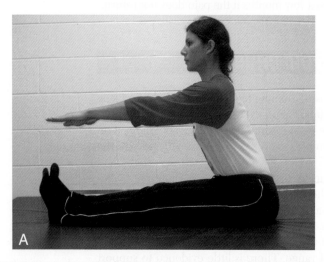 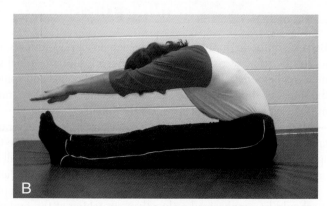

■ **FIGURE 15.15 A.** When stretching the hamstring muscles an increased load to the spine can be prevented by maintaining a neutral spine curve. **B.** Flexing the spine while attempting to stretch the hamstring muscles puts the back at risk. The increased excursion of the hands is due to spinal motion and not a greater stretch of the hamstring muscles. Stretching in this position should be avoided.

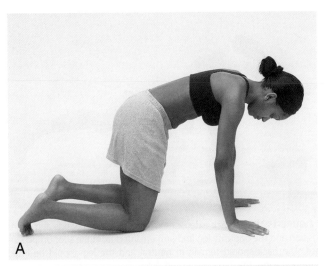

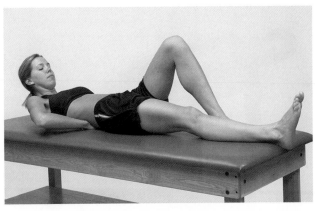

■ **FIGURE 15.17** The curl-up is performed by raising the head and shoulders from the supporting surface. The hands are placed under the lumbar spine to help stabilize and maintain a neutral spine. Note the position of the legs to also help stabilize the spine. (Reprinted from Oatis CA. *Kinesiology—The Mechanics and Pathomechanics of Human Movement*. Baltimore: Lippincott Williams & Wilkins, 2004.)

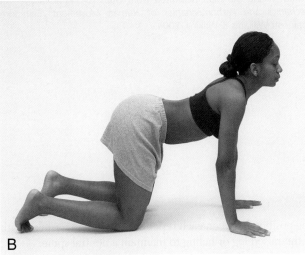

■ **FIGURE 15.16** The flexion/extension exercise is performed first by cycling through full spinal flexion **(A)** to full extension **(B)**. The emphasis is on spinal mobility and not stretching into the ends of each range. (Reprinted from Oatis CA. *Kinesiology—The Mechanics and Pathomechanics of Human Movement*. Baltimore: Lippincott Williams & Wilkins, 2004.)

Side Bridge

No single exercise challenges all the abdominal muscles and spinal stabilizers. The side bridge exercise is done next to train the internal and external obliques, transverse abdominis, and quadratus lumborum muscles. It is also performed maintaining a neutral spine. The athlete lifts from the supporting surface to bear weight on the feet and supporting forearm (Fig. 15.18) and holds for 8 seconds. If this position is difficult, the athlete can support the body with the knees. Repetitions are completed on one side and repeated on the other side.

Back Extensor Exercise

This exercise is also commonly referred to as the birddog. The starting position is on hands and knees with the hands directly under the shoulders and the knees in line with the hips. As in the above exercises, this one is also done maintaining the neutral position of the spine. One leg and the opposite arm are raised from the supporting surface and held for 8 seconds (Fig. 15.19). All repetitions are done on one side and then repeated on the other side. To make the exercise more challenging, the athlete can sweep the arm and leg together

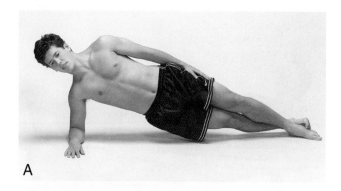

A

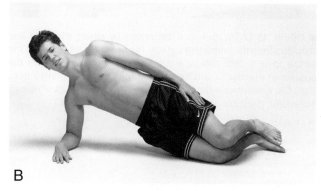

B

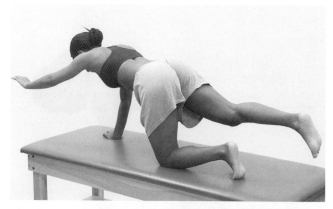

■ **FIGURE 15.19** The back extensor exercise begins in a hands and knees position and the opposite leg and arm are lifted from the supporting surface. The back should remain in neutral and the leg should be lifted without hiking the hip. (Reprinted from Oatis CA. *Kinesiology—The Mechanics and Pathomechanics of Human Movement.* Baltimore: Lippincott Williams & Wilkins, 2004.)

■ **FIGURE 15.18 A.** This is the end position for the side bridge after lifting from the supporting surface. If this position is too challenging, the distal support can be at the knees, **B.** The athlete can progress to the support at the feet. (Reprinted from Oatis CA. *Kinesiology—The Mechanics and Pathomechanics of Human Movement.* Baltimore: Lippincott Williams & Wilkins, 2004.)

under the torso rather than returning to the starting position between each repetition. Common mistakes with this exercise include hiking the hip on the side of the raised leg or failing to maintain a neutral spine.

SUMMARY

- The skull and three layers of meninges provide protection for the brain. Despite this protection, the brain can be injured in several ways during sports participation.
- Concussion is the most common sports related brain injury. Often symptoms are ignored or not recognized. Coaches and athletes must learn how to recognize the signs and symptoms and be aware of the possibly serious consequences of returning to play prematurely.
- Intracranial hemorrhage is bleeding inside the skull. It is the most severe type of athletic head injury and the leading cause of death following an athletic head injury. Rapid and aggressive treatment is needed to prevent a fatal outcome.
- The spinal column provides protection to the spinal cord and provides a partly rigid and partly flexible axis for the body and a pivot for the head.
- Spinal cord injuries are relatively rare in athletics, but catastrophic. Injury to the spinal cord can result in permanent paralysis or death. An athlete who is down on the field should never be moved until spinal cord injury is ruled out.
- Low back pain is common in athletes. Muscle strains, ligament sprains, herniated discs, sacroiliac joint dysfunction and spondylolysis are common causes of pain. These conditions are often a result of excessive loading over time rather than a single incident.
- Maintaining a neutral spine position with activity, avoiding the extreme end ranges of motion, and conditioning the structures that support the spine can help athletes protect their backs from injury. Three exercises that target key spinal stabilizers with minimal spinal loading form the foundation of a low back exercise program.

References

1. Centers for Disease Control and Prevention. *Sports-related Recurrent Brain Injuries: United States. MMWR* 1997;46:224–227. Available online at http://www.cdc.gov/mmwr/preview/mmwrhtml/00046702.htm. Accessed January 25, 2007.
2. Cooper MT, McGee KM, Anderson DG. Epidemiology of athletic head and neck injuries. *Clin Sports Med* 2003;22:427–443.
3. Bailes JE, Hudson V. Classification of sport-related head trauma: a spectrum of mild to severe injury. *J Athl Train* 2001;36:236–243.
4. McCrory P, Johnston K, Meeuwisse W, et al. Summary and agreement statement of the 2nd International Conference on Concussion in Sport, Prague 2004. *Clin J Sport Med* 2005;15:48–55.
5. Collins MW, Iverson GL, Lovell MR, et al. On-field predictors of neuropsychological and symptom deficit following sports-related concussion. *Clin J Sport Med* 2003;13:222–229.
6. Zemper ED. Two-year prospective study of relative risk of a second cerebral concussion. *Am J Phys Med Rehabil* 2003;82:653–659.
7. Lovell M, Collins M, Bradley J. Return to play following sports-related concussion. *Clin Sports Med* 2004;23:421–441.
8. American College of Sports Medicine. Concussion (mild traumatic brain injury) and the team physician: a consensus statement. Available online at www.acsm-msse.org. Accessed January 25, 2007.
9. Bailes JE, Cantu RC. Head injury in athletes. *Neurosurgery* 2001;48:26–46.
10. Knapik JJ, Marshall SW, Lee RB, et al. Mouthguards in sport activities: history, physical properties and injury prevention. *Sports Med* 2007;37:117–144.
11. Mihalik JP, McCaffrey MA, Rivera EM, et al. Effectiveness of mouthguards in reducing neurocognitive deficits following sports-related cerebral concussion. *Dent Traumatol* 2007;23:14–20.
12. Cross KM, Serenelli C. Training and equipment to prevent athletic head and neck injuries. *Clin Sports Med* 2003;22:639–667.
13. Aubry M, Cantu R, Dvorak J, et al. Summary and agreement statement of the first International Conference on Concussion in Sport, Vienna 2001. *Br J Sports Med* 2002;36:6–10.
14. Cantu RC. Guidelines for return to contact sports after a cerebral concussion. *Phys Sportsmed* 1986;14(10):75–83.
15. Sports Medicine Committee, Colorado Medical Society. *Guidelines for the Management of Concussion in Sports.* May 1990 (revised May 1991).
16. Quality Standards Subcommittee of the American Academy of Neurology. Practice parameter: the management of concussion in sports (summary statement). *Neurology* 1997;48:581–585.
17. McClincy MP, Lovell MR, Pardini J, et al. Recovery from sports concussion in high school and collegiate athletes. *Brain Inj* 2006;20:33–39.
18. Gusckiewicz KM, Bruce SL, Cantu RC, et al. National Athletic Trainers' Association position statement: management of sport-related concussion. *J Athl Train* 2004;39:280–297.
19. Webbe FM, Barth JT. Short-term and long-term outcome of athletic closed head injuries. *Clin Sports Med* 2003;22:577–592.
20. Ghiselli G, Schaadt G, McAllister DR. On-the-field evaluation of an athlete with a head or neck injury. *Clin Sports Med* 2003;22:445–465.
21. Cantu RC. Recurrent athletic head injury: risks and when to retire. *Clin Sports Med* 2003;22:593–603.
22. McCrory P. Does second impact syndrome exist? *Clin J Sport Med* 2001;11:144–149.
23. Cantu RC. Athletic head injuries. *Clin Sports Med* 1997;16:531–542.
24. National Spinal Cord Injury Statistical Center. Spinal cord injury: facts and figures at a glance. June 2006. Available online at www.spinalcord.uab.edu. Accessed February 9, 2007.
25. Eddy D, Congeni J, Loud K. A review of spine injuries and return to play. *Clin J Sport Med* 2005;15:453–458.
26. Dimberg EL, Burns TM. Management of common neurologic conditions in sports. *Clin Sports Med* 2005;24:637–662.
27. Trainor TJ, Wiesel SW. Epidemiology of back pain in the athlete. *Clin Sports Med* 2002;21:93–103.
28. Bono CM. Low-back pain in athletes. *J Bone Joint Surg Am* 2004;86:382–396.
29. Greene HS, Cholewicki J, Galloway MT, et al. A history of low back injury is a risk factor for recurrent back injuries in varsity athletes. *Am J Sports Med* 2001;29:795–800.
30. Trainor TT, Trainor MA. Etiology of low back pain in athletes. *Curr Sports Med Rep* 2004;3:41–46.
31. Battié MC, Videman T. Lumbar disc degeneration: epidemiology and genetics. *J Bone Joint Surg Am* 2006;88 Suppl 2:3–9.
32. Baker RJ, Patel D. Lower back pain in the athlete: common conditions and treatment. *Prim Care Clin Office Pract* 2005;32:201–229.
33. Eck JC, Riley LH. Return to play after lumbar spine conditions and surgeries. *Clin Sports Med* 2004;23:367–379.
34. Prather H. Sacroiliac joint pain: practical management. *Clin J Sport Med* 2003;13:252–255.
35. McCleary MD, Congeni JA. Current concepts in the diagnosis and treatment of spondylolysis in young athletes. *Curr Sports Med Rep* 2007;6:62–66.
36. Lawrence JP, Greene HS, Grauer JN. Back pain in athletes. *J Am Acad Orthop Surg* 2006;14:726–735.
37. Micheli LJ, Curtis C. Stress fractures in the spine and sacrum. *Clin Sports Med* 2006;25:75–88.
38. McGill SM. Low back exercises: prescription for the healthy back and recovery from injury. In: *ACSM's Resource Manual for Guidelines for Exercise Testing and Prescription,* 4th ed. Baltimore: Lippincott Williams & Wilkins, 2001.
39. McGill SM. *Ultimate Back Fitness and Performance.* Waterloo, Ontario, Canada: Wabuno Publishers, 2004.
40. McGill SM. *Low Back Disorders: Evidence-Based Prevention and Rehabilitation.* Champaign, IL: Human Kinetics, 2002.

16

Emergency Situations on the Field and Beyond

Upon reading this chapter, the coach should be able to:

1. Implement emergency and catastrophic plans.

2. Value the importance of cardiopulmonary resuscitation and first aid training.

3. Describe the elements of a primary survey and differentiate it from the secondary survey.

4. Discuss the signs and symptoms of shock and emergency treatment.

5. Control bleeding in an emergency situation using standard precautions.

6. Discuss whether an injured athlete should be moved and possible means of conveyance.

On a beautiful fall afternoon the West High soccer team was on the practice field. At West High an athletic trainer covers the home games and sees athletes in the training room, but is not on the field at each practice. The team finished their warmup and the players were rotating through drill stations and playing 5 minute 6-on-6 games when the unthinkable happened. Two players went up to head the ball when they collided in mid-air. One fell to the ground and was not moving. Coach Maroni quickly ran over to the athlete. Pieces of information from her first aid and CPR training were racing through her mind. She thought about the primary survey and what she might need to do. As she approached the athletes she saw blood on the forehead of the athlete who had collapsed. In her 10 years of coaching she had not experienced a serious injury with her athletes. At that moment she was feeling thankful that she had continued to take refresher courses in first aid and CPR. As the first person on the scene, what does the coach need to do? What needs to be immediately assessed? How should she control the bleeding? Should she call for help or transport the athlete?

Despite our best efforts to prevent injuries and accidents, some will occur. Therefore, we must plan ahead and be prepared for an athletic emergency when it arises. Athletic emergencies not only result from trauma to previously well athletes, but can arise when a previously recognized medical problem is aggravated (e.g., asthma, diabetes, or heart condition) or with the onset of a previously undiagnosed medical problem. Because there are times when coaches may be the first person on the scene, they should be trained and certified to provide cardiopulmonary resuscitation (CPR) and standard first aid. Full instruction in first aid and CPR is beyond the scope of this book. CPR and first aid guidelines are updated periodically. Readers are referred to the resources at the end of the chapter.

THE EMERGENCY PLAN

Most injuries that occur in athletics are relatively minor. On occasion, injuries occur that can be limb-threatening or life-threatening; they are unpredictable and can occur without warning (1). Having an emergency plan in place is essential for the well-being of the athletes and to help protect the institution or organization in case of legal action. Both the National Collegiate Athletic Association (NCAA) (2) and the National Federation of State High School Associations (3) have recommended that their member institutions develop an emergency plan for their athletic programs. In 2002, the National Athletic Trainers Association published a position statement on emergency planning in athletics (1):

NATIONAL ATHLETIC TRAINERS' ASSOCIATION POSITION STATEMENT

Emergency Planning in Athletics

The following is a summary of the 12 items in the statement:

1. Each institution or organization that sponsors athletic activities must have a written emergency plan that is comprehensive, yet flexible enough to be adapted to any situation.
2. The written plan should be distributed to athletic trainers and athletic training students, team and attending physicians, safety personnel, administrators, and coaches. Local emergency medical services personnel should be consulted in the plan development.
3. The emergency plan identifies the personnel who will carry out the plan and their qualifications. Sports medicine professionals, officials and coaches should be trained in automatic external defibrillation, cardiopulmonary resuscitation, first aid, and prevention of disease transmission.
4. Emergency equipment to carry out the plan should be specified and the location of the equipment should be indicated. The equipment should be appropriate for the level of training of the personnel who will use it.
5. The plan must include a clear mechanism for communication to appropriate emergency care service providers and specify the mode of transportation for the injured participant.
6. The emergency plan must be venue specific with each activity site having a defined plan.
7. The emergency plan should include the facilities to which the injured individual will be taken for care and the facilities should be notified in advance of scheduled events. Personnel from these facilities should be involved in the plan development.
8. Responsibility for documenting actions taken during the emergency should be specified as well as evaluation of the emergency response and training of institutional personnel.
9. The emergency plan should be reviewed and rehearsed annually, but may need to be done more frequently. Changes to the plan as the result of the reviews and rehearsals should be documented.
10. All personnel involved in the organization and sponsorship of athletic activities share the professional responsibility to provide emergency care, including the development and implementation of the emergency plan.
11. All personnel involved in the organization and sponsorship of athletic activities share a legal duty to develop, implement and evaluate an emergency plan for all sponsored activities.
12. The emergency plan should be reviewed by the administration and legal counsel of the sponsoring organization or institution.

Considerations in Plan Development

There are four basic components of the emergency plan: personnel, communication, equipment, and transportation.

PERSONNEL

The personnel involved in the emergency plan carry out four basic roles (4). The first and most important role is the immediate care of the injured athlete. The most qualified individual on the scene should assume this role and others should yield to those with the most appropriate training.

The second role is retrieving of emergency equipment and anyone on the team with knowledge of the types and location of equipment can assume this role. Coaches, athletic training students, and managers can assume this role.

Activating the emergency medical services (EMS) system is the third role and is necessary when emergency transportation is not already onsite at the event. As soon as the situation is considered an emergency or life-threatening, the EMS system should be activated. While anyone on the team can assume this role, a person who is calm under pressure and can communicate well on the telephone as well as being familiar with the location and address would be the best choice.

Once EMS has been activated the fourth role is to meet the EMS personnel and direct them to the scene. This individual should have keys for any locked gates or doors that could block access or slow the arrival of the EMS personnel. Coaches, athletic trainers, or managers can serve in this role.

Those involved in carrying out the emergency plan should be able to adapt to various situations presented in various sports and venues. Having more than one individual assigned to each of the above outlined roles allows the emergency team to function even if some individuals are not present.

COMMUNICATION

Access to a working telephone, cell phone, or other communication device is essential. The working order of the device needs to be checked prior to each practice or competition. The plan should include a backup communication system in case the primary device fails. A list of emergency phone numbers, street address, and directions to the site should be posted with the communication system or in a readily available location. Venue maps should include the location of telephones. If a number needs to be dialed to reach an outside line, that number should be clearly posted. The plan should also include other types of communication, such as warning signals that might be used for hazardous weather as well as the all-clear signal.

EQUIPMENT

All equipment that might be needed in an emergency should be readily accessible and in good working condition. This equipment may include, but is not limited to an automatic external defibrillator (AED), bag-valve mask, barrier mask, biohazardous waste supplies, splints, backboard, and tools to remove a face mask from a helmet. Personnel should be trained in advance in the proper use of the equipment. The equipment needs to be checked regularly to ensure that it is in working order and the personnel should regularly rehearse the use of the equipment. The available equipment should be appropriate for the level of training of the emergency personnel and the venue. The National Athletic Trainers' Association strongly encourages the availability of an AED in every setting (5). The survival rate following cardiac arrest is much greater if the heart can be quickly defibrillated (shocked), and this can be accomplished with the AED.

FOCAL POINT

Sudden Cardiac Death

Sudden cardiac death, also known as sudden cardiac arrest, is a result of an abrupt loss of heart function. This is the leading cause of death in young athletes (1). Athletes are considered healthy individuals and their sudden death is catastrophic for their families, friends, and teammates.

The most common causes of sudden cardiac death are undiagnosed cardiovascular disease and commotio cordis (2). Commotio cordis is a disturbance of the heart that is a result of a low impact and nonpenetrating blow to the chest wall. The blow usually does not cause any structural damage and the disturbance can occur even when a chest protector is worn. The presumed cause of the disturbance is the blow occurring during a vulnerable period in the heart cycle that results in a ventricular arrhythmia and cardiac arrest (3).

(continues)

Sudden Cardiac Death *(continued)*

Whenever an athlete suddenly collapses and is unresponsive, maintain a high suspicion of sudden cardiac arrest and immediately activate the emergency plan. Early initiation of CPR and use of an AED increase the chance that the athlete will survive (1).

1. Drezner JA, Courson RW, Roberts WO, et al. Inter-association task force recommendations on emergency preparedness and management of sudden cardiac arrest in high school and college athletic programs: a consensus statement. *J Athl Train* 2007;42:143–158.
2. Maron BJ. Sudden death in young athletes. *N Engl J Med* 2003;349:1064–1075.
3. Madias C, Maron BJ, Weinstock J, et al. Commotio cordis: sudden cardiac death with chest wall impact. *J Cardiovasc Electrophysiol* 2007;18:115–122.

TRANSPORTATION

The emergency plan needs to address the transportation of those injured or ill. An ambulance should be onsite for high-risk events. EMS response time should be a factor in determining the need for onsite ambulance coverage. Also to be considered is the level of transportation service that is available (basic or advanced life support and equipment available) and the level of training of the ambulance personnel. If an ambulance is onsite it should be located where it can have a clear route for entering and exiting the venue. In an emergency situation the athlete should be transported to a facility that has the necessary staff and equipment to deliver appropriate care. An athlete in an unstable condition should not be transported in a vehicle that does not have appropriate life support equipment. Should an emergency care provider leave the venue to transport an athlete, there needs to be a plan to ensure that the site remains supervised.

Implementation of the Emergency Plan

Once the plan has been developed, it must be implemented. There are three basic steps to implementation (1).

The first step in the implementation process is to put the plan in a written format that can be readily followed by all the emergency team members. It can be written using many different formats including a flow sheet or a list of numbered and bulleted points. The various sports, venues, and activity levels will have different locations, types of equipment, and communication devices that need to be reflected in the plan. Separate plans can be written for different situations or the main plan can be modified for each venue. See Figure 16.1 for an example of a venue specific emergency protocol.

Education is the second step. Everyone who will be using the plan must be familiarized with it. Each member of the emergency team needs a written copy of the plan and should have documentation of his or her roles and responsibilities in emergency situations. A copy of the plan that is specific to each venue should be posted in a prominent place and be available at a telephone at each site.

The final step is rehearsing the emergency plan and procedures. This provides an opportunity for all team members to learn the plan, maintain their emergency skills, and communicate about the plan with the other team members. The rehearsal can be done at an annual training, but may need to be reviewed throughout the year as personnel and procedures change.

CATASTROPHIC INCIDENTS

In addition to the emergency plan, having a plan to deal with catastrophic incidents is important to provide optimum care and support for all involved (2). Similar to the emergency plan, the catastrophic incident plan requires advance preparation. Catastrophic incidents can occur anywhere and include the sudden death of an athlete, coach, staff member, or fan due to an accident, illness, or a disabling and/or quality of life altering injury such as a spinal cord injury with complete or partial paralysis.

Sample Venue-Specific Emergency Protocol

_____ University Sports Medicine Football Emergency Protocol

1. Call 911 or other emergency number consistent with organization policies
2. Instruct emergency medical services (EMS) personnel to "report to _____ and meet _____ at _____ as we have an injured student-athlete in need of emergency medical treatment."
   University Football Practice Complex: _____ Street entrance (gate across street from _____) cross street: _____Street
   University Stadium: Gate _____ entrance off _____ Road
3. Profice necessary information to EMS personnel:
   • name, address, telephone number of caller
   • number of victims; condition of victims
   • first-aid treatment initiated
   • spedific directions as needed to locate scene
   • other information as requested by dispatcher
4. Provide appropriate emergency care until arrival of EMS personnel: on arrival of EMS personnel, provide pertinent information (method of injury, vital signs, treatment rendered, medical history) and assist with emergency care as needed

Note:
   • sports medicine staff member should accompany student-athlete to hospital
   • notify other sports medicine staff immediately
   • parents should be contacted by sports medicine staff
   • inform coach(es) and administration
   • obtain medical history and insurance information
   • appropriate injury reports should be completed

Emergency Telephon Numbers
_____ Hopspital   _____ - _____
_____ Emergency Department   _____ - _____
University Health Center   _____ - _____
Campus Police   _____ - _____

Emergency Signals

Physician: arm extended overhead with clenched fist
Paramedics: point to location in end zone by home locker room and wave onto field
Spine board: arms held horizontally
Stretcher: supinated hand in front of body or waist level
Splints: hand to lower leg or thigh

■ **FIGURE 16.1** Sample venue-specific emergency protocol. (Reprinted with permission from Andersen JC, Courson RW, Kleiner DM, et al. National Athletic Trainer's Association position statement: emergency planning in athletics. _J Athl Train_ 2002;37(1):99–104.)

The plan should define what the organization includes as a catastrophic incident and identify the persons who make up the management team and their roles. The action plan should include a chain of command and the actions that will take place following the incident. The plan should list who gets notified and the procedures for notification. Long-term follow-up, including counseling services, should also be included in the plan.

FOCAL POINT

Dealing with Tragedy

You cannot watch the news or read the newspaper without hearing about a tragedy. Sometimes the catastrophic incident hits close to home. Incidents of high school or college athletes dying suddenly on the playing field or in traffic accidents occur fairly frequently. Fortunately, larger scale incidents are less frequent.

In the early 1970s, the Marshall University football team perished in a plane crash. More recently, in 2001, a charter plane carrying some members of the Oklahoma State University basketball team crashed, killing all

(continues)

Dealing with Tragedy *(continued)*

onboard. By the time the other plane carrying the rest of the team arrived back home from the away game, news reports were already on the air about the disaster.

At the time, there was no plan for how to handle such an emergency. They do have a plan in place now. In the immediate aftermath of such a tragedy making decisions on how to proceed can be difficult. By having a plan in place the chain of command and duties are clearly spelled out which can speed the process of notifying all the parties involved, initiating counseling services and handling all the other details. The plan establishes guidelines and procedures for coping with the aftermath of any situation that traumatically affects the athletes and athletic department staff. Incidents can include sudden death on the playing field, suicide, auto accidents, debilitating injury, or attacks.

EXPECTATIONS OF THE COACH

The coach is an integral member of the emergency team and in many instances can be the first responder to an emergency. The coach must be familiar with the emergency action plan, know his or her role in the plan, and be ready to provide CPR and/or first aid until more qualified personnel are on site. Figure 16.2 is a card that can be carried by the coach and referred to in emergency situations.

In the case of a catastrophic injury the coach may also have multiple roles. These may include notifying the director of athletics, assistant coaches, and/or team members as well as providing support and assistance to athletes and families.

CPR AND FIRST AID CERTIFICATION

According to the NCAA, certification in CPR, first aid, and prevention of disease transmission should be required of all athletics personnel associated with practices, competitions, and other training and conditioning activities (2). All coaches, whether regulated by NCAA or not, should obtain these certifications in the interest of their athletes. Other members of the sports medicine team have the primary responsibility for the care of injured athletes and under no circumstances should coaches practice medicine or another discipline without a license. However, coaches must be ready to provide appropriate care as a first responder until licensed health care professionals are on the scene.

THE UNCONSCIOUS ATHLETE

In situations where there is an unconscious athlete and the coach has no other members of the sports medicine team present, emergency medical assistance should be contacted immediately. The athlete could have a life-threatening injury and needs to be assessed immediately with the primary survey discussed below. If the athlete is wearing a helmet, do not remove it. If CPR is needed, the face mask can be cut away or a CPR mask with a breathing tube can be slipped under the face mask. These tools should be present at the site of practice and games. Athletic trainers carry this equipment. If athletic trainers will not be at the site, the coach should ensure there is ready access to these tools in case of an emergency.

Cut out card along solid line and fold on dotted lines.

National Athletic Trainers' Association

Coach
Emergency Action Card

● **COACHES ROLE IN EMERGENCY:** **CHECK → CALL → CARE**

1. Approach, but do not move injured person – maintain position.
2. Immediate CHECK of athlete or spectator.
   Airway – Breathing – Circulation – Bleeding)
3. CALL emergency phone number & give proper directions to site.
   (Police – EMS – Fire)
4. Make sure you have someone in charge of directing emergency vehicles to field.
5. CARE for injured person.
   (CPR – Rescue Breathing – Control Bleeding – Immobilize)
6. NEVER leave an injured person alone. Stay until EMS arrives to the scene.
7. EMERGENCY SUPPLY NEEDS:
   First Aid Kit – Phone – Blankets for Warming – AED Unit

Important Note: All athletic league coaches should be required to be trained and certified in CPR & First Aid. AED training should be required for those athletic leagues with AED units on property.

● **ATHLETIC TEAM MEDICAL HISTORY CONDITION REPORT:**

Names of athletes with possible medical conditions
(parent contact information – conditions, allergies & medications)

1. _____
2. _____
3. _____
4. _____

● **ATHLETIC FIELD LOCATIONS/DIRECTIONS:**

Names/addresses and directions of athletic field locations

1. _____
2. _____
3. _____
4. _____

● **IMPORTANT EMERGENCY CONTACTS & PHONE NUMBERS:**

EMERGENCY **911** OR (_ _ _) _ _ _ – _ _ _ _
LOCAL HOSPITAL ER: (_ _ _) _ _ _ – _ _ _ _
FACILITY SUPERVISOR NAME: _____ _ _ _ – _ _ _ _
ATHLETIC TRAINER NAME: _____ _ _ _ – _ _ _ _
ATHLETIC LEAGUE DIRECTOR NAME: _____ _ _ _ – _ _ _ _

● **ATHLETIC FIELD LOCK COMBINATIONS/KEY LOCATIONS OR OTHER INFORMATION:**

1. _____
2. _____
3. _____
4. _____

■ **FIGURE 16.2** Coach Emergency Action Card. This card can be copied and carried by the coach for use in emergency situations. (Courtesy of the National Athletic Trainers' Association.)

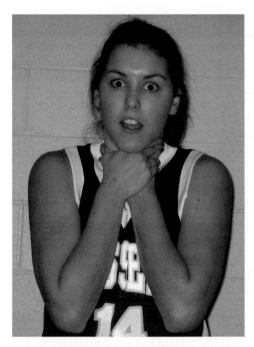

■ **FIGURE 16.3** Universal choking sign.

PRIMARY AND SECONDARY SURVEY

The primary survey is the immediate assessment of the injured athlete to determine if there are life-threatening problems requiring a rapid response. Once the athlete is stabilized, or life-threatening problems are ruled out, the secondary survey is done to gather further information about the injury or condition. As a first responder the coach should be most concerned with the primary survey. A secondary survey can often wait until a licensed health care professional is available.

Elements of the Primary Survey

If an athlete is unconscious and the coach is the only one at the scene, the first step is to send for emergency medical assistance. Then the primary survey can begin, which is essentially checking for vital signs or the ABCs:

A—airway
B—breathing
C—circulation

Additionally, the athlete should be checked for severe bleeding and shock. While coaches are not expected to fully assess the ABCs, they should be able to recognize when they are not normal.

AIRWAY

The airway in a conscious athlete can be checked by listening for gasping or choking noises. Ask the athlete, can you speak? If speech is possible the airway is likely open. If the athlete cannot speak and is displaying the universal choking sign of hands placed at the throat (Fig. 16.3), back blows and abdominal thrusts (Fig. 16.4) are needed to displace the object that is blocking the airway.

If the athlete is unconscious and not breathing, the head must be positioned using the head tilt/chin lift technique (Fig. 16.5) to open the airway. If the athlete is still not breathing after opening the airway (Fig. 16.6), rescue breathing is initiated.

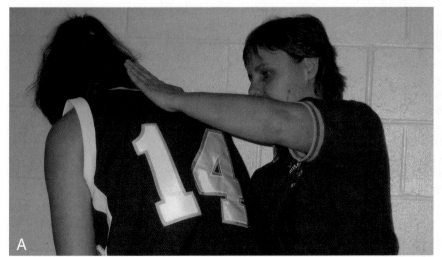
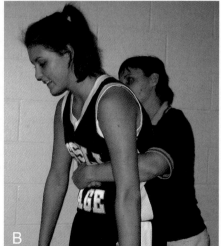

■ **FIGURE 16.4** Alternate 5 back blows **(A)** with 5 abdominal thrusts **(B)** to attempt to dislodge an object obstructing the airway. With a fisted hand placed just above the navel, the thrust is in an inward and upward direction.

Anaphylaxis and Epinephrine Administration

Anaphylaxis is a severe allergic reaction that can cause life-threatening swelling and obstruction of the airways. Emergency medical personnel should be contacted as soon as anaphylaxis is suspected. Epinephrine administration is the cornerstone of emergency management of severe allergic reactions. Athletes with known severe allergic reactions to insect stings, certain foods, or other substances will likely have an epinephrine auto-injector (EpiPen) prescribed by their physician (1). These athletes should have their medication readily available at all times. To ensure this, a back-up dose can be kept with the medical kit of the team's athletic trainer or, in situations where there is no athletic trainer, it could be kept with the emergency kit the coach brings to practices. Since the medication has an expiration date, the date should be checked periodically to ensure the product can still be used when needed. If the medication is expired or looks cloudy, it should NOT be used.

Coaches should seek training in the use of the auto injector in case the athlete needs assistance with self-administration or is unable to do so and there is no athletic trainer or medical personnel present. As long as the medication has been prescribed by a physician, this assistance is appropriate, however, checking the laws of the state in which you reside is advised. For minors, consent from the player's parent to assist with injection should be obtained prior to the start of the season. Always determine whether the athlete has already taken the medication. Never administer another dose unless directed to do so by EMS. Following administration of the medication, the athlete should be transported to a medical facility for follow-up. The beneficial effects of the epinephrine can be of short duration and additional medication at the hospital may be needed (2). When EMS personnel arrive, give them the used auto-injector.

1. National First Aid Science Advisory Board. *Circulation.* 2005;112:IV-196–IV-203. Available online at http://circ.ahajournals.org/cgi/content/full/112/24_suppl/IV-196. Accessed November 19, 2007.
2. American Red Cross. *First Aid: Responding to Emergencies*, 4th ed. Yardley, PA: Stay Well, 2006.

BREATHING

If the athlete is conscious and you have determined the airway is open, listen for wheezing or other breathing difficulties and the rate of breathing (respiration). Does the athlete appear to be breathing too fast or too slow? Is the breathing shallow? Typical resting breathing rates can be found in Table 16.1. An athlete who has been active will have an elevated breathing rate which should return to normal within a few minutes. To determine breathing rate, count the number of times the chest and abdomen rise with inspiration for a period of 15 or 30 seconds and multiply by 4 or 2 respectively. If the athlete is having breathing difficulties send for emergency medical assistance.

CIRCULATION

Circulation can be checked by taking the pulse (heart rate) at the radial artery at the wrist or the carotid artery in the neck (Fig.

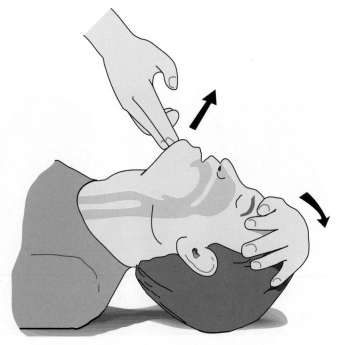

■ **FIGURE 16.5** Opening the airway: push down on the forehead with one hand and lift the chin using 2 to 3 fingers of the other hand. (LifeART image © 2008 Lippincott Williams & Wilkins. All rights reserved.)

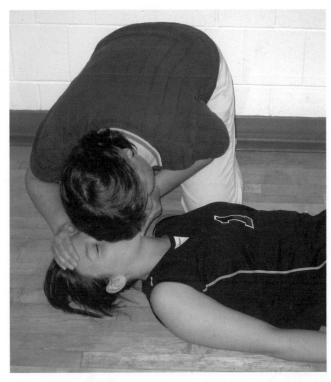

■ **FIGURE 16.6** Look, listen, and feel for breathing. Look for movement of the chest while listening for sounds of breathing and feeling for expiration on your face.

16.7). Fingers, and not the thumb, should be used to feel the pulse since the thumb has its own pulse. Count the number of beats in 15 or 30 seconds and multiply by 4 or 2 respectively. Typical resting heart rates can be found in Table 16.2. Athletes often have lower than average resting heart rates. The heart rate will be elevated following activity, but should return to resting level within a few minutes. When taking the pulse also feel for the regularity and strength of the beat.

In addition to checking the pulse, circulation can be assessed by evaluating the appearance of the skin, lips, and nail beds. If they seem blue, there is likely a circulation problem. If that occurs or if the heart rate is irregular, faint, or too fast, send for emergency medical assistance.

Elements of the Secondary Survey

After completing the primary survey and determining that there are no life-threatening emergencies, the coach may need to conduct a secondary survey if no other licensed health care professional is present. The secondary survey is done to determine the site and severity of the injury and to help decide if and how the athlete will be transported from the playing field. A more thorough secondary survey can be done later by the athletic trainer and/or physician.

As with the primary survey a systematic approach can be used to ensure a thorough assessment. The HIT acronym can be helpful in remembering the steps (6).

H—History
I—Inspection
T—Touch

HISTORY

History is the gathering of relevant information about the injury or illness. The athlete is asked about what happened including what was heard or felt when the incident occurred. This helps identify the type of injury and location. This information guides the inspection in the next step.

INSPECTION

A visual inspection is made of the injured area and it is compared to the uninjured part of the body. A deformity, swelling, and discoloration can be readily apparent on visual inspection. This information helps to further pinpoint the site and nature of the injury.

TABLE 16.1 Resting Breathing Rates	
Age Group	**Breathing Rate at Rest (beats per minute)**
Children 1–10	20–40
Children over 10 and adults	10–20

TOUCH

Touch, or palpation, is the third step in which the injured region is gently felt to gather additional information. An area that may not show any visible signs of injury can be very tender to touch, indicating damage to internal structures. Palpation should be done by starting away from the suspected injured site and gently moving towards the injured area with a light touch of the fingertips. Palpation can reveal point tenderness, skin temperature, and deformity. Sensation can also be determined by asking the athlete if your touch is being felt.

Once all the information is gathered the coach will have a better idea about the seriousness of the injury, the immediate first aid that might be necessary, and if and how the athlete should be removed from the playing field.

MANAGING SHOCK

Shock is the result of insufficient delivery of oxygen to the tissues. There are different types of shock, depending on the cause, but the signs, symptoms, and treatment are similar. In athletics, trauma and hemorrhage are common causes. Shock can be considered under two broad categories: compensatory and progressive. In compensatory shock the athlete's body is able to compensate for the shock and there may not be any overt evidence of shock. In more severe cases or when interventions are delayed or inadequate the body cannot compensate and clinical manifestations become evident. This can be considered progressive shock.

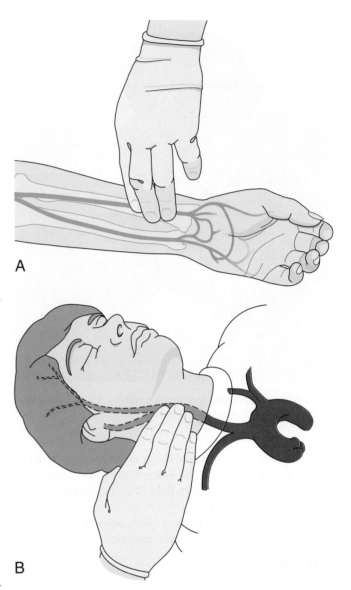

■ **FIGURE 16.7 A.** Radial pulse. The radial artery is palpated near the wrist on the thumb side of the forearm. Note the use of fingers (not thumb). **B.** Carotid pulse. Use gentle pressure to palpate the carotid pulse on either side of the neck. (LifeART image © 2008 Lippincott Williams & Wilkins. All rights reserved.)

TABLE 16.2 Resting Heart Rates	
Age Group	**Heart Rate at Rest (beats per minute)**
Children 1–10	70–120
Children over 10 and adults	60–100
Well-trained athletes	40–60

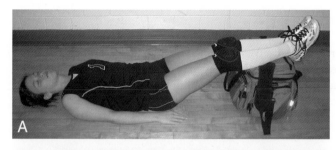
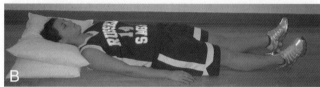

■ **FIGURE 16.8** Positioning for shock. **A.** If a spinal injury is not suspected, position with the legs elevated 8 to 12 inches. **B.** Elevate the head for a suspected head injury (if a spinal injury is not suspected). Once positioned, cover the athlete to keep warm.

Signs and Symptoms

Shock is often indicated by the presence of the following, which typically appear in the order presented below (7):

- Altered mental status
  - restlessness
  - anxiety
  - combativeness
  - progressive deterioration of level of consciousness
- Pale, cool, moist skin
- Nausea and vomiting
- Vital sign changes
  - Rapid, weak pulse
  - Rapid, shallow respirations progressing to slow, labored respirations
  - Decreased blood pressure

In compensatory shock, changes in breathing and blood pressure are not usually evident. The heart rate will be increased and the skin will be cool, pale, and moist. Mild anxiety can also be present.

Emergency Treatment

The first person on the scene should call for additional help and initiate simple emergency treatment. The individual should be kept warm and in most situations positioned so the legs are elevated about 8 to 12 inches to facilitate blood return to the heart (Fig. 16.8A). Any bleeding should be stopped. The positioning depends on the injury. For example, if there is a suspected head injury the head and shoulders should be elevated (Fig. 16.8B). If there is a suspected spinal injury the athlete should not be moved, and a fractured leg should not be elevated until it is immobilized (8).

Someone in shock or with any serious injury should not be given food or drink as it could cause nausea and vomiting. This could result in aspiration (inhalation) of foreign material into the lungs. If surgery is needed food and liquid can cause complications (9).

CONTROLLING BLEEDING

Injuries can result in both external and internal bleeding. While external bleeding is obvious, internal bleeding is not unless it is visible through a body opening. Internal bleeding in the muscles, which appears as a bruise, is generally not dangerous. However, bleeding within a body cavity is very serious and difficult to detect. If an athlete sustains an internal injury, medical attention is required for observation and treatment.

There are three types of external bleeding: arterial, venous and capillary.

1. Arterial: loss of blood from an artery and is characterized by bright red blood that spurts with each heart beat. This is the most serious type of bleeding.
2. Venous: loss of blood from a vein and is characterized by dark blood that flows steadily.
3. Capillary: loss of blood from the small capillaries that are located near the surface of the skin and is characterized by a slow flow of blood.

Severe bleeding is known as hemorrhage and can lead to shock and death if not properly treated. Stopping the bleeding is essential. While waiting for emergency assistance the coach may need to take steps to control the bleeding.

Techniques to Manage Bleeding

Bleeding is commonly controlled by using direct pressure. When trained health care professionals are not able to control severe bleeding with direct pressure and elevation, they may use pressure points. Pressure is placed on the artery where it is close to an underlying bone to help diminish blood flow through the artery. Standard precautions (see below) must be used when exposed to someone's blood and bodily fluids.

DIRECT PRESSURE

Using direct pressure is the most common and effective way to control bleeding (7). Ideally, a sterile dressing is applied over the wound and direct pressure is applied with a gloved hand (Fig. 16.9). If you do not have a glove or appropriate barrier, you can have the injured athlete apply pressure with his or her hand (9). Clean cloth can be used if sterile gauze is not available. A dressing should not be removed once

FROM THE ATHLETIC TRAINING ROOM

Safely Removing Contaminated Gloves

Protecting yourself by wearing gloves when handling potentially infectious body fluids must be followed by proper removal of the gloves to avoid any contact with what may now be on the outside surface of the gloves. Only touch "dirty to dirty" and "clean to clean" surfaces. The outer surface of the gloves is considered dirty and the inside surface and your hands are considered clean. When finished handling a wound, take care to remove the gloves prior to touching any other surface. Below is the method currently taught by the American Red Cross for safely removing contaminated gloves (1).

Step 1—Partial Removal of First Glove
Partially remove one glove by pinching it at the wrist with the other gloved hand being careful to touch only the outside surface.

Carefully pull the glove toward the fingertips without removing it completely. The glove will turn inside out as you pull it away.

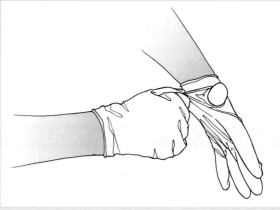

Step 2—Removal of Second Glove
Similar to what was done with the first glove, pinch the outside surface of the second glove with your partially gloved hand. Carefully pull the second glove toward the fingertips letting it turn inside out and completely remove it.

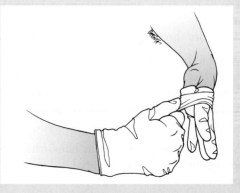

(continues)

Safely Removing Contaminated Gloves *(continued)*

Step 3—Finishing Glove Removal
With your free hand, only touching the clean interior surface of the gloves, grasp both gloves and completely remove the first glove.

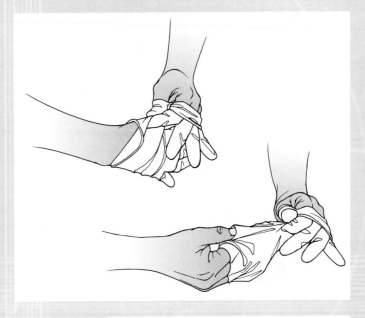

Step 4—Cleanup
Discard the gloves in an appropriate container for biohazardous waste. Wash your hands thoroughly with soap and water. If not possible, use a waterless gel hand cleaner until you are able to wash with soap and water.

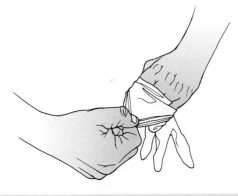

1. American Red Cross. *First Aid: Responding to Emergencies*, 4th ed. Yardley, PA: StayWell; 2006.

it is placed because removal may destroy clots that have formed. If the dressing becomes soaked with blood additional layers should be applied over it.

ELEVATION

Elevation is used by health care professionals along with direct pressure to control bleeding as long as a fracture is not suspected. Elevating the limb above the level of the heart allows gravity to help reduce the blood pressure in the limb and slows the bleeding.

BLOODBORNE PATHOGENS AND STANDARD (UNIVERSAL) PRECAUTIONS

Bloodborne pathogens are disease causing microorganisms that are transmitted through blood or blood components, sexual contact, and perinatally from mother to infant. Human immunodeficiency virus (HIV), hepatitis B virus (HBV), and hepatitis C virus (HCV) are ones of primary concern in athletics. While they are of concern, the risk of acquiring a bloodborne infection during a sporting event is negligible (10,11). The terms standard and universal precautions are often used synonymously. Universal precautions is the term that was first introduced and now the term standard precautions expands the elements of universal precautions into a standard of care designed to protect individuals from pathogens that can be spread by blood or any other body fluid, secretion, or excretion (except sweat).

There is a higher concentration in blood of HBV than HIV and HBV is more stable in the environment (12). HBV is 50 to 100 times more infectious than HIV

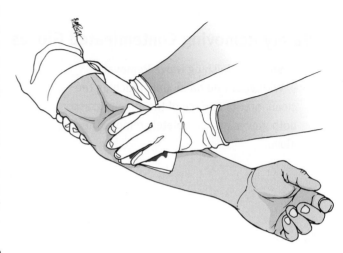

■ **FIGURE 16.9** Direct pressure to control bleeding. Note the gloved hands.

(13). Because HBV can be transmitted via inanimate objects, the risk of HBV transmission in sports is probably greater than other bloodborne infections. Athletes who participate in contact and collision sports and those who travel to regions of the world where HBV is endemic may also be at higher risk (14).

Avoidance of high risk sexual behaviors, sharing needles, and sharing personal articles that could contaminate mucous membranes along with HBV inoculation and practicing standard precautions can help prevent transmission (15). Personal choices related to sexual behavior and illicit drug use with shared needles for injection of steroids, hormones, and vitamins put athletes at greater risk than participation in athletics (12). Ongoing educational programs should teach athletes about these diseases and their prevention. Cuts, sores, and open wounds in the oral cavity can be a means of transmission. Therefore, athletes should have their own water containers and not share toothbrushes and other oral appliances. Transmission of HBV is reduced with inoculation (15,16). Athletes, those who train them, treat their injuries, and handle their equipment can all be inoculated for HBV to further reduce the incidence of transmission.

Universal precautions, as defined by the Centers for Disease Control, are practices designed to prevent transmission of bloodborne pathogens when providing first aid or health care (17). With these precautions, blood and other body fluids of all individuals are considered potentially infectious. Using precautions with everyone is a nondiscriminatory practice. Because the theoretical risk of infection in sport is through contact with blood or body fluids containing blood, prevention of transmission should focus on bleeding injuries. The following practices should be employed in the athletic setting to reduce the possibility of virus transmission (18).

1. All athletics personnel (coaches, athletic trainers, equipment managers, student managers) should be trained in standard precautions including first aid, infection control, and access and use of supplies. Supplies include gloves (nonlatex for those with latex allergies); eye and clothing protection; bleach and/or disinfectant; and biohazard containers for soiled clothing and towels, gloves and dressings, and needles and other sharp instruments.

2. All wounds should be treated prior to an event or as they occur during an event. An occlusive dressing should be used that can withstand the forces of training or competition. This limits contamination to others from the wound and covers a point of entry.

3. If bleeding occurs during an event, in addition to stopping the bleeding and covering the wound, all blood should be cleansed from the skin, hair, and nails of the athlete and the uniform should be changed if soiled with blood. Changing a uniform is not required if only small amounts of dried blood are present since that does not pose a risk for transmission of bloodborne pathogens (19). An athlete should only be returned to play if the wound is completely covered and there is no bleeding through or around the dressing.

4. Gloves used to treat the wound should be disposed of prior to touching other surfaces and hands should be washed.
5. Any surface that was contaminated with a blood spill should be cleaned with a bleach solution (1:10 bleach/water) or commercial disinfectant that kills bloodborne pathogens. These agents are not intended for direct contact with skin or uniforms.
6. Soiled uniforms and other contaminated linens that are normally washed should be placed in a designated, labeled container to prevent secondary contamination. Laundry personnel should handle these items with gloves and launder so they are disinfected.

FROM THE ATHLETIC TRAINING ROOM

Community-Acquired MRSA Infections (CA-MRSA)

Staphylococcus aureus, commonly known as staph, is a bacteria that is carried on the skin or in the nose of healthy people. Methicillin-resistant *Staphylococcus aureus* (MRSA) is a type of staph that is resistant to antibiotics. While 25% to 30% of the population has staph colonized (present, but not causing infection) in the nose, approximately 1% is colonized with MRSA (1).

While staph infections, including MRSA, most frequently occur in hospital and healthcare settings, they are present elsewhere. When MRSA is acquired outside of the health care arena it is known as community-acquired MRSA (CA-MRSA). Staph, including MRSA, can cause simple skin infections that look like a pimple or boil. They can also cause redness, swelling, and pain or have pus and drainage. More serious infections can lead to pneumonia or infections in the bloodstream.

CA-MRSA can develop from person-to-person contact, sharing of towels and other personal items, and contact with contaminated equipment and surfaces such as mats and pads. The best way to prevent infection is good hygiene and avoiding contact with drainage from skin lesions. These infections could easily spread among team members if proper precautions are not taken. The following are among the things that can be done to help prevent MRSA infections (2):

1. Hands should be cleaned regularly by washing thoroughly with soap and water or with an alcohol-based hand sanitizer.
2. Showering immediately following activity should be encouraged.
3. Whirlpools and common tubs should not be used with open wounds, scrapes or scratches.
4. Skin lesions should be cleaned and appropriately covered before participation.
5. Towels, razors and athletic gear should not be shared.
6. Athletic gear and towels should be washed after each use.
7. Active skin lesions should be evaluated by appropriate medical personnel.
8. Contact with other people's wounds or bandages should be avoided.

1. Centers for Disease Control and Prevention. *Community-Associated MRSA Information for the Public.* Available online at http://www.cdc.gov/ncidod/dhqp/ar_mrsa_ca_public.html. Accessed November 19, 2007.
2. National Athletic Trainers' Association. *Official statement from the National Athletic Trainers' Association on Community-Acquired MRSA Infections (CA-MRSA).* March 1, 2005. Available online at http://www.nata.org/publicinformation/docs/MRSA_Statement.pdf. Accessed November 19, 2007.

MOVING AND TRANSPORTING THE INJURED ATHLETE

A primary role of the coach is to minimize injury to the athletes. When an injury does occur, risk of further injury by moving the athlete must be avoided. Unless trained in first aid and safe methods of transport, the coach should not attempt to move a seriously injured athlete except for life-threatening conditions. At the beginning of the season the coach can instruct the team not to move an injured teammate and can reinforce this throughout the season. While their intentions may be good, teammates may exacerbate injuries by moving the injured athlete. Many injuries require immobilization or splinting before the athlete can be moved safely. This is best done by trained emergency personnel.

To Move or not to Move a Critically Injured Athlete

In cases of serious and life-threatening injuries emergency medical assistance should be called and the athlete kept still until assistance arrives. However, there may be situations when the coach is the only person on the scene and prior to the arrival of emergency assistance the athlete must be moved because of life-threatening conditions or there is danger of further harm without moving the athlete. An unconscious athlete who is not breathing or without a pulse and is lying on the stomach or side must be moved to the supine (face up) position for immediate administration of CPR. In cases of environmental emergencies such as tornadoes, hurricanes, lightening, fire, flooding, or a dangerous traffic scene such as might occur when involved in an accident while traveling to a game, an injured athlete may need to be immediately moved because of potential further harm by remaining. Whenever an injured, unconscious athlete is moved, assume that there could be a head or spine injury and always immobilize the head, neck, and back to the best of your ability.

ONE PERSON DRAG

If you need to move an unconscious athlete by yourself to a safer environment, the one person drag can be used (Fig. 16.10). Squat facing the athlete's head and place your hands under the armpits as you cradle the head with your forearms. Slowly drag the athlete to a safer location trying to keep the head and neck aligned with the spine. To protect your back, maintain the normal curve of your spine.

ONE PERSON ROLL

If you are faced with the situation of an athlete needing to be repositioned for rescue breathing, CPR, or drainage of vomit and no other help is immediately available, you can use the one person roll. If the athlete is in the prone (face-down) position and in need of rescue breathing or CPR, the individual needs to be rolled to supine (Fig. 16.11).

If an unconscious athlete is vomiting, he or she should be positioned on the side to allow drainage and prevent choking. If the athlete is supine, the individual must be rolled in a similar manner to a side-lying position.

Moving Athletes with Suspected Spinal Injury

In cases of a suspected spinal injury, the athletic trainer and/or emergency management personnel should be summoned immediately and no attempt should be made to move the athlete until they arrive, except in the situations noted above. A four or more person rescue team is used to move the athlete to a spine board with one

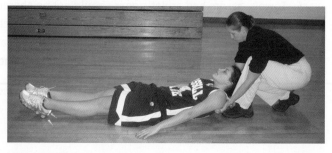

■ **FIGURE 16.10** The one-person drag can be used to move an athlete in an emergency situation.

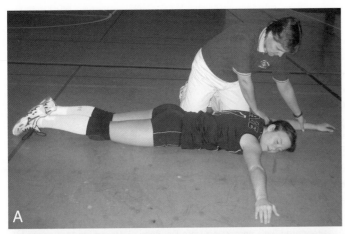

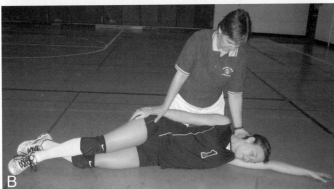
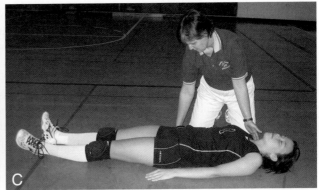

■ **FIGURE 16.11** One person roll to position athlete for CPR. **A.** Position yourself near head and place the arms as illustrated. **B.** Cradle the head with one hand to help stabilize the neck and use your other hand at the hip to roll the athlete toward you. **C.** Continue to roll to supine and reposition the overhead arm to the side. Roll head, neck, and back in unison.

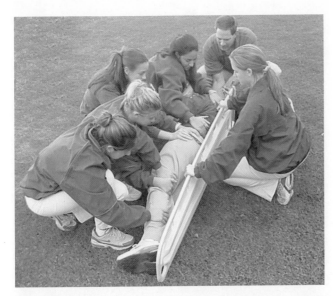

■ **FIGURE 16.12** Log roll to move athlete onto a stretcher. (Reprinted with permission from Del Rossi G, Horodyski M, Powers ME. A comparison of spine-board transfer techniques and the effect of training on performance. *J Athl Train* 2003;38(3):99–104.)

person serving as the leader and directing movement to ensure that the head and neck are stabilized and that the body is moved as one unit. A log-roll technique, rolling the athlete to one side to place the board and then rolling the athlete back onto the board, is a method commonly used (Fig. 16.12). Another method is the lift-and-slide technique where the athlete is lifted off the surface as a unit with support at the head, torso and legs and the stretcher is slid underneath and the athlete lowered onto the stretcher (Fig. 16.13). A coach could be asked to help with these maneuvers. A recent study comparing the techniques found that head motion was better restricted with the lift-and-slide method (20). The subjects in the study did not have injuries so further investigation is needed to determine which technique is better when there is instability in the neck.

Moving Athletes with Noncritical Injuries

Athletes with noncritical injuries can be moved in various ways. If a fracture is suspected, the athlete should not be moved until the limb is splinted to prevent any further damage to the limb. Emergency personnel should be summoned. They will use a variety of splints depending on the nature of the injury. A stretcher is a safe method to move an athlete a short distance following a suspected fracture or other serious injury.

With less severe injuries athletes can be assisted off the playing field with the support of one or two individuals holding the

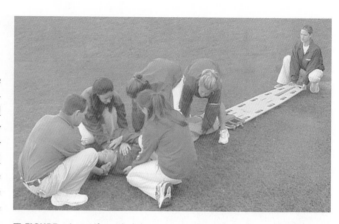

■ **FIGURE 16.13** Lift and slide technique to place athlete on stretcher. (Reprinted with permission from Del Rossi G, Horodyski M, Powers ME. A comparison of spine-board transfer techniques and the effect of training on performance. *J Athl Train* 2003;38(3):99–104.)

athlete around the waist and the athlete's arms holding on to the shoulder of those giving assistance (Fig. 16.14). When greater assistance is needed or a longer distance needs to be covered than can be done with ease using the walking assist, a carrying assist can be used (Fig 16.15). Two people grasp each other's forearm and the athlete sits on the forearms holding on around the shoulders and those giving assistance support the back with the free hand. Before using either of these techniques the athlete needs to be carefully assessed to be sure there are no major injuries.

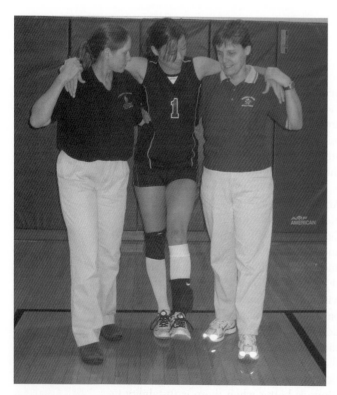

■ **FIGURE 16.14** Two person walking assist for noncritically injured athlete.

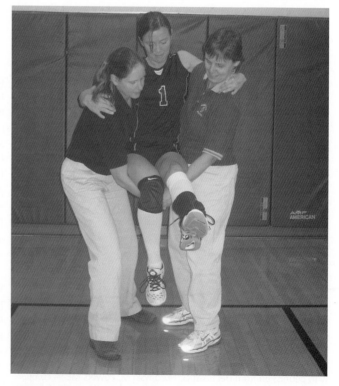

■ **FIGURE 16.15** Two person carrying assist for noncritically injured athlete who needs additional support.

Use of Crutches

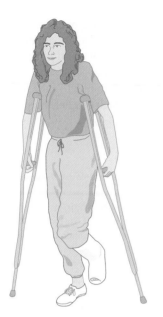

■ **FIGURE 16.16** Correct body position with crutches. Note the space between the top of the crutches and the axilla (arm pit). To help prevent blisters, there is padding on the contact points which are the axillary supports and hand grips. (LifeART image © 2008 Lippincott Williams & Wilkins. All Rights Reserved.)

Following an injury that requires nonweight-bearing or partial weight-bearing on the injured lower extremity, an athlete is fitted with crutches (Fig. 16.16). While issuing and fitting crutches is beyond the scope of practice for the coach, knowledge of their appropriate use can be helpful in ensuring that the athlete complies with safe use of the crutches. A common faulty practice in the use of axillary crutches is to hang on the axillary support (top piece of the crutch). This can put excessive pressure on the nerves that pass through the axilla (armpit) and can result in muscle weakness and diminished sensation from the nerve damage (21).

When using crutches on stairs, the crutches remain with the injured limb. When going up stairs the sound limb goes first followed by the crutches with the injured limb. When going downstairs, the crutches and injured limb go first followed by the sound limb. The phrase, up with the "good" and down with the "bad," can be used to remember which limb goes first when going up and down stairs.

SUMMARY

- Athletic injuries and other emergencies can arise at any time. Because the coach can often be the first person on the scene, knowledge of emergency procedures is essential as well as training in CPR and first aid.
- An emergency plan that includes personnel, communication, equipment, and transportation should be in place for the well-being of the athletes and to help protect the institution or organization in case of legal action. The plan should be in writing, everyone who will be using the plan must be familiarized with it, and the plan should be rehearsed.
- A plan to deal with catastrophic incidents, such as the sudden death or disabling injury of an athlete or coach, should also be in place and the plan should include the chain of command and the actions that will take place following the incident. The coach may have multiple roles in the plan including notifying the director of athletics, assistant coaches, and/or team members as well as providing support and assistance to athletes and families.
- Following an injury a primary survey is done to determine if there are life-threatening problems requiring a rapid response. Once the athlete is stabilized or life-threatening problems are ruled out the secondary survey is done to gather further information about the injury or condition. While neither is a primary responsibility of the coach, as a first responder the coach may need to conduct a primary survey.
- The primary survey includes checking the ABCs (airway, breathing, circulation) and checking for bleeding and shock.
- Trauma and hemorrhage are common causes of shock. While waiting for assistance someone suffering from shock should be kept warm and in most situations the legs should be elevated higher than the heart.
- Bleeding can usually be controlled with direct pressure over the wound.
- Blood may contain pathogens such as HIV (human immunodeficiency virus), HBV (hepatitis B virus), and HCV (hepatitis C virus). Precautions should be taken to prevent transmission. Athletes are far more likely to acquire these viruses through risky personal behavior than through sports participation.

- Under most circumstances the coach should not move a seriously injured athlete and should wait until assistance arrives. If an injured, unconscious athlete must be moved in an emergency situation, assume there could be a head or spine injury and try to first immobilize the head, neck and back. An athlete with noncritical injuries can be assisted off the field with a walking or carrying assist.
- Following a lower extremity injury that requires limited weight-bearing, an athlete may need to use crutches to unweight the limb. By knowing proper crutch technique the coach can help ensure that the athlete uses the crutches safely.

References

1. Anderson JC, Courson RW, Kleiner DM, et al. National Athletic Trainer's Association position statement: emergency planning in athletics. *J Athl Train* 2002;37:99–104.
2. National Collegiate Athletic Association. *Sports Medicine Handbook 2007–2008.* Available online at http://www.ncaa.org/library/sports_sciences/sports_med_handbook/2007-08/2007-08_sports_medicine_handbook.pdf. Accessed November 19, 2007.
3. Shultz SJ, Zinder SM, Valovich TC. *Sports Medicine Handbook.* Indianapolis, IN: National Federation of State High School Associations, 2001.
4. Courson R, Navitskis L, Patel H. Emergency-action planning. *Athl Ther Today* 2005;10(2):7–15.
5. National Athletic Trainer's Association. *Official Statement—Automated External Defibrillators.* Available online at http://www.nata.org/statements/official/AEDofficialstatement.pdf. Accessed November 19, 2007.
6. Flegel MJ. *Sport First Aid: A Coach's Guide to Preventing and Responding to Injuries,* 3rd ed. Champaign, IL: Human Kinetics, 2004.
7. Limmer D, O'Keefe MF, Dickinson ET. *Emergency Care,* 10th ed. Upper Saddle River, NJ: Pearson Education, Inc., 2005.
8. Prentice WE, Arnheim DD. *Essentials of Athletic Injury Management,* 6th ed. New York, NY: McGraw Hill, 2005.
9. American Red Cross. *First Aid: Responding to Emergencies,* 4th ed. Yardley, PA: StayWell, 2006.
10. Dorman JM. Contagious diseases in competitive sport: what are the risks? *J Am Coll Health* 2000;49:105–109.
11. Pirozzolo JJ, LeMay DC. Blood-borne infections. *Clin Sports Med* 2007;26:425–431.
12. Mast EE, Goodman RA, Bond WW, et al. Transmission of blood-borne pathogens during sports: risk and prevention. *Ann Intern Med* 1995;122:283–285.
13. World Health Organization. *Fact sheet N°204: Hepatitis B.* Available online at http://www.who.int/mediacentre/factsheets/fs204/en/print.html. Accessed November 19, 2007.
14. Kordi R, Wallace WA. Blood borne infections in sport: risks of transmission, methods of prevention, and recommendations for hepatitis B vaccination. *Br J Sports Med* 2004;38:678–684.
15. Centers for Disease Control and Prevention. *Hepatitis B Fact Sheet.* July 27, 2007. Available online at http://www.cdc.gov/ncidod/diseases/hepatitis/b/fact.htm. Accessed November 19, 2007.
16. American Academy of Pediatrics. Human immunodeficiency virus and other blood-borne viral pathogens in the athletic setting. *Pediatrics* 1999;104:1400–1403.
17. Centers for Disease Control and Prevention. *Universal Precautions for Prevention of Transmission of HIV and Other Bloodborne Infections.* Available online at http://www.cdc.gov/ncidod/dhqp/bp_universal_precautions.html. Accessed November 19, 2007.
18. National Association of Intercollegiate Athletics. *Medical Guidelines.* Available online at http://naia.cstv.com/member-services/training/medical.htm. Accessed November 19, 2007.
19. Mast EE, Goodman RA. Prevention of infectious disease transmission in sports. *Sports Med* 1997;24:1–7.
20. Del Rossi G, Horodyski M, Powers ME. A comparison of spine-board transfer techniques and the effect of training on performance. *J Athl Train* 2003;38:204–208.
21. Raikin S, Froimson MI. Bilateral brachial plexus compressive neuropathy (crutch palsy). *J Orthop Trauma* 1997;11:136–138.

CPR and First Aid Resources

American Red Cross
http://www.redcross.org/services/hss/courses/

American Heart Association
http://www.americanheart.org/cpr

National Safety Council
http://www.nsc.org/

Psychology and Sports Injuries

Upon reading this chapter, the coach should be able to:

1. Explain the psychological factors that increase risk of injury.
2. Understand how feelings of excess stress can interfere with peak performance and increase risk of injury.
3. Explain and recommend appropriate stress management practices to athletes to prevent and cope with injury.
4. Discuss the importance of developing good mental focus and awareness to increase peak performance and prevent injury.
5. Encourage your athletes to train hard and work through the discomfort of appropriate overload, but take injury symptoms seriously.
6. Understand the range of emotions athletes may experience following sports injuries.
7. Provide appropriate emotional support and give direction to injured players to encourage good rehabilitation program adherence.
8. Help recovering athletes train safely and effectively so that they may overcome anxieties about returning to play.

Gabe's arm was broken during an ice hockey game early in the season in his junior year in college. The break was complicated and painful, and Gabe was told to stay off the ice for at least 6 weeks. When he asked the athletic trainer whether he would be able to play in any of the games later in the season, the athletic trainer looked at him sadly and said, "We'll have to see. We don't want you to experience another collision and reinjury." Gabe was pretty sure the answer was athletic training code for "No."

Riding the exercise bike in the training room was incredibly boring compared to being on the ice. Gabe's legs and spirit both tired quickly. After several days, Gabe developed a bad cold and stayed away from the training room for over 3 weeks. He did not go to very many of the hockey games, as he could not stand sitting on the side lines. When he went to parties with the team he felt left out and distant from his teammates. He wondered why the coach never emailed to ask how he was doing. A month after his injury, 10 pounds heavier, and with atrophied muscles, Gabe did not even feel at home in his body. Depressed and lonely, Gabe could not think of anything he really enjoyed in life, and thought about dropping out of college.

We tend to discuss injury as something that happens to a part of the body, as a physical occurrence, with physical causes and physical symptoms. In fact, that is what we have done during the last four chapters, because understanding the physical nature of sports injuries is critical to your work as a coach. But the physical aspect of a sport injury is only a part of the story, just as the athlete's body is only part of the athlete. Every coach knows that an athlete's thoughts, feelings, and spirit all contribute to sport performance, and are important parts of every athlete. While the physical part of the athlete and of the injury is the most visible, it is important to consider the whole athlete when studying sports medicine.

This chapter provides a brief overview of the psychological forces that help you understand sports injuries. We will begin with a consideration of the psychological factors that have been found to contribute to the occurrence of injuries, and a discussion of what a coach can do to help athletes compete with more focus and awareness. Standard mental training procedures are easy to incorporate into your practices, and will both improve your athletes' performance and decrease risk of injury. In addition, coaches can create an emotional climate that encourages athletes to understand potential injury symptoms, rather than projecting the idea that pain should always be ignored, or that injured athletes are sissies or wimps. You can encourage your athletes to train hard and work through the discomfort of appropriate overload, but still take injury symptoms seriously. Athletes who hide symptoms and play while injured often run the risk of a more serious injury later in the season.

Your job is to train athletes and prepare them for contests, and the athlete's job is to follow your directions regarding training and competition. What is the coach's role once an athlete has sustained an injury and can no longer compete? An injury interrupts this relationship, and suddenly you can no longer train the athlete, and the athlete can no longer look to you for instruction. Yet you may remain an important person in that athlete's life. You must take on a new role and coach in a new way. The show must go on, and most of your time will still go to training the rest of your team, but you can continue to support your injured player in several important ways. The next section in this chapter will help you better understand what your injured athletes are going through emotionally. We will discuss how athletes respond to injury, and the many ways, both good and bad, that athletes attempt to cope with sports injury. We will offer suggestions for ways that coaches can be helpful during the rehabilitation process.

Once your injured athlete has completed rehabilitation and is cleared to play, you may both wish you could pick up where you left off weeks, or even months, earlier. But the athlete who has returned to play is not the same person you were previously coaching. Athletes returning to play need your help to get back into physical and mental condition and ready for competition. This can be a very difficult period for athletes and their coaches, as athletes cope with the fear of reinjury, and the discouragement of deconditioning and the loss of their place on the team. You may feel frustrated that they are not playing as well as they used to, and wonder whether they are worth your effort. We will discuss what a coach can do to help returning players regain skill and confidence, and to train for peak performance.

PSYCHOLOGICAL FACTORS INFLUENCE AN ATHLETE'S RISK OF INJURY

Injury happens. Every athlete (and indeed, every person) is at some risk of sustaining an injury. Many factors have been shown to increase an athlete's risk of injury. Physical differences explain why some athletes on your team are more likely to sustain injuries than others; some athletes are simply more prone to tendonitis and other overuse injuries, even though their technique is correct and you train them appropriately. And of course, many injuries boil down to bad luck: athletes are playing fine but in one heartbeat they "land wrong" and tear their ACLs, or collide and sustain a concussion. In addition to physical characteristics and bad luck, researchers have found that certain psychological factors predispose some athletes to a higher risk of injury. The factors which have the most research support include high levels of negative stress, high levels of performance anxiety, negative mood, and poor coping skills (1).

High Levels of Negative Stress

Several researchers have found associations between high levels of stress and an increased risk of injury (2,3). The effect of stress levels on sport performance and injury risk depends upon the volume of stress in athletes' lives, and whether that stress is perceived to be positive or negative (1).

The word "stress" means different things to different people (4,5). Athletes use the word stress to refer to both sources of stress (called stressors in the psychology literature) and their physical and psychological response to stressors. In most people's minds, the two are intertwined: you have too much work to do, you feel stressed.

Coaches must realize that athletes vary in response to a given stress load. Situations some athletes find stimulating and challenging can put other athletes "over the edge." To a great extent, an athlete's perception of stress determines his or her stress response. In other words, if athletes *feel* stressed, even if you do not think they have too many demands being placed on them, they are stressed, and may experience negative stress effects, such as trouble sleeping, difficulty concentrating, and so forth.

Stress can pile up in an athlete's life in many ways. Overtraining and underrecovery create stress. Stress from other areas of an athlete's life in turn contributes to the symptoms of overtraining. Student-athletes often feel that they have too much to do in too little time, and complain of too much pressure. Even positive demands (for example, being asked to play an important role on the team, participating in exciting tournaments, or enjoying visits from off-campus friends) can create stress as athletes' schedules become too packed. Positive demands also require accommodation and adjustment, which in turn can create feelings of stress.

Especially toxic to an athlete's health and performance, however, are negative stressors. An athlete who perceives stressors as negative tends to view the sources of stress as being largely uncontrollable and as having a high probability of leading to negative outcomes (6). Stressors may be negative because of their content (e.g., the death of a loved one is almost universally regarded as a negative stressor) or because of a person's perception. Many situations can be perceived to be positive, neutral, or negative. Consider a game away from campus that will require extra travel time. One athlete might be thinking, "Yes! A chance to get away!" while another might be stressing out about less time to complete a paper due the following day. By definition, negative stress feels worse and is experienced as more problematic than positive stress. Not surprisingly, the physical and emotional responses to negative stress differ significantly from the response to positive stress, and are more likely to lead to stress-related health problems (7) as well as sports injury (2).

High Levels of Performance Anxiety

Anxiety is an emotional manifestation of stress characterized by fear and worry about the future. Anxiety is not necessarily a bad thing. An appropriate level of anxiety improves sport performance (8). It stimulates athletes to train and prepare for competition. Anxiety stimulates a stress response that speeds reflexes, increases strength and endurance, and sharpens thought. Athletes with the "right" amount of anxiety experience excitement and challenge as they face competition (9).

But when anxiety levels are too high, performance suffers and risk of injury increases (Fig. 17.1) (10,11). Athletes who are too anxious have difficulty focusing during competition and are less likely to make good decisions (8). They experience anxiety as distress and fear (9).

Many factors contribute to excessive levels of performance anxiety in athletes, and a coach has little control over most of them. Be sure your emotional tone is supportive and encouraging rather than derogatory or threatening. Athletes' parents and friends may put a lot of pressure on them to win. If you coach young athletes, and one of your athletes is very anxious and still living at home, a word to the parents might be appropriate. If you have athletes whose levels of anxiety interfere with performance (or life), refer them for counseling with a sports psychologist, if available, or other psychology professional. As they learn to reduce anxiety levels their performance may improve and they will also reduce risk of injury. They will also be a lot happier! Stress management techniques may also reduce anxiety levels in over-anxious athletes.

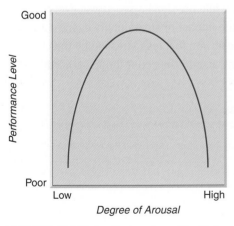

■ **FIGURE 17.1** Yerkes-Dodson Law. The Yerkes-Dodson Law, named after the psychologists who proposed this model in 1908, describes the relationship between arousal and performance (11). An athlete's performance of a given task improves as physiological arousal increases until some optimal point, after which performance declines as arousal continues to increase. Yerkes and Dodson noted that the optimal level of arousal varies with the type of task being performed and that higher levels of arousal seem to be more detrimental as the complexity of the task increases.

Do Certain Personality Traits Help Protect an Athlete from Injury?

Psychologists have long wondered why some people seem especially prone to the negative effects of stress while others seem to sail through the day with a workload that would overwhelm most. Researchers have come up with a profile of people who do a good job of balancing life's many demands without falling prey to the negative health effects of too much stress. One of the terms used to describe this type of personality is hardy (1). Research on athletes supports the notion that athletes who score high on measures of hardiness tend to be less prone to injury (2,3).

The following variables are components of the hardiness profile:

- Sense of control: Hardy people have a sense of control over the things that happen in their lives, or at least feel as though they have some options, as opposed to feeling helpless and hopeless in the face of stress.
- Sense of commitment: Hardy people feel a sense of commitment to the important people, activities, and values in their lives, such as their families, friends, school, work, and/or sport team. Hardy people are committed to personal values that help carry them through rough times, as opposed to feeling alienated and uninvolved.
- Sense of challenge: Hardy people see change and demands as challenges to be met rather than as obstacles standing in their way.
- Social support: Hardy people feel that there are others they can turn to for help. Social support refers not only to friends and family, but to acquaintances and helpful resources such as health services, counseling services, advisors, and so forth.
- Physical activity: Athletes are covered here! People who engage in regular physical activity tend to be more resistant to the negative effects of stress than their sedentary peers.

Other variables that appear to help protect athletes from the negative effects of stress include:

- Sense of optimism: Optimistic people see fewer sources of stress in life, while pessimists see stress everywhere they look. Optimism reduces feelings of stress, and thus buffers the impact of stressful life events (2).
- Positive self-esteem: When you believe you will be able to cope with stress, you feel less stressed by the circumstances of your life. Positive self-esteem increases your sense of control, and thus contributes to hardiness (2).

1. Kobasa SC, Maddi SR, Kahn S. Hardiness and health: a prospective study. *J Pers Soc Psychol* 1982;42:168–177.
2. Ford IW, Eklund RC, Gordon S. An examination of psychosocial variables moderating the relationship between life stress and injury time-loss among athletes of a high standard. *J Sports Sci* 2000;18(5):301–312.
3. Williams JM, Andersen MB. Psychosocial antecedents of sport injury: Review and critique of the stress and injury model. *J Appl Sport Psychol* 1998;10:5–25.

Negative Mood

Mood refers to a person's emotional state. A negative mood is usually experienced as a form of stress, and often attributed to excess stress. In a study by Galambos and colleagues (12), mood scores helped to predict risk of injury in a sample of 845 elite male and female athletes from a variety of sports. Higher injury rates were associated with higher scores for anger, fatigue, tension, and depression on a questionnaire measuring mood profile (12).

Many coaches have observed how mood can influence an athlete's performance. Just as anxiety can be helpful in appropriate amounts, anger, tension, and aggression can be experienced as energizing by many athletes. Too much anger, however, interferes with decision making and focus, and may cause reckless behavior that might lead to injury.

Fatigue and depression tend to go hand in hand. Fatigue and depression lower quality of life and drive to perform (13). Fatigue and depression are common stress symptoms, and may increase when vulnerable athletes feel excessively stressed.

Poor Coping Skills

Coping refers to a person's attempts to deal with a stressful situation. Psychologists generally divide coping responses into two categories: problem-focused coping that includes efforts to cope directly with the source of stress by changing it; and emotion-focused coping that includes efforts to reduce the person's feelings of stress, without dealing directly with the source of stress (Fig. 17.2) (14).

Consider student-athletes worried about a research paper. Problem-focused coping would include taking steps to get the paper written: going to the teacher for help, getting help from a tutor or writing assistant, doing some research at the library or online, organizing one's notes, and so forth. Problem-focused coping should always be the first line of defense against sources of stress, when possible.

But the student-athlete may still feel stressed even though he has taken steps to complete the paper. Emotion-focused coping includes things people do to reduce feelings of stress, such as talking to a friend, listening to music, taking a walk, playing sports, or watching a funny movie. Taking breaks to do fun things should be part of a student-athlete's (and everyone's) life.

Good coping skills allow athletes to deal effectively with sources of stress, while poor coping skills mean ineffective responses to difficult situations and higher stress levels. In some cases, athletes' attempts to cope with stress can make matters worse: substance abuse, aggressive behavior, driving too fast, and other harmful behaviors may reduce feelings of stress temporarily but lead to negative outcomes in the future, including an increased risk of injury.

Why Does Stress Increase Injury Risk?

Stress may increase injury risk in several ways. First, people under stress experience a narrowing of the peripheral visual field (2); this means they have less visual information reaching their brain. Under stress, a person feels overwhelmed, and the body tries to accommodate this problem by reducing the input of information to help a person cope. An athlete's vision is very important for performance. Athletes must be aware of what is going on around them in order to make good decisions regarding play and negotiating the sport environment. Factors in the peripheral visual field may also lead to injury if an athlete becomes aware of them too late: for example, players rushing in from the side or obstacles in the environment.

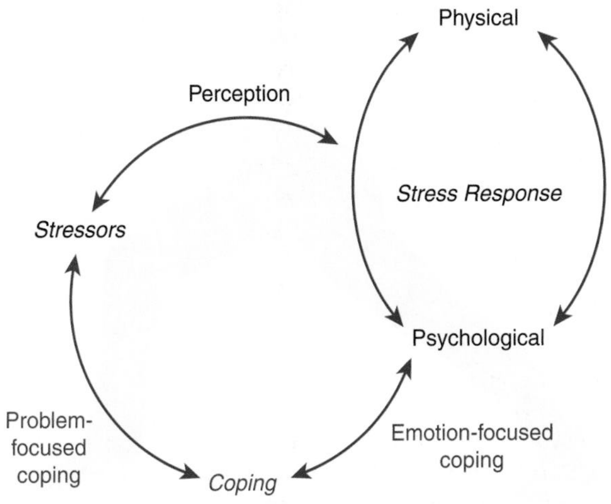

Second, people under stress have poorer concentration and focus because they are distracted. Sports psychologists emphasize the importance of an optimal mind set during sport training and competition, where athletes are totally in the moment and focusing on their sport. When you are "in the game" you make better decisions and respond more appropriately. When you are not "paying attention" you make poorer decisions, do not respond appropriately, and are more likely to sustain an injury (2).

Muscle tension is a symptom of excess stress, and occurs as the body prepares to fight or flee. Muscle tension is especially likely to contribute to back, shoulder, and neck pain both on and off the field. Muscle tension may increase risk of injury (2) and make existing injury more painful (15).

■ FIGURE 17.2 Coping responses. Problem-focused coping responses attempt to deal directly with the source of stress. Emotion-focused coping responses attempt to reduce a person's feelings (both physical and psychological) of stress.

Excess stress can contribute to the problems of overtraining and under-recovery, and increase injury risk. Overtraining can result not only from the physical stress of too much overload, but from a combination of too much training plus stress from other areas of life, including relationship, academic, and financial stress.

Improving Stress Management Skills May Reduce Injury Risk

If excess stress increases risk of sport injury, then helping athletes reduce feelings of stress should reduce injury risk. A great deal of research supports the benefit of stress reduction on a variety of psychological and physical variables (5,16). While only a few well-controlled studies have been conducted on athletes, these suggest that teaching stress management skills to athletes has beneficial effects. Stress management has been shown to reduce feelings of depression and fatigue in competitive athletes (17) and to reduce the frequency of injury and illness (18). Some stress management techniques are similar to the mental training techniques used by sports psychologists and coaches, and not only reduce stress, but improve focus and performance.

What is stress management, and how can coaches encourage their athletes to deal more effectively with stress? Stress management refers to any collection of techniques that help people cope more effectively with stress, and usually involves helping people change both their thoughts and their behavior (19,20). Examples of stress management approaches include the following (5,19–22).

- Time management—People who improve their ability to set goals, make plans for reaching those goals, organize their time, and schedule activities according to priorities feel more in control of their lives, and consequently less stressed.
- Study skills and organization—Students can reduce feelings of stress by learning how to take notes, study, take exams, and complete assignments more effectively.
- Problem-solving—Stressors are problems, and learning to solve problems more creatively and effectively increases one's sense of control and reduces feelings of stress.
- Communication skills—Effective communication improves a person's ability to deal with stressors, create effective solutions, and cultivate social support.
- Healthy lifestyle—Adequate sleep, good nutrition, and other common sense health behaviors not only improve athletic performance but reduce stress as well.
- Cognitive restructuring—Cognitive restructuring means examining your thoughts, and replacing stress-provoking thoughts with more realistic, constructive ones. For example, some people "catastrophize," or make mountains out of mole hills. These people can learn to examine their thoughts, and catch themselves when they are making too big a deal out of small issues. With practice, people can learn to correct their thinking so that it is more accurate and encourages productive behavior.
- Relaxation and stress reduction techniques—Breathing exercises, relaxation, visualization, meditation, and other techniques can reduce feelings of stress and the negative health effects of excess stress, and help athletes feel better.

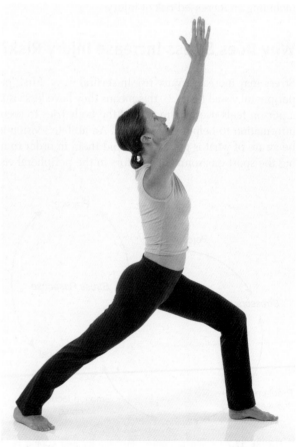

■ **FIGURE 17.3** Yoga warrior pose. Yoga and other mind-body physical activities reduce feelings of stress with a focus on mindful awareness and breathing.

This list of topics is obviously more than a coach could include in a season's practice schedule! Instead, put your athletes in touch with resources in your school and community that can help them do a better job of coping with stress. You can also emphasize the importance of developing a balanced, healthy lifestyle and coping with problems before they feel out of control. You can also refer troubled athletes to professional help. Here are some of the ways coaches can help their athletes handle stress more effectively, and in turn improve playing ability and reduce injury risk.

- Invite your athletic trainer, guidance counselor, or other member of the counseling staff to give a brief presentation on stress management topics you feel would be the most helpful to members of your team. Maybe your athletic director or athletic training staff would hold a session for all team athletes. These sessions could be mandatory but outside of practice time.
- Endorse the importance of a balanced lifestyle. Student athletes need to hear from you that good nutrition, adequate rest, and good health are important for peak performance. Athletes who are nourished and well-rested are more resistant to the negative effects of stress.
- Become an expert on the resources available at your institution to student-athletes. Encourage your athletes to make use of tutoring services, writing assistance services, time management workshops, and whatever else might be helpful. Does your school offer stress management or stress reduction classes or workshops? If you do not work in a school setting, find out about resources available in your community.
- Encourage your athletes to pursue stress reduction options out of season as well. Maybe they would like to try yoga, tai chi, and other physical activities that would balance their sport training and provide mental training along with physical conditioning (Fig. 17.3).
- Include visualization and mental focus exercises as part of team practices and preparation for competition (See Focal Point: Mental Training).
- Refer athletes who appear to be overly anxious, depressed, or stressed to a counseling professional.

FOCAL POINT

Mental Training

Sports psychologists encourage coaches to do all they can to help athletes develop a focused, competitive mindset that enhances peak performance (1). Perhaps you have taken a sports psychology course, or studied sports psychology as part of a coaching certification program. Many coaches take time in their practices or before contests to lead some sort of visualization exercise to help their athletes prepare for a productive practice or get ready for a competition. Your goal in these exercises is to teach an athlete to be in the moment, in the sport, and not distracted by extraneous worries and thoughts.

Mental training exercises work best when they are practiced regularly. If you use these exercises, use them with most practices, not just when athletes are really wound up and distracted before an important contest. An example of a mental training exercise is the following.

At the beginning of practice, before warm-up, have your athletes sit or lie in a comfortable position and pay attention to their breathing. Have them scan their bodies for tension, working from their toes to their heads, naming feet, legs, hips, back, abdomen, stomach, chest, shoulders, arms, hands, neck, jaw, forehead, etc., giving a minute after each for the athlete to focus and relax. Encourage athletes to imagine extraneous thoughts as being written in the sand on a beach by the ocean, and to imagine the breath as waves. With inhalation the wave energy builds. With exhalation the wave breaks on the shore and washes the words away.

(continues)

Mental Training *(continued)*

Once athletes are relaxed, you can ask them to recall a successful sport experience and relive it in their mind's eye. Ask them to recall what the scene looked like, sounded like, felt like. Tell them to replay the scene, and to re-experience the determination, focus, and thrill of that success.

You may also wish to have athletes visualize a sport skill they are seeking to improve, visualizing its perfect execution. Again ask them to imagine how the skill looks, sounds, and feels in their body.

Finish your mental training exercise by encouraging athletes to maintain their focus and awareness in the upcoming practice or game to enhance their training, learning, and peak performance.

1. Murphy S. *The Sport Psych Handbook*. Champaign: Human Kinetics, 2005.

A Coach's Attitude Can Influence Injury Risk

Pain is a part of sport training and competition for most people. Who is not familiar with the adage "No pain, no gain?" Early in their careers most athletes learn to tolerate some discomfort as part of their training. As coaches urge their athletes on to greater levels of exertion, pain may be part of the sport experience (23). A good coach, however, should teach athletes to differentiate pain that may signal the development of an injury from the muscle pain that signals fatigue. Indeed, much of the impetus for more rigorous certification standards for coaches has evolved from concern about the high rates of injury in athletes at all levels of competition (24). As emphasized throughout this book, injury prevention is an important part of your job.

The emotional tone you set regarding the meaning of pain can have repercussions on how your athletes experience pain, and learn to work through some level of fatigue. Teaching athletes to get tough and work hard can be a good thing. But if you direct athletes to ignore symptoms that may indicate a developing injury, you may inadvertently increase injury risk for your athletes.

Hopefully this book has helped you understand which pains indicate that your athlete needs medical attention, and has helped you understand the importance of working with your medical staff to determine appropriate treatment and limitations for injured athletes. You do not need to halt practice and gush over every athlete who gets a side stitch to screen him or her for appendicitis; but you do need to take serious symptoms seriously.

We have heard many stories from athletes who were afraid to report injury symptoms to their coaches. They feared intimidation and humiliation, and felt that their coaches thought that injuries indicated weakness. These athletes often played while injured and in a great deal of pain. Some went on to sustain more serious injuries when their original pain was ignored or not taken seriously. One of the most sobering stories we have heard came from Anna, a former high school distance runner. She was on her way to breaking her state cross country records when she developed back pain. Although the pain limited her running somewhat, and she cut back on her weekly mileage, she was so determined to set a record that she did not admit to anyone the amount of pain she was enduring. Naturally, her coach and parents urged her on as well, despite the pain, as the season was almost over. Anna continued her miles and miles of training, running through intense pain, but finally conceded that the pain was too great. She was forced to rest and did not compete in the state finals. Ruptured disks and severe pain led to back surgery and the fusion of four vertebrae, which eventually relieved the pain but put an end to Anna's cross-country career.

Over time, most coaches get to know the pain tolerance of their athletes. You have probably worked with athletes who always had some pain or other, but no serious injuries. They may have had low pain thresholds and a bit of hypochondria. You may have seen other athletes continue competing with sprained ankles, severe shin splints, and muscle strains to finish an important game. Good sense lies somewhere between these two extremes. Coaches must be good listeners and observers and refer athletes who may have symptoms of a serious or developing injury without treating these athletes with condescension or disrespect.

PSYCHOLOGICAL RESPONSE TO SPORT INJURY

Most coaches have experienced a sport injury themselves at some point in their athletic careers. When you have been through an experience yourself, it can help you understand what someone else now going through that same experience might be feeling. Having experienced injury, you may be able to feel sympathy for your athlete who is unable to participate fully in the life of the team. But you may also project your feelings onto your athletes and assume you understand what they are feeling when, in reality, they may be feeling something totally different.

Many researchers have studied athletes' emotional responses to injury (1,25–29). Responses are as varied as athletes themselves, and it is impossible to devise one model that fits all. In general, athletes feel a wide range of intense, negative emotions following injury that may become milder as they succeed in their rehabilitation programs, begin to feel more in control of their injuries, and develop more hope about returning to play.

It is important to note, however, that some athletes find injury a somewhat positive experience. Injury may take the pressure off of athletes who are anxious about upcoming competitions. Injury may be a relief to athletes looking for a way to leave sport gracefully despite the insistence of friends, family members, teammates, or coaches.

But studies show that, no surprise, the vast majority of athletes, about 90% experience negative emotions following sports injuries (25). Most athletes feel some combination of frustration, anger, boredom, depression, fear, anxiety, confusion, and loneliness after injury. These negative emotions not only feel bad, but can interfere with athletes' determination to return to play, and their adherence to their rehabilitation programs. Negative emotions may also interfere with athletes' success in school and work, and with their personal relationships.

Athletes respond to injury in many different ways, and their response depends upon a number of factors, including the nature of the injury, the athlete's personal situation, and the meaning of sport participation in that athlete's life (1).

The Nature of the Injury

Obviously, the more serious the injury, the more the injury disrupts the athlete's sport participation and life in general. An athlete's response generally becomes more negative the more painful and disruptive the injury (27). It is bad enough having sport cut out of your life. Now add constraints on mobility, missed classes because of medical appointments and transportation difficulties, trying to get to physical therapy appointments with a busy academic schedule, work piling up, pain and pain medications interfering with your concentration: you get the picture. In some cases, athletes have trouble getting meals and conquering other simple tasks, such as cleaning and laundry.

An athlete's psychological response to injury is influenced by the athlete's perception of the injury (29). The information received from the medical team and the coach contributes strongly to this perception. For example, does the medical team seem concerned, uneasy, or worried? What prognosis do they give? Will surgery be required? Athletes need information about their injuries, but they also need hope. Coaches should note that even relatively minor injuries may be very worrisome if prognosis is uncertain or poor. Chronic injuries that do not seem to heal can be a big problem too, and athletes with chronic injuries often practice and compete with significant levels of pain (30). Season and career-ending injuries are especially difficult for most athletes (31).

The Athlete's Personal Situation

Many personal factors influence an athlete's psychological response to a sport injury, and we will just mention a few here. The timing of the injury in terms of the sport season and in terms of the athlete's sport career strongly influences the athlete's (and coach's) reaction to injury. An athlete may recover from a fairly minor injury in the early part of the season, and still be able to play in the more important games later in the season. An injury during an athlete's freshman year may not seem as significant as the same injury that occurs during the end of senior year, at the end of the player's eligibility, and presumably when the athlete has come to play a more important role on the team (32).

An athlete's personality and stress hardiness influence the athlete's response to injury (27). Feeling in control of rehabilitation and recovery reduces feelings of stress. Athletes who feel strong positive social support not only from their team but from other friends, family, and groups in their lives tend to feel less stressed (29).

Research suggests that, in general, younger athletes are more traumatized by a given injury than more mature athletes, and show higher rates of mood disturbances (33–36). They also appear to be more vulnerable to negative feedback from coaches, teammates, parents, and others.

Athletic Identity and the Importance of Sport

The more strongly people identify themselves with the role of athlete, and the more important sport is in their lives, the more they will suffer psychologically from sports injuries. Life without sport participation may feel boring or depressing, and athletes side-lined with injury may struggle with a changing sense of identity, especially when injuries are serious. When people put all their life-satisfaction eggs in one basket, and the basket falls, their life may feel broken into pieces. The following story illustrates just such a situation.

"Sports have always been the center of my life. I started playing soccer when I was 6, and it quickly became something I identified with. When I was meeting people in college, one of my first pieces of identifying information was 'I am on the soccer team.' People in my dorm called me 'Soccer Lisa.'

"During my first 3 years in college, soccer continued to be one of the most important things in my life. I started all three seasons and created a niche on campus that allowed me to feel both comfortable and confident. But at the end of my third season, I received a career-ending concussion in the conference finals.

"When the doctor told me I could no longer play soccer I was absolutely devastated. I was so angry and frustrated. This was my life and it should have been my choice. For 7 months I experienced intense periods of depression and anxiety. I was losing what made me who I was and I no longer had any control over my life."

How Can Coaches Help?

Coaches do not diagnose injury or supervise the rehabilitation process, but they can still provide valuable assistance to athletes during the rehabilitation process (37). Coaches should offer sympathy and urge injured athletes to put as much energy into their rehabilitation as they would be putting into team practices and competitions. It will not take a lot of your time to provide some emotional support for your injured athletes, and this time may even help build team spirit among the remaining athletes if you play your cards right, and get the whole team involved. After all, sports participation is not just about winning; it is about people. Because you coach the whole person, you do not suddenly end your relationship with your athlete just because he or she is no longer an active participant on your team. Your actions demonstrate to the injured athlete, and also to the whole team, that you have consideration, respect, and positive regard for the people on your team. Here are a few ideas for how coaches can "coach" an injured athlete.

- Take advantage of the fact that athletes are accustomed to taking direction from you. Direct your injured athletes to work with their health care providers, physical therapists, and athletic trainers to follow rehabilitation instructions thoroughly and completely.
- Express confidence in the medical team, and in the athlete's abilities to follow rehabilitation procedures.

- Express optimism about the athlete's chances to return to the team following rehabilitation. Without promising them their old positions back, tell athletes you will work with them once they are back at practice to help them rebuild fitness and skills.
- If you know of athletes (even in other sports) who have returned to play after a similar injury, ask the healed athlete to visit the injured athlete to commiserate, share stories, and offer hope.
- Ask your captains to organize help for the injured player. Encourage teammates to help with transportation, and to visit the injured player. Can someone help with notes for the classes the athlete has missed? Such altruism will help build positive team spirit, as the team pitches in for a good cause.
- Model a nonjudgmental attitude toward injury. Teammates and coach should offer positive or neutral comments to the injured athlete. "We miss seeing you." "How's rehab going?" Not, "When are you coming back from your vacation? We lost the last game because you got injured. You've ruined our chances in next week's tournament." "Come on back and play. Can't you take a little pain?"
- If your athletes are performing rehabilitation in the athletic training room, stop by occasionally and cheer them on. Speak with the athletic trainer to get an update on their adherence, and remark to the athlete on this. They will know you are watching. Praise good adherence, and admonish slackers to pick up the pace.
- When possible, ask injured players to meet with the team at the start of practice, and then send them to the training room for their workout while you work with the rest of your team. Keep them with the team as much as their physical condition and your practice plan allows.
- Should injured players come to competitions and watch? You may want to leave this up to the injured athlete. Some find this too depressing; others like being involved in the life of the team. Some injured players can help team managers with their jobs, help with stats, and even help coach less experienced players. Use your judgment as to what would work best for your injured athletes and your team.
- With the other coaches and personnel in your program, advocate for the best possible athletic training staff and facilities. It is great to know your injured athletes are in good hands, and receiving the best possible care.

PSYCHOLOGY AND SPORTS INJURY REHABILITATION

A great deal of research has shown that psychological factors contribute to athletes' adherence to sports injury rehabilitation, and to their eventual treatment outcome (38,39). Athletes can take advantage of this, and use mental training techniques to manage pain, visualize successful adherence to rehabilitation and return to play, and reduce feelings of stress and negative mood. Although coaches do not directly supervise sports injury rehabilitation, they should be knowledgeable about the psychological factors that contribute to an athlete's successful sport injury rehabilitation.

Rehabilitation Program Adherence

Rehabilitation programs only aid recovery from sports injuries if athletes follow their rehabilitation instructions. Yet many athletes find rehabilitation programs very boring compared to sports participation, and have difficulty sticking to their rehabilitation programs. Adherence becomes even more difficult if athletes experience pain during rehabilitation procedures, if rehabilitation sessions are difficult to schedule or attend, or if athletes will be out of play and in rehabilitation for extended periods of time.

Psychological factors can enhance or impede rehabilitation adherence (38). Especially problematic are negative emotions such as fear, anxiety, and depression, and feelings of isolation. While some negative emotions are to be expected, athletes who seem to dwell continuously in these negative states should be referred to counseling. If you think your injured athletes are overly negative, talk to their athletic trainers or other health care providers to see if they are seeing the same things. They can help you evaluate whether the athlete is mostly negative in front of you, or if the negative emotions are more pervasive. They may also be willing to help refer the troubled athlete to counseling.

Feelings of excess stress and negative emotions exert a double whammy during sports injury rehabilitation. First, they can weaken the immune system and interfere with the healing process (40). And second, they decrease an athlete's drive to participate fully in the rehabilitation process (41). Injured athletes can easily be overcome by an inertia that makes summoning the energy to perform rehabilitation routines difficult.

Adherence improves when athletes take an active part in the rehabilitation process. A sense of control decreases feelings of stress and helps athletes keep trying, even in the face of difficulties (42). Some of the most successful strategies for increasing adherence include the following.

EDUCATION

Health care providers should educate athletes about their injuries and be sure athletes understand rehabilitation instructions. Athletes should not be overwhelmed with negative information, however, and some athletes prefer not to have too much information. Education should focus on answering athletes' questions, and explaining the facts of the injury and the most productive ways of treating these injuries. In one study, a group of injured athletes watched a video that explained upcoming surgery and rehabilitation for their ACL injuries (43). The video followed an athlete who underwent surgery, participated in rehabilitation, and recovered successfully from the injury. This group was compared to a group that received information but did not view the video. Athletes in the video group reported greater confidence in their ability to perform the rehabilitation program and walk after their surgery. They also had earlier recoveries than the other group (43). Coaches and providers must encourage athletes to hope for the best, and to view good adherence to rehabilitation instructions as the way to achieve the best possible outcome. Athletes must believe in the efficacy of their rehabilitation programs.

GOAL SETTING

Goal setting improves rehabilitation adherence (42). Small, achievable goals help athletes feel like they are making progress, and help them feel in control of the rehabilitation process. Athletic trainers and other health care providers should include injured athletes in the process of goal setting. Rehabilitation goals might include achievements like being able to support weight on an injured foot, achieve a certain degree of flexion in the injured joint, complete a certain number of exercise repetitions, or whatever makes sense for that injury.

POSITIVE SELF-TALK

Athletes should try to focus on the positive: rehabilitation achievements, positive activities, helpful friends and teammates, and tell themselves they are doing everything possible to get better. Positive self-talk improves mood and increases rehabilitation adherence (26,44). The power of belief has amazing healing potential. While self-talk alone may not heal a difficult injury, it won't hurt; it might help; and the athlete will certainly feel better in the process, and avoid the negative emotions that can interfere with healing and adherence to rehabilitation instructions.

SOCIAL SUPPORT

Support from family, friends, teachers, coaches, teammates, and health care providers enhances rehabilitation adherence (45). Social support may take the form of friendly remarks or offers of help that make injured athletes feel better and build self-confidence.

Coaches and health care providers often do not realize how the little things they say and do can have a huge impact on an athlete, as the following story illustrates.

"When I was injured playing basketball last year, I was really worried about my slow progress coming back from the injury. The athletic trainers were always very business-like and didn't talk to me much. I tried to find the hidden meanings behind the words they said, and behind their facial expressions and tone of voice. What weren't they telling me? Was I doing OK?

"I remember one day my coach came into the training room while I was icing my leg before exercise. He didn't even make eye contact with me, but rushed in, spoke with one of the athletic trainers, seemed kind of angry, then stalked out. I wondered if they were talking about me, if I wasn't making good progress, or if something else was wrong they weren't telling me about. It put me in a bad mood for the rest of the day."

Little things can make a big difference. Taking a few minutes to fire off a supportive email or make a quick phone call can change your injured athlete's day. Stop by the training room occasionally and ask how things are going. Say something positive that shows your athlete that you care.

Mental Training Can Enhance Sports Injury Rehabilitation

Much has been written about mental training techniques to help athletes cope with injury (1,39). Research lends a great deal of support regarding the benefits of these techniques to reduce stress and pain, and increase rehabilitation adherence. Coaches rarely have the time to work with individual injured athletes to teach mental training techniques. But if you have taught mental training techniques to the athletes on your team, they may be able to modify imagery exercises to help reduce pain or visualize healing if they become injured. You might be able to give them simple written instructions that they can follow at home if they already have some skill in this area. Athletes who already have some skill in mental training techniques will be more likely to use healing imagery successfully during injury rehabilitation (46,47).

Some athletic trainers teach relaxation and imagery exercises to the athletes in their care. If this is the case at your institution, it is important for you to endorse these practices so that the athlete takes them seriously. Athletes who do not believe these techniques can be helpful are reluctant to practice them (48,49).

FOCAL POINT

Mental Training for Sports Injury Rehabilitation

Athletes can practice mental training exercises to encourage positive self-talk, stress reduction, pain management, and maximum participation in their rehabilitation programs (1–3). Athletes should practice daily for at least 10 to 15 minutes. They can use the mental training guidelines from Focal Point: Mental Training above, beginning with a deep relaxation, and then simply add a positive visualization that reinforces their personal goals and addresses their individual needs. Some examples include the following.

- Rehabilitation adherence: Athletes may imagine themselves performing the behaviors leading to successful adherence, such as making time to attend therapy sessions or performing prescribed exercises. Visualizations should include a focus on positive emotions and successful rehabilitation.
- Stress reduction: Athletes may imagine themselves doing things they enjoy. If return to play is a realistic goal, visualize this. If not, athletes should find other positive things in their lives on which to focus.
- Healing: Athletes may visualize the injury site becoming healed and healthy. They might visualize bones knitting together, ligaments become stronger, inflammation dissipating, or whatever fits their injury.
- Pain management: Athletes may visualize their pain as a bright light that is gradually becoming dimmer, a tight knot loosening, a stormy sea becoming calm, or an angry dog becoming peaceful. Athletes may be able to imagine sensations of pain as numbness or pressure, or to imagine the pain as somewhere outside their bodies.

1. Brown C. Injuries: The psychology of recovery and rehab. In: Murphy S. *The Sport Psych Handbook*. Champaign IL: Human Kinetics, 2005:215–235.
2. Crossman J. *Coping with Sports Injuries: Psychological Strategies for Rehabilitation*. Oxford: Oxford University Press, 2001.
3. Driediger M, Hall C, Callow N. Imagery use by injured athletes: a qualitative analysis. *J Sci Med Sport* 2006;24(3):261–271.

FROM THE ATHLETIC TRAINING ROOM

Complementary Techniques for Pain Management

Pain is one of the most difficult symptoms of sports injuries. In general, pain tells you that something is wrong. Pain can be a useful message from your body that tells you to stop what you are doing to prevent further harm. You take off tight shoes to prevent a blister from getting worse or rest an ankle that has been sprained.

Athletes with serious injuries often experience a great deal of pain. Pain is complicated because many factors influence a person's perception of pain beyond the physical injury (1). Pain medications, both over-the-counter and prescription, provide some relief in most cases. But many athletes try to limit pain medication because of side effects such as gastric distress or drowsiness.

Many nondrug therapies can help reduce pain, both alone and in conjunction with appropriate medication, when medication alone is not enough to eliminate pain. Some of the most promising therapies include the following:

- Psychological counseling: counseling may help lessen pain by helping to reduce negative emotions such as anxiety and fear, which can intensify sensations of pain. Counseling can also reduce pain by helping people feel more in control (2).
- Relaxation techniques: techniques such as meditation and self-hypnosis may reduce pain by reducing physiological arousal and relaxing tight muscles (3)
- Acupuncture: the physiological effects of acupuncture are still under investigation, but it is gaining support as an effective treatment for reducing pain (Fig. 17.4) (4).
- Massage therapy: massage therapies may help by increasing feelings of comfort, improving blood flow, and/or inducing muscle relaxation (5).

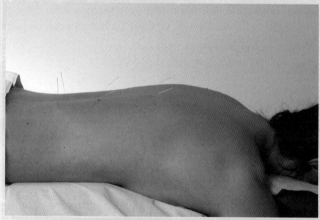

■ **FIGURE 17.4** Patient receiving acupuncture treatment. Acupuncture is an ancient healing tradition in which very fine gauge needles are inserted at specific anatomical sites to treat disease and relieve pain.

1. Roessler KK. Sport and the psychology of pain. In: Loland S, Skirstad B, Waddington I. *Pain and Injury in Sport: Social and Ethical Analysis*. London: Routledge, 2006:34–48.
2. Kerns RD, Thorn BE, Dixon KE. Psychological treatments for persistent pain: an introduction. *J Clin Psychol* 2006;62(11):1327–1332.
3. Tan G, Alvarez JA, Jensen MP. Complementary and alternative medicine approaches to pain management. *J Clin Psychol* 2006;62(11):1419–1432.
4. Vas J, Mendez C, Perea-Milla E, et al. Acupuncture as a complementary therapy to the pharmacological treatment of osteoarthritis of the knee: randomised controlled trial. *Br Med J* 2004;329:1216.
5. Centers for Disease Control. *Effective Complementary and Alternative Medicine (CAM) Treatments*. Available online at http://www.cdc.gov/prc/research-projects/special-interest-projects/effective-complementary-alternative-medicine-treatments.htm. Accessed November 20, 2006.

(continues)

When Athletes May Not Return to Play

Sometimes athletes do not fully recover from injuries, despite excellent medical care and dedicated adherence to rehabilitation instructions. Coping with catastrophic injury can be an overwhelming endeavor. What can coaches do when the athlete sustains a career-ending injury, or is getting somewhat better, but may never achieve the physical condition needed to return to play on your team?

We have no magic answers for this difficult question. Retiring from athletics can be difficult, even under the best of circumstances, especially for people who have invested a great deal of their lives in sport participation, and who have developed a strong athletic identity (50). Retirement from sport is more difficult when it comes suddenly, and is due to factors outside of the athlete's control (51), which is often the case with career-ending sport injuries. Athletes may experience emotional health problems during this transition, including identity crisis, decreased self-confidence, depression, and anxiety (52).

Although there may not be a great deal a coach can do to help athletes through this difficult situation, you can offer sympathy and understanding, and guide your ex-athletes to helpful resources. If you have athletes who may not return to play following sports injuries, keep the following suggestions in mind.

- Hold out hope as long as possible. While some injuries are obviously career-ending, the recovery from other injuries is hard to predict. Athletes need hope to stick to their rehabilitation programs and get through the difficult weeks and months ahead.
- Work with your medical team to evaluate each athlete's situation. And remember that there is always some uncertainty in every prognosis. Time will tell whether your athlete will be able to rejoin your team.
- Encourage your institution's athletic program to offer "life after sport" planning for all athletes. Only a small minority of college athletes go on to play professional sports after college. Collegiate athletes should participate in career planning activities throughout their college years, and do well academically so they will be prepared for success in the years following college. One section of the NCAA CHAMPS/Life Skills program focuses on career development (53).
- When possible, give your injured athletes a job that continues a connection to the team, if they are interested. Can they help coach other athletes? Help with team management?
- Encourage your ex-athletes to develop other interests, or other ways to remain involved in their sport. Can they referee? Announce? Assist team managers? Are there ways they can use their sport knowledge to help others? Are there opportunities to teach or coach at local schools and youth programs?
- Offer understanding and sympathy. Refer athletes to counseling services to help with the emotional difficulties of transitioning out of sport. Your athletic training staff may be able to help.

RETURN TO PLAY

Although athletes in rehabilitation look forward to returning to active sport participation, once they are finally cleared to play they may have mixed feelings about returning (54). Many athletes report that they worry about reinjury and not being able to participate at their pre-injury level (55). Their injuries may be healed, but athletes may leave the athletic training room overweight, deconditioned, and discouraged.

Research suggests that elite and other highly competitive athletes may have the most difficulty returning to play (56,57). They may have a harder time returning to their prior level of conditioning and playing ability, and realize they are not where they used to be in these areas. In addition, they may feel the stakes are higher, and be more afraid of failing to meet high expectations (their own and others').

Sport psychologists Leslie Podlog and Robert Eklund recently reviewed the literature on the psychosocial aspects of a return to sport following injury, and described three important factors that strongly influence the return to play process (58). They call the first factor competence (58). Athletes must rebuild their feelings of competence, overcoming fear of reinjury and fear of being unable to return to pre-injury playing ability. The second factor is autonomy (58). In their model, autonomy refers to athletes having autonomy in decisions regarding when and how they return to play. In general, athletes who report feeling pressured to return to play tend to show less favorable outcomes, including greater rates of re-injury, and lower levels of confidence and performance. Athletes who report returning to sport more slowly and with less pressure generally show more favorable outcomes, and more satisfaction with their return to play. Relatedness is the third factor exerting a strong influence on the return to play process. By relatedness, Podlog and Eklund mean social support and assistance from sources such as friends, teammates, physical therapists, and coaches (58). Relatedness helps to smooth the transition back to play. On the other hand, athletes who feel alienated and isolated from others report a more difficult recovery period.

Consider these factors as you develop strategies to help previously injured athletes return to play. Your job is to take your returning athletes and train them appropriately to help them recover their physical condition, skill level, and the psychological drive that helped them succeed as athletes. This transformation from injured athlete to starting player does not happen overnight, and you must help your athletes start slowly and progress gradually so they experience the success necessary to rebuild their self-confidence.

Start your returning athletes with a physical conditioning program that builds from the work your athletes were doing with their physical therapists or athletic trainers. Add sport-specific drills when your athletes are ready. Let them work in parallel with the team until they are ready to join in. Sports skills should be rehearsed in low pressure practice situations to begin with, slowly progressing to practicing with the team. The intensity of participation should increase gradually as athletes become stronger and more skilled, and become less fearful of reinjury. Returning athletes should not compete until they are performing during practice at levels equivalent to those of competition (1).

Sounds easy. But coaches must realize that these weeks of conditioning may be especially stressful for many athletes. You can help contribute to a successful return to play in many ways, including the following.

- Discuss your training strategies with your athletes. Good communication will let them know you realize they need to start slowly and rebuild self-confidence. When they understand your strategies, they will be less fearful and will participate more fully.
- Set realistic expectations. Athletes are relieved to hear you don't expect them to return to play immediately.
- Increase self-efficacy with role models. Ask athletes who have recovered and returned to play from similar injuries to talk to your returning athletes. When returning athletes see that others have overcome similar injuries, they will feel more confident in their own ability to do so.
- Let returning athletes set the pace for their return to play. When athletes feel in control of the return to play process, they feel less stressed, and are less likely to become reinjured.

SUMMARY

- Psychological factors can influence an athlete's risk of injury. In particular, high levels of negative stress, high levels of performance anxiety, negative mood, and poor coping skills increase injury risk.
- Stress seems to increase injury risk in several ways. People under stress may experience a narrowing of the peripheral visual field; have poorer concentration and focus; experience increased muscle tension; and are at increased risk of overtraining and under-recovery.
- Stress management refers to techniques and practices that help people cope more effectively with stress and reduce physiological arousal. Stress management techniques usually involve teaching people how to change both their thinking and their behavior.
- Coaches must develop the ability to encourage their athletes to train hard and work through the discomfort of appropriate overload. At the same time, coaches must teach athletes to take injury symptoms seriously, since early diagnosis and treatment often prevents injuries from becoming more serious.
- A small minority of athletes may experience a positive response to becoming injured (e.g., relief at being able to quit sport participation). However, most athletes experience a negative psychological response to injury. These negative feelings may interfere with adherence to rehabilitation instructions, school and work performance, personal relationships, and quality of life.
- An athlete's psychological response to injury depends upon many variables, including the nature of the injury, the timing of the injury in terms of the season and the athlete's sport career, the athlete's personal situation and personality, his perceived level of social support, and the importance of sport in the athlete's life.
- Coaches can support injured athletes during the rehabilitation process in many ways. They should direct athletes to follow rehabilitation instructions, express confidence in the athlete and in the medical team, maintain supportive contact with the injured athlete, and encourage team captains to organize support for the injured player.
- Many injured athletes have difficulty sticking to their rehabilitation programs. Good patient education, goal setting, positive self-talk, and social support can improve program adherence.
- Mental training can enhance sports injury rehabilitation adherence and reduce pain.

- When athletes experience a catastrophic injury that may end their sport career, coaches should hold out hope for return to sport as long as possible. When it is clear the athlete will not return to your team, express sympathy and understanding, and guide him or her to helpful resources.
- Athletes may experience increasing levels of anxiety as they prepare to return to play. Many fear re-injury and a failure to perform at their previous level.
- Athletes who return to sport after extensive rehabilitation and conditioning show higher levels of perceived competence and feel more in control of their sport participation. Athletes who feel higher levels of social support from friends, teammates, medical personnel, and coaches report greater success in their return to sport.
- Coaches should start returning athletes with a physical conditioning program that builds on their rehabilitation programs, and progress to sport-specific drills and practice with the team as returning athletes are ready. Athletes should not compete until they are performing during practice at levels equivalent to those of competition.

References

1. Brown C. Injuries: The psychology of recovery and rehab. In: Murphy S. *The Sport Psych Handbook 2005.* Champaign IL: Human Kinetics, 2005:215–235.
2. Williams JM, Andersen MB. Psychosocial antecedents of sport injury: Review and critique of the stress and injury model. *J Appl Sport Psychol* 1998;10:5–25.
3. Mann DP, Lacke C. The impact of life stress on athletic injury in female college-aged lacrosse players. *J Athl Train* 2001;36(2): S–55.
4. Geisler G, Leith LM. Sources of stress in student-athletes: An exploratory study of intercollegiate soccer players in Canada, Germany, and Japan. *Bul Ins Health Sport Sci Univ Tsukuba* 2007;30:63–74.
5. Brehm BA. *Stress Management: Increasing Your Stress Resistance.* New York: Addison, Wesley, Longman, 1998.
6. Dienstbier RA. Behavioral correlates of sympathoadrenal reactivity: The toughness model. *Med Sci Sports Exerc* 1991;23: 846–852.
7. Fusilier M, Manning MR. Psychosocial predictors of health status revisited. *J Behav Med* 2005;28(4):347–359.
8. Balague G. Anxiety: from pumped to panicked. In: Murphy S. *The Sport Psych Handbook.* Champaign IL: Human Kinetics, 2005: 73–93.
9. Bauman J. Returning to play: the mind does matter. *Clin J Sport Med* 2005;15(6):432–435.
10. Junge A. The influence of psychological factors on sports injuries. *Am J Sports Med* 2000;28, Suppl:S-10.
11. Yerkes RM, Dodson JD. The relation of strength of stimulus to rapidity of habit formation. *J Comp Neur Psychol* 1908;18: 459–482.
12. Galambos SA, Terry PC, Moyle GM, et al. Psychological predictors of injury among elite athletes. *Br J Sports Med* 2005;39: 351–354.
13. Thayer RE. *Calm Energy: How People Regulate Mood with Food and Exercise.* Oxford: Oxford University Press, 2001.
14. Lazarus RS, Folkman S. *Stress, Appraisal, and Coping.* New York: Springer, 1984.
15. Roessler KK. Sport and the psychology of pain. In: Loland S, Skirstad B, Waddington I. *Pain and Injury in Sport: Social and Ethical Analysis.* London: Routledge, 2006:34–48.
16. Hammerfald K, Eberle C, Grau M, et al. Persistent effects of cognitive-behavioral stress management on cortisol responses to acute stress in healthy subjects—a randomized controlled trial. *Psychoneuroendocrinology* 2006;31(3):333–339.
17. Perna FM, Antoni MH, Kumar M, et al. Cognitive-behavioral intervention effects on mood and cortisol during athletic training. *Ann Behav Med* 1998;20:92–98.
18. Perna FM, Antoni MH, Baum A, et al. Cognitive behavioral stress management effects on injury and illness among competitive athletes: a randomized clinical trial. *Ann Behav Med* 2003;25(1):66–73.
19. Gaab J, Sonderegger L, Scherrer S, et al. Psychoneuroendocrine effects of cognitive-behavioral stress management in a naturalistic setting—a randomized controlled trial. *Psychoneuroendocrinology* 2006;31(4):428–438.
20. Williams JM, Scherzer CB. Injury risk and rehabilitation: psychological considerations. In: Williams JM. *Applied Sport Psychology: Personal Growth to Peak Performance.* New York: McGraw-Hill, 2006:565–594.
21. Seaward BL. *Managing Stress: Principles and Strategies for Health and Well-Being.* Boston: Jones & Bartlett, 2005.
22. Murphy S. *The Sport Psych Handbook.* Champaign IL: Human Kinetics, 2005.
23. Loland S, Skirstad B, Waddington I. *Pain and Injury in Sport: Social and Ethical Analysis.* London: Routledge, 2006.
24. Koester MC. Youth sports: a pediatrician's perspective on coaching and injury prevention. *J Athl Train* 2000;35(4):466–470.
25. Cramer Roh JL. Psychology/counseling: a universal competency in athletic training. *J Athl Train* 2000;35(4):458–465.
26. Crossman J. Managing thoughts, stress, and pain. In: Crossman J. *Coping with Sports Injuries: Psychological Strategies for Rehabilitation.* Oxford: Oxford University Press, 2001:128–147.
27. Granito VJ. Athletic injury experience: a qualitative focus group approach. *J Sport Behav* 2001;24(1):63–82.

28. Weiss MR. Psychological aspects of sport-injury rehabilitation: a developmental perspective. *J Athl Train* 2003;38(2):172–175.
29. Wiese-Bjornstal D, Smith A, Shaffer S, et al. An integrated model of response to sport injury: Psychological and sociological dynamics. *J Appl Sport Psychol* 1998;10:46–69.
30. Shuer ML, Dietrich MS. Psychological effects of chronic injury in elite athletes. *West J Med* 1997;166:104–109.
31. Kerr GA, Miller PS. Coping strategies. In: Crossman J. *Coping with Sports Injuries: Psychological Strategies for Rehabilitation.* 2001 83-102). Oxford: Oxford University Press, 2001:83–102.
32. Saunders P. *The Relationship Between Emotional Response to Athletic Injury and Rehabilitation Adherence.* Senior thesis, 2004, Trinity College.
33. Brewer BW. Developmental differences in psychological aspects of sport-injury rehabilitation. *J Athl Train* 2003;38(2):152–153.
34. Newcomer RR, Perna FM. Features of posttraumatic distress among adolescent athletes. *J Athl Train* 2003;38(2):163–166.
35. Tripp DA, Stanish WD, Reardon G, et al. Comparing postoperative pain experiences of the adolescent and adult athlete after anterior cruciate ligament surgery. *J Athl Train* 2003;38(2):154–157.
36. Udry E, Shelbourne KD, Gray T. Psychological readiness for anterior cruciate ligament surgery: describing and comparing the adolescent and adult experiences. *J Athl Train* 2003;38(2):167–171.
37. Podlog L, Eklund RC. Professional coaches' perspectives on the return to sport following serious injury. *J Appl Sport Psychol* 2007;19(2):207–225.
38. Brewer BW. Psychology of sports injury rehabilitation. In: Tenenbaum G, Eklund RC. *Handbook of Sport Psychology.* Hoboken: John Wiley & Sons, 2007:404–424.
39. Crossman J. *Coping with Sports Injuries: Psychological Strategies for Rehabilitation.* Oxford: Oxford University Press, 2001.
40. Segerstrom SC, Miller GE. Psychological stress and the human immune system: A meta-analysis study of 30 years of inquiry. *Psychol Bull* 2004;130:601–630.
41. Middel M. Using mind power for healing. *Phys Sportsmed* 1996;24(7):27.
42. Evans L, Hardy L. Injury rehabilitation: a goal-setting study. *Res Q Exerc Sport* 2002;73(3):310–319.
43. Maddison R, Prapavessis H, Clatworthy M. Modeling and rehabilitation following anterior cruciate ligament reconstruction. *Ann Behav Med* 2006;31(1):89–98
44. Gordon S, Potter M, Hamer P. The role of the physiotherapist and sport therapist. In: Crossman J. *Coping with Sports Injuries: Psychological Strategies for Rehabilitation.* Oxford: Oxford University Press, 2001:62–82.
45. Udry E. The role of significant others: social support during injuries. In: Crossman J. *Coping with Sports Injuries: Psychological Strategies for Rehabilitation.* Oxford: Oxford University Press, 2001:148–156.
46. Short SE, Tenute A, Feltz DL. Imagery use in sport: mediational effects for efficacy. *J Sci Med Sport* 2005;23(9):951–960.
47. Driediger M, Hall C, Callow N. Imagery use by injured athletes: a qualitative analysis. *J Sci Med Sport* 2006;24(3):261–271.
48. Francis SR, Andersen MB, Maley P. Physiotherapists' and male athletes' views on psychological skills for rehabilitation. *J Sci Med Sport* 2000;3:17–29.
49. Myers CA, Peyton DD, Jensen BJ. Treatment acceptability in NCAA Division I football athletes: Rehabilitation intervention strategies. *J Sport Behav* 2004;27(2):165–169.
50. Webb WM, Nasco SA, Riley S, et al. Athlete identity and reactions to retirement from sports. *J Sport Behav* 1998;21(3):338–363.
51. Taylor J, Ogilvie B. Career transition among athletes: is there life after sports? In: Williams JM. *Applied Sport Psychology: Personal growth in Performance.* Mountain View: Mayfield, 2001:480–496.
52. Stephan Y, Bilard J, Ninot G, et al. Repercussions of transition out of elite sport on subjective well-being: a one-year study. *J Appl Sport Psychol* 2003;15:354–371.
53. NCAA. *CHAMPS Life Skills Program.* Available online at http://www1.ncaa.org/eprise/main/membership/ed_outreach/champs-life_skills/program.html. Accessed November 20, 2006.
54. Brewer BW, Petitpas AJ. Returning to self: The anxieties of coming back after injury. In: Andersen MB. *Sport Psychology in Practice.* Champaign IL: Human Kinetics, 2005:93–108.
55. Podlog L, Eklund RC. Assisting injured athletes with the return to sport transition. *Clin J Sport Med* 2004;14(5):257–259.
56. Johnston LH, Carroll D. Coping, social support and injury: changes over time and the effect of level of sports involvement. *J Sport Rehabil* 2000:9:290–303.
57. Morrey MA, Stuart MJ, Smith AM, et al. A longitudinal examination of athletes' emotional and cognitive responses to anterior cruciate ligament injury. *Clin J Sport Med* 1999;9:63–69.
58. Podlog L, Eklund RC. The psychosocial aspects of a return to sport following serious injury: A review of the literature from a self-determination perspective. *J Sport Exerc Psychol* 2007;8(4):535–566.

Index

Page numbers followed by *f* or *t* indicate material in figures or tables, respectively.

A

Overtraining *(continued)*
periodized training and, 86–92
two-way communication and, 83–84
research on, 79–80
stress/stressors in, 80, 80*f*, 82–85, 83*f*–85*f*, 337, 340
symptoms of, 79*t*
Overtraining syndrome (OTS), 80
Overuse injuries, 22–24, 236
factors in, 22
increase in, 22
prevention of, 13*t*, 22–24
contextual interference and, 23
distributed practice and, 23
good technique and, 24
gradual progress and, 24
random practice and, 23
repetition reduction and, 23
running shoes and, 74
sport specialization and, 22, 78
stress fractures as, 25
tissue damage in, 13*t*
training errors and, 22
Overweight, definition of, 169, 169*f*
Overweight athletes, 180
Overweight kids, 179
Oxidative stress, antioxidants and, 155–157
Oxygen
in aerobic energy system, 103–106, 105*f*
maximum consumption of, 106, 113, 114

P

Pain management, 243
complementary techniques for, 348
mental training for, 347
NSAIDs for, 238
Pain-spasm cycle, 240
Pain tolerance, 342–343
Palmar aponeurosis, 265*f*
Palmar interossei, 267*t*
Palmaris brevis, 265*f*
Palmaris longus, 265*f*
Palmar plate injuries, 268
Palpation, 324
Parietal bone, 295*f*
Pars interarticularis stress fracture, 308*f*, 309
Passive range of motion, 243, 244*f*
Passive warm-up, 16
Patella, 231*f*, 279
Patella dislocation, 280
Patella tendon graft, for ACL reconstruction, 30
Patella tracking, 283
Patellofemoral pain syndrome, 283
Peak flow values, 220
Pectineus, 274*t*

Pectoralis major, 233*f*, 253*f*
function of, 255*t*
strength training of, 125*t*
Pectoralis minor, 253*f*
Pedicle, 302*f*
Peer pressure, positive, 209
Pelvic girdle, 273
Pelvis, 231*f*
female
and ACL injury, 33, 33*f*
and patella tracking, 283
Pennington, Bill, 78
PEP Program, 37
Performance anxiety, 337, 337*f*
Performance enhancing drugs, 214–215
Performance enhancing supplements, 214–217
Performance tests, 86
Pericranium, 295*f*
Periodized training, 86–92
annual plan in, 87–90, 87*f*, 88*f*, 89*f*, 90*f*
combined programs, 126–127
competitive season in, 88*f*, 90, 90*f*, 127, 129*t*
concepts of, 86–87
endurance, 124–127, 129*t*
general preparation in, 88*f*, 90, 90*f*
history of, 86
macrocycles in, 90*f*, 91, 91*f*
microcyles in, 91–92, 91*f*, 92*f*
in problem (fall) sports, 127
specific preparation in, 88*f*, 90, 90*f*
strength, 124–127
training phases in, 88–89, 88*f*
transition/rest in, 88*f*, 90–91, 90*f*
Periostitis, 286
Peripheral visual field, stress and, 339
Peroneal nerve, 285. *See* Fibular nerve
Peroneus brevis, 285, 285*f*, 286*t*. *See* Fibularis brevis
Peroneus longus, 233*f*, 285, 285*f*, 286*t*. *See* Fibularis longus
Peroneus tertius, 284, 286*t*. *See* Fibularis tertius
Personality, and injury risk, 338
Perturbation training, for ACL rehabilitation, 41
Phalanges
foot, 231*f*, 284, 284*f*
hand, 231*f*, 264, 264*f*
Phosphagen energy system, 101–102, 105*t*
characteristics of, 105*t*
contributions by sport, 108, 110*t*
recovery, 81, 82*t*
recovery of, 81, 82*t*
time-based zone of, 108, 108*f*, 109*t*
training of, 110–111, 111*t*
utilization of, prediction of, 107–109
Phosphocreatine, 81, 101–102. *See also* Phosphagen energy system

Phosphorus, dietary/nutritional, 143, 159
Physical evaluation, preparticipation, 247–248
Pia mater, 294, 295*f*
Piercings, safety of, 66
Piriformis, 274*t*
Pisiform, 264*f*
Plantar fasciitis, 288–289, 290*f*
Plantar flexion, 284, 285*f*, 286*t*
Plantaris, 285*f*
Plate portions, 162, 162*f*
Playing surface, 56–58
and ACL injury, 42, 57
cushioning of, 57–58
friction on, 25, 42, 57, 64, 75
and injury prevention, 24, 26
and injury risk, 57–58
regularity of, 57
temperature on, 50
and tibial stress injuries, 286
and turf toe, 289–290
Plyometrics
and ACL injury, 21, 35, 39–41, 41*f*, 42*f*
and ankle sprain, 21
and ATP-PC energy system, 110–111
box height in, 138
depth jumping, 35, 39, 41*f*, 137–138, 137*t*
general considerations in, 137–138
high-intensity, 39–41
level, 35, 39, 42*f*
and power, 134–138
progression of, 137, 137*t*
upper body, 138
Pneumonia, 201*f*
Podlog, Leslie, 349
Popliteal bursa, 234*f*
Popliteal ligaments, 280
Popliteal surface, 279*f*
Portion sizes, 175, 175*f*, 182
Positive self-talk, 346
Postconcussion syndrome, 294, 300
Posterior compartments, thigh, 284–285, 285*f*
Posterior cruciate ligament (PCL), 280–281, 281*f*
Posterior longitudinal ligament, 303, 304*f*
Posterior talofibular ligament, 290*f*
Posterior tibiofibular ligament, 290
Posture, and ACL injury, 34
Potassium loss/replacement, 53–54, 159
Power
aerobic training and, 138
definition of, 117
restoration, in rehabilitation, 244–245
vs. strength, 117–118
Power clean, 134–135
Power eating, 161–165
Power endurance, 126